RSSDI
Yearbook of
Diabetes 2020

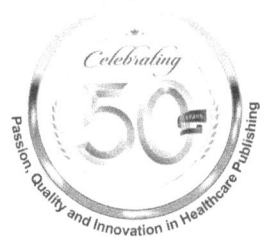

RSSDI
Yearbook of Diabetes 2020

Editor-in-Chief

Sujoy Ghosh MD (Med) DM (Endo) FRCP FACE
Professor
Department of Endocrinology
Institute of Post Graduate Medical
Education and Research
Kolkata, West Bengal, India

Associate Editor

Sayantan Ray MD DM
Consultant Endocrinologist
Medica Superspeciality Hospital
Kolkata, West Bengal, India

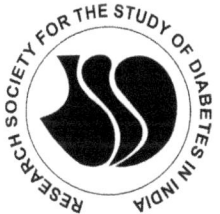

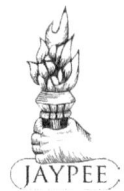

JAYPEE BROTHERS MEDICAL PUBLISHERS
The Health Sciences Publisher
New Delhi | London

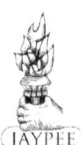 **Jaypee Brothers Medical Publishers (P) Ltd**

Headquarter
Jaypee Brothers Medical Publishers (P) Ltd
4838/24, Ansari Road, Daryaganj
New Delhi 110 002, India
Phone: +91-11-43574357
Fax: +91-11-43574314
Email: jaypee@jaypeebrothers.com

Overseas Office
J.P. Medical Ltd
83 Victoria Street, London
SW1H 0HW (UK)
Phone: +44 20 3170 8910
Fax: +44 (0)20 3008 6180
Email: info@jpmedpub.com

Website: www.jaypeebrothers.com
Website: www.jaypeedigital.com

© 2021, Jaypee Brothers Medical Publishers

The views and opinions expressed in this book are solely those of the original contributor(s)/author(s) and do not necessarily represent those of editor(s) of the book.

All rights reserved. No part of this publication may be reproduced, stored or transmitted in any form or by any means, electronic, mechanical, photocopying, recording or otherwise, without the prior permission in writing of the publishers.

All brand names and product names used in this book are trade names, service marks, trademarks or registered trademarks of their respective owners. The publisher is not associated with any product or vendor mentioned in this book.

Medical knowledge and practice change constantly. This book is designed to provide accurate, authoritative information about the subject matter in question. However, readers are advised to check the most current information available on procedures included and check information from the manufacturer of each product to be administered, to verify the recommended dose, formula, method and duration of administration, adverse effects and contraindications. It is the responsibility of the practitioner to take all appropriate safety precautions. Neither the publisher nor the author(s)/editor(s) assume any liability for any injury and/or damage to persons or property arising from or related to use of material in this book.

This book is sold on the understanding that the publisher is not engaged in providing professional medical services. If such advice or services are required, the services of a competent medical professional should be sought.

Every effort has been made where necessary to contact holders of copyright to obtain permission to reproduce copyright material. If any have been inadvertently overlooked, the publisher will be pleased to make the necessary arrangements at the first opportunity. The **CD/DVD-ROM** (if any) provided in the sealed envelope with this book is complimentary and free of cost. **Not meant for sale.**

Inquiries for bulk sales may be solicited at: jaypee@jaypeebrothers.com

RSSDI Yearbook of Diabetes 2020

First Edition: **2021**

ISBN: 978-93-90595-28-0

Contributors

EDITOR-IN-CHIEF

Sujoy Ghosh MD (Med) DM (Endo) FRCP FACE
Professor
Department of Endocrinology
Institute of Post Graduate Medical
Education and Research
Kolkata, West Bengal, India

ASSOCIATE EDITOR

Sayantan Ray MD DM
Consultant Endocrinologist
Medica Superspeciality Hospital
Kolkata, West Bengal, India

SECTION AUTHORS

Ajitesh Roy MD (Gen Med)
DM (Endo)
Assistant Professor, Department
of Endocrinology, Vivekananda
Institute of Medical Science
Kolkata, West Bengal, India

Amit Gupta DNB MNAMS FACE
FICP FRCP (Glasg, Edin)FACP (USA)
PGD-Diab (Cardiff UK) DFID (CMC
Vellore) F-Diab (Diabetes India) FGSI
FIMSA FIACM
Director, Centre for Diabetes Care
Greater Noida, Uttar Pradesh, India

Amritava Ghosh MD (Med)
DM (Endo)
Assistant Professor and
Faculty-in-charge, Department
of Endocrinology and
Metabolism, All India Institute of
Medical Sciences
Raipur, Chhattisgarh, India

Anand Moses MD FRCP
Emeritus Professor
Professor of Diabetology
The Tamil Nadu Dr MGR Medical
University
Chennai, Tamil Nadu, India

Anuj Maheshwari MD FICP
FIACM FIMSA FRSSDI FACP (USA)
FACE (USA) FRCP (London, Edinburgh)
Professor and Head
Department of General Medicine
Babu Banarasi Das University
Lucknow, Uttar Pradesh, India

Archana Sarda MD (Med)
Consultant Diabetologist
Founder
UDAAN, an NGO for Children
with Diabetes
Aurangabad, Maharashtra,
India

Banshi Saboo MD PhD FRCP
MNAMS
Fellow American College of
Endocrinology (FACE)
Fellow International College of
Nutrition (FICN - Canada)
Diabetologist
Endocrine and Metabolic
Physician
President - RSSDI
Honorary Diabetologist H. E. The
Governor of Gujarat
Ahmedabad, Gujarat, India
Scientific Chairman: RSSDI 2019

Bikash Bhattacharjee MBBS
GDIPDC MDC (Australia)
Director and Senior Consultant
Diabetologist
Sun Valley Diabetic Care and
Research Centre
Guwahati, Assam, India

Contributors

Brij Mohan Makkar MD FIAMS FICP FRCP (Glasg, Edin) FACP FACE FRSSDI
Senior Diabetologist and Obesity Specialist, Dr Makkar's Diabetes and Obesity Centre
New Delhi, India

Chitra Selvan MD (Med) DM (Endo)
Associate Professor
Ramaiah Medical College
Bengaluru, Karnataka, India

Ch Vasanth Kumar MD
Senior Consultant Physician
Apollo Hospitals
President Elect. RSSDI
Founder and President
Diabetes and You Society
Faculty and Examiner
Medvarsity
Hyderabad, Telangana, India
Organizing Chairman: RSSDI 2016

Indira Maisnam MD DM FRCP FACE
Consultant Endocrinologist
RG Kar Medical College
Kolkata, West Bengal, India

Jothydev Kesavadev MD
Chairman, Jothydev's Diabetes Research Centre
Thiruvananthapuram, Kerala, India

Jugal Kishor Sharma MD (Med) FICP FACP FACE FRCP (London, Edin, Glasg, Ireland) FRSSDI FIACM FIMSA FGSI Fellow Diabetes India, FISH
Medical Director
Central Delhi Diabetes Centre
New Delhi, India

Mithun Bhartia MRCP (UK) CCT (Endo, UK)
Consultant Endocrinologist
Apollo Hospital
Guwahati, Assam, India

Neeta Deshpande MD FRCP
Consultant Diabetologist and Bariatric Physician
Belgaum Diabetes Centre
Professor and Head
Department of Medicine
MM Dental College
Associate Professor-Medicine
USM-KLE International Medical Program
Belgaum, Karnataka, India

Partha P Chakraborty MD DM (Endo) DNB (Endo) FACE FICP
Clinical Tutor
Department of Endocrinology and Metabolism
Medical College
Kolkata, West Bengal, India

Pratap Jethwani MD (Med)
PG Diploma Diabetes FRSSDI FDiab India
Director and Consultant Diabetes Specialist
Jethwani Diabetes Care Center
Jethwani Hospital,
Rajkot, Gujarat, India

Purvi Chawla MBBS
MS (Pharm Sci, USA) PG (Diab, UK)
Consultant Diabetologist and Director of Clinical Research
Lina Diabetes Care and Mumbai Diabetes Research Centre
Hon. Consultant Diabetologist
Bhartiya Arogya Nidhi and Mahavir Hospitals
Mumbai, Maharashtra, India

Rajeev Chawla MD F Diab FRSSDI FACP (USA) FRCP (Edin) FACE (USA)
Senior Consultant Diabetologist Director
North Delhi Diabetes Centre
Rohini, New Delhi, India

Rakesh Kumar Sahay MD DNB (Med) DM (Endo)
Professor and Head
Department of Endocrinology
Osmania Medical College and Osmania General Hospital
Hyderabad, Telangana, India

Rana Bhattacharjee MD (Med) MRCP DM (Endo) FICP FRCP FACE
Assistant Professor
Department of Endocrinology and Metabolism
Institute of Post Graduate Medical Education and Research
Kolkata, West Bengal, India

Sanjay Agarwal MD FACE
Director
Aegle Clinic - Diabetes Care
Head
Department of Medicine and Diabetes, Ruby Hall Clinic
Senior Consultant in Diabetes and Medicine
Jehangir Hospital
Secretary - RSSDI
Pune, Maharashtra, India

Sanjay Reddy MD
Consultant Diabetologist
Center for Diabetes and Endocrine Care, Fortis Hospital, Cunningham Road
Vice President
Primer Academy of Medical Sciences (PAMS)
Bengaluru, Karnataka, India

Shalini Jaggi Dip Diab (UK) Dip Endo (UK) FRSSDI FRCP (London, Glasg, Edin)
Consultant Diabetologist and Director
Lifecare Diabetes Centre
New Delhi, India

Soumik Goswami MD (Med) DM (Endo)
RMO cum Clinical Tutor
Department of Endocrinology
Nilratan Sircar Medical College
Kolkata, West Bengal, India

Sreenivasa Murthy L MD
FRCP (Edin, Glasg) FRSSDI FICP
Professor and Head of Unit
Department of General Medicine
Dr B R Ambedkar Medical College (BRAMC)
Senior Consultant Physician and Diabetologist, Lifecare Hospital and Research Centre
Bengaluru, Karnataka, India

Sudhir Bhandari MD DNB FRCP (London) FRCP (Edinburgh) FACP FACE (Fellow American College of Endocrinology) FISC FRSSDI FELLOW OF DIABETES INDIA (FDI)
Senior Professor in Upgraded Department of Medicine
Principal and Controller
SMS Medical College and Hospital
Jaipur, Rajasthan, India

Sunil Surajprasad Gupta MD FACE FRCP (London, Edinburgh and Glasgow) FACP FICP FRSSDI
Director, Sunil's Diabetes Care n' Research Centre Pvt Ltd
Nagpur, Maharashtra, India

Vijay Kumar Panikar MD FCPS DNB FRCP (London)
Consultant Endocrinologist
Department of Endocrinolgy and Diabetes
Lilavati Hospital
Mumbai, Maharashtra, India

Vijay Viswanathan MD PhD FRCP (London and Glasgow)
Head and Chief Diabetologist
Prof M Viswanathan Diabetes Research Centre
Chennai, Tamil Nadu, India

Message from the RSSDI President

Dear Readers,

Greetings from RSSDI!

I hope this will find you in the best of your health and good spirit.

As a President of Research Society for the Study of Diabetes in India (RSSDI), it gives me immense pleasure to launch the yet another version of RSSDI Yearbook, 2020.

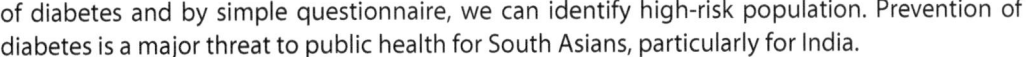

As you all know, diabetes, today, is a major concern of society as well as health sector. Various studies have shown that it is a preventable disorder, or at least, it can be delayed. There are definite risk factors of diabetes and by simple questionnaire, we can identify high-risk population. Prevention of diabetes is a major threat to public health for South Asians, particularly for India.

It is evidently proven that early diagnosis and screening of diabetes help in preventing complications of diabetes and, therefore, the healthcare professionals needs to be trained in management and prevention of diabetes.

I congratulate Dr Sujoy Ghosh for coming out with *RSSDI Yearbook, 2020*. I am sure it will help healthcare professionals to upgrade their knowledge about management and prevention of diabetes as well as related complications. The contents of the book are designed to appropriately keeping the need of the time in mind and contain all the topics from diagnosis to pathophysiology to management and prevention as well.

I write this foreword with immense pleasure and I am sure it will be a useful book for readers.

Banshi Saboo MD PhD FRCP MNAMS
President—RSSDI
Diabetologist, Endocrine and Metabolic Physician
Honorary Diabetologist H. E. The Governor of Gujarat
Ahmedabad, Gujarat, India
Scientific Chairman: RSSDI, 2019

Message from the RSSDI Secretary

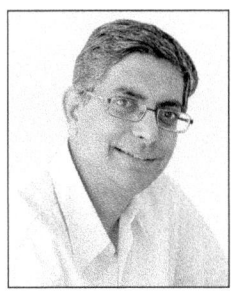

I would like to congratulate Dr Sujoy Ghosh, the executive committee of Research Society for the Study of Diabetes in India (RSSDI), and scientific team to bring out such a comprehensive 2020 RSSDI Yearbook. This is the second volume of the book and a much-awaited scientific compilation in diabetes.

In this changing landscape of information, we need to keep abreast with latest developments in diabetes. This book breaks down the information in various segments, making reading easy. Reviews and commentaries have been covered well from articles, which span from all prestigious peer reviewed journals with high-impact factor.

I urge all clinicians working in the field of diabetes to read this book. It has cutting edge information, which will assist you to take informed decisions in management of patients, in line, with world opinion. To all researchers, articles by fellow colleagues give an insight to thoughts of leaders in research world.

The book has been printed with easy reading fonts and colors with good take home messages. It is an invaluable asset to your library.

Happy Reading!!

Sanjay Agarwal MD FACE
Honorary Secretary—RSSDI
Director, Aegle Clinic—Diabetes Care
Head, Department of Medicine and Diabetes
Ruby Hall Clinic
Senior Consultant in Diabetes and Medicine
Jehangir Hospital
Pune, Maharashtra, India

Preface

Incidentally, yearbooks in different specialties are available for almost all specialties and sub-/superspecialties of medical sciences. However, a Yearbook of Diabetes by the Research Society for the Study of Diabetes in India (RSSDI) is unique. Considering that a large number of articles related to diabetes are published every year that it is a formidable task of putting together a yearbook on diabetes.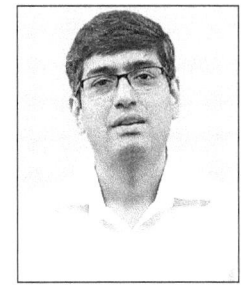

Clinicians, both primary care and specialists often attend conferences and clinical meetings with the expectation to update their understanding of diabetology. Clinical service delivery makes it difficult for most to keep abreast with all the studies newly published.

The most important publications are summarized in an easy-to-read format for the physician published. The RSSDI is one of the biggest organizations in the field of diabetology worldwide and is, therefore, the appropriate organization to take up this responsibility.

We decided to screen all diabetes related (major publications, from major journals) published articles between 1st July, 2019 and 30th June, 2020. We screened over 4,000 original articles and then divided up the selected articles into 8 subsections and wrote up a critical appraisal of all the selected ones. Abstracts of the articles were re-written to avoid any copyright issue.

I was fortunate to be working with an outstanding team of doctors, including a dynamic editorial team consisting of a mix of a physician, diabetologists, and endocrinologists. The entire writing team of doctors for the book has done a wonderful job, that too at such short notice.

I am highly indebted to all the members of the executive committee of RSSDI led by Dr Banshi Saboo and Dr Sanjay Agarwal.

I am also extremely grateful to Dr Sayantan Ray, the associate editor of this book, without his help this book would not have been possible.

The entire process of completion of this book has been a roller-coaster journey. The book would never have seen the light of day without the determination, help, support, and guidance that I received from Mr Sabyasachi Hazra of Jaypee Brothers Medical Publishers (P) Ltd.

Finally, I would like to thank all my colleagues at work and my family who have been a constant source of support and encouragement.

I dedicate this book to all those who involved in the management of patients with diabetes and hope this helps in improvement of patient care and outcome.

Long live RSSDI.

Sujoy Ghosh

Content

Section 1: Basic Science
Soumik Goswami, Sreenivasa Murthy L, Rakesh Kumar Sahay, Vijay Viswanathan

1. Liver Iron Concentration is an Independent Risk Factor for the Prediabetic State in β-thalassemia Patients ... 1
2. Nonalcoholic Fatty Liver Disease, Insulin Resistance, and Ceramides ... 2
3. Taking a Brown Adipose Tissue to the Chains of Diabetes ... 4
4. The *TCF7L2* Locus: A Genetic Window into the Pathogenesis of Type 1 and Type 2 Diabetes ... 5
5. Glycemic Index of Wheat and Rice are Similar when Consumed as Part of a North Indian Mixed Meal ... 7
6. *MACF1* Gene Variant rs2296172 is Associated with Type 2 Diabetes Susceptibility in Mizo Population from Northeast India ... 8
7. Copeptin, a Surrogate Marker for Arginine Vasopressin Secretion, is Positively Associated with Glucagon ... 10
8. PAX Proteins and Their Role in Pancreas ... 11
9. What has Zinc Transporter 8 Autoimmunity Taught us About Type 1 Diabetes? ... 13

Section 2: Epidemiology
Chitra Selvan, Jugal Kishor Sharma, Anand Moses, Vijay Kumar Panikar

1. Association of Maternal Lactation with Diabetes and Hypertension: A Systematic Review and Meta-analysis ... 15
2. Prevalence and Predictors of Osteopenia and Osteoporosis in Patients with Type 2 Diabetes Mellitus: A Cross-sectional Study From a Tertiary Care Institute in North India ... 16
3. Autoantibody Reversion: Changing Risk Categories in Multiple-autoantibody-positive Individuals ... 18
4. Incidence and Associations of Chronic Kidney Disease in Community Participants with Diabetes: A 5-year Prospective Analysis of the EXTEND45 Study ... 19
5. Establishment and Validation of a Risk Prediction Model for Early Diabetic Kidney Disease Based on a Systematic Review and Meta-analysis of 20 Cohorts ... 21

6. Every Fifth Individual with Type 1 Diabetes Suffers from an
   Additional Autoimmune Disease: A Finnish Nationwide Study — 22
7. Absence of Islet Autoantibodies and Modestly Raised Glucose Values at
   Diabetes Diagnosis Should Lead to Testing for MODY: Lessons from a
   5-year Pediatric Swedish National Cohort Study — 24
8. Effect of Age at Menarche on Microvascular Complications
   Among Women with Type 1 Diabetes — 26
9. Geographic Variation and Associated Covariates of Diabetes Prevalence in India — 28
10. Sex Differences in the Burden of Type 2 Diabetes and Cardiovascular Risk
    Across the Life Course — 30
11. Incidence of New-onset Diabetes and Post-transplant Metabolic Syndrome
    after Liver Transplantation - A Prospective Study from South India — 31
12. Use of Antihyperglycemic Medications in U.S. Adults: An Analysis of the
    National Health and Nutrition Examination Survey — 33
13. Why are South Asians Prone to Type 2 Diabetes? A Hypothesis Based on
    Underexplored Pathways — 34
14. Prevalence and Clinical Characteristics of Individuals with Newly Detected Lean
    Diabetes in Tamil Nadu, South India: A Community-based Cross-sectional Study — 36
15. Prevalence of Diabetes Mellitus in 2019 Novel Coronavirus: A Meta-analysis — 37
16. Vitamin D Supplementation and Prevention of Type 2 Diabetes — 38
17. Prognostic Significance of Long-term HbA1c Variability for All-cause Mortality
    in the ACCORD Trial — 40
18. Evaluating the Performance of the Indian Diabetes Risk Score in
    Different Ethnic Groups — 42

Section 3: Comorbidities
Amritava Ghosh, Shalini Jaggi, Mithun Bhartia, Bikash Bhattacharjee

1. Usefulness of Routine Fractional Flow Reserve for Clinical Management of
   Coronary Artery Disease in Patients with Diabetes — 44
2. The Long-term Effects of Metformin on Patients with Type 2
   Diabetic Kidney Disease — 46
3. Impact of Treating Oral Disease on Preventing Vascular Diseases: A Model-based
   Cost-effectiveness Analysis of Periodontal Treatment Among Patients
   with Type 2 Diabetes — 48
4. Risk of Rapid Kidney Function Decline, All-cause Mortality, and
   Major Cardiovascular Events in Nonalbuminuric Chronic Kidney Disease
   in Type 2 Diabetes — 49
5. Performance of Plasma Biomarkers and Diagnostic Panels for
   Nonalcoholic Steatohepatitis and Advanced Fibrosis in Patients with Type 2 Diabetes — 51
6. Time in Range is Associated with Carotid Intima-media Thickness in Type 2 Diabetes — 53

Section 4: Complications
Indira Maisnam, Amit Gupta, Neeta Deshpande, Brij Mohan Makkar

1. Reduced Pancreatic Polypeptide Response is Associated with Early Alteration of Glycemic Control in Chronic Pancreatitis — 56
2. Young-onset Type 2 Diabetes and Younger Current Age: Increased Susceptibility to Retinopathy in Contrast to other Complications — 58
3. Dipeptidyl Peptidase 4 Inhibitors and the Risk of Bullous Pemphigoid among Patients with Type 2 Diabetes — 60
4. Seroprevalence and Risk Factors Associated with HBV and HCV Infection among Subjects with Type 2 Diabetes from South India — 62
5. Prevalence and Patterns of Cardiac Autonomic Dysfunction in Male Patients with Type 2 Diabetes Mellitus and Chronic Charcot's Neuroarthropathy: A Cross-sectional Study from South India — 64
6. Longitudinal Associations between Depression and Diabetes Complications: A Systematic Review and Meta-analysis — 66
7. Bone Histomorphometry in Young Patients with Type 2 Diabetes is Affected by Disease Control and Chronic Complications — 68
8. Teriparatide [Recombinant Human Parathyroid Hormone (1-34)] Increases Foot Bone Remodeling in Diabetic Chronic Charcot Neuroarthropathy: A Randomized Double-blind Placebo-controled Study — 70

Section 5: Type 1 Diabetes Mellitus
Ajitesh Roy, Archana Sarda, Banshi Saboo, Ch Vasanth Kumar

1. Immune Checkpoint Inhibitor-induced Type 1 Diabetes: A Systematic Review and Meta-analysis — 75
2. Serum Urate Lowering with Allopurinol and Kidney Function in Type 1 Diabetes — 77
3. Profile of Auto-antibodies (Disease Related and Other) in Children with Type 1 Diabetes — 80
4. Biomarker Panels Associated with Progression of Renal Disease in Type 1 Diabetes — 82
5. Effect of Continuous Glucose Monitoring on Glycemic Control in Adolescents and Young Adults with Type 1 Diabetes: A Randomized Clinical Trial — 84
6. Continuous Glucose Monitoring in People with Type 1 Diabetes on Multiple-dose Injection Therapy: The Relationship between Glycemic Control and Hypoglycemia — 86
7. The Efficacy of Technology in Type 1 DM: A Systemic Review, Network Meta-analysis, and Narrative Synthesis — 88
8. Use of Sensor-integrated Pump Therapy to Reduce Hypoglycemia in People with Type 1 Diabetes: A Real-world Study in the UK — 90

Section 6: Gestational Diabetes Mellitus
Rana Bhattacharjee, Purvi Chawla, Sunil Surajprasad Gupta, Rajeev Chawla

1. Prevention of Gestational Diabetes Mellitus in Overweight or Obese Pregnant Women: A Network Meta-analysis — 95
2. Maternal Age and the Risk of Gestational Diabetes Mellitus: A Systematic Review and Meta-analysis of Over 120 Million Participants — 96
3. Gestational Diabetes Mellitus in HIV-infected Pregnant Women: A Systematic Review and Meta-analysis — 98
4. Continuous Glucose Monitoring in Pregnancy: Importance of Analyzing Temporal Profiles to Understand Clinical Outcomes — 99
5. Urinary and Serum Angiogenic Markers in Women with Pre-existing Diabetes During Pregnancy and their Role in Pre-eclampsia Prediction — 101

Section 7: Drugs and Therapeutics
Sayantan Ray, Pratap Jethwani, Anuj Maheshwari, Sudhir Bhandari

1. Effect of Dapagliflozin on Worsening Heart Failure and Cardiovascular Death in Patients with Heart Failure with and without Diabetes — 105
2. Glycemic Efficacy and Safety of Glucagon-like Peptide-1 Receptor Agonist on Top of Sodium-glucose Cotransporter-2 Inhibitor Treatment Compared to Sodium-glucose Cotransporter-2 Inhibitor Alone: A Systematic Review and Meta-analysis of Randomized Controlled Trials — 107
3. Once-weekly Insulin for Type 2 Diabetes without Previous Insulin Treatment — 109
4. Efficacy and Safety of the Glucagon Receptor Antagonist RVT-1502 in Type 2 Diabetes Uncontrolled on Metformin Monotherapy: A 12-Week Dose-ranging Study — 111
5. Optimization of Metformin in the GRADE Cohort: Effect on Glycemia and Body Weight — 113
6. Combined GLP-1, Oxyntomodulin, and Peptide YY Improves Body Weight and Glycemia in Obesity and Prediabetes/Type 2 Diabetes: A Randomized, Single-blinded, Placebo-controlled Study — 114
7. Hypoglycemia is Reduced with Use of Inhaled Technosphere® Insulin Relative to Insulin Aspart in Type 1 Diabetes Mellitus — 116
8. Systematic Review and Meta-analysis of Clinical Trials Examining the Effect of Hyperbaric Oxygen Therapy in People with Diabetes-related Lower Limb Ulcers — 118
9. Oral Semaglutide and Cardiovascular Outcomes in Patients with Type 2 Diabetes — 119
10. Effects of Probiotic Supplementation during Pregnancy on Metabolic Outcomes: A Systematic Review and Meta-analysis of Randomized Controlled Trials — 121
11. Dapagliflozin in Patients with Heart Failure and Reduced Ejection Fraction — 122
12. Associations between Metformin Use and Vitamin B12 Levels, Anemia, and Neuropathy in Patients with Diabetes: A Meta-analysis — 124
13. Risk of Severe Hypoglycemia and its Impact in Type 2 Diabetes in DEVOTE — 126

14. Switching to Degludec is Associated with Reduced Hypoglycemia, Irrespective of Definition Used or Patient Characteristics: Secondary Analysis of the ReFLeCT Prospective, Observational Study — 127

15. A Survey of Physician Experience and Treatment Satisfaction using Fast-acting Insulin aspart in People with Type 1 or Type 2 Diabetes — 128

16. A Randomized Trial Evaluating the Efficacy and Safety of Fast-acting Insulin Aspart Compared with Insulin Aspart, Both in Combination with Insulin Degludec with or without Metformin, in Adults with Type 2 Diabetes (Onset 9) — 130

17. Oral Semaglutide versus Empagliflozin in Patients with Type 2 Diabetes Uncontrolled on Metformin: The PIONEER 2 Trial — 131

18. Efficacy, Safety, and Tolerability of Oral Semaglutide versus Placebo Added to Insulin with or without Metformin in Patients with Type 2 Diabetes: The PIONEER 8 Trial — 133

19. Effectiveness and Safety of Insulin Glargine 300 U/mL in Insulin-naïve Patients with Type 2 Diabetes after Failure of Oral Therapy in a Real-world Setting — 135

20. An Assessment of Physician Reasons for Prescribing Insulin Lispro 200 units/mL in Germany — 136

21. Cardiovascular and Kidney Outcomes of Linagliptin Treatment in Older People with Type 2 Diabetes and Established Cardiovascular Disease and/or Kidney Disease: A Prespecified Subgroup Analysis of the Randomized, Placebo-controlled CARMELINA® trial — 138

22. Linagliptin and Cardiorenal Outcomes in Asians with Type 2 Diabetes Mellitus and Established Cardiovascular and/or Kidney Disease: Subgroup Analysis of the Randomized CARMELINA® Trial — 139

23. Efficacy and Safety of Remogliflozin Etabonate, a New Sodium-glucose Cotransporter-2 Inhibitor, in Patients with Type 2 Diabetes Mellitus: A 24-Week, Randomized, Double-blind, Active-controlled Trial — 141

24. An Open-label, Single-period, Two-stage, Single Oral Dose Pharmacokinetic Study of Remogliflozin Etabonate Tablet 100 and 250 mg in Healthy Asian Indian Male Subjects Under Fasting and Fed Conditions — 143

25. Efficacy of Empagliflozin on Heart Failure and Renal Outcomes in Patients with Atrial Fibrillation: Data from the EMPA-REG OUTCOME Trial — 144

26. Effect of Empagliflozin on Left Ventricular Mass in Patients with Type 2 Diabetes Mellitus and Coronary Artery Disease: The EMPA-HEART CardioLink-6 Randomized Clinical Trial — 146

27. Suboptimal Glycemic Control among Subjects with Diabetes Mellitus in India: A Subset Analysis of Cross-sectional Wave-7 (2016) Data from the International Diabetes Management Practices Study (IDMPS) — 148

28. A Practitioner's Toolkit for Insulin Motivation in Adults with Type 1 and Type 2 Diabetes Mellitus: Evidence-based Recommendations from an International Expert Panel — 149

29. Impact of Baseline Characteristics and Beta-cell Function on the Efficacy and Safety of Subcutaneous Once-weekly Semaglutide: A Patient-level, Pooled Analysis of the SUSTAIN 1-5 Trials — 151

30. Efficacy and Safety of Once-weekly Semaglutide versus Daily Canagliflozin as Add-on to Metformin in Patients with Type 2 Diabetes (SUSTAIN 8): A Double-blind, Phase 3b, Randomized Controlled Trial — 153

Section 8: Newer Technologies and Future Directions
Partha P Chakraborty, Sanjay Reddy, Jothydev Kesavade, Sanjay Agarwal

1. Effects of Continuous Glucose Monitoring on Metrics of Glycemic Control in Diabetes: A Systematic Review with Meta-analysis of Randomized Controlled Trials — 160
2. Clinical Targets for Continuous Glucose Monitoring Data Interpretation: Recommendations from the International Consensus on Time in Range — 162
3. Diabetes Digital App Technology: Benefits, Challenges, and Recommendations. A Consensus Report by the European Association for the Study of Diabetes (EASD) and the American Diabetes Association (ADA) Diabetes Technology Working Group — 163
4. Systematic Review of Randomized Controlled Trials Evaluating Glycemic Efficacy and Patient Satisfaction of Intermittent-scanned Continuous Glucose Monitoring in Patients with Diabetes — 165
5. Serum Tenascin-C is Independently Associated with Increased Major Adverse Cardiovascular Events and Death in Individuals with Type 2 Diabetes: A French Prospective Cohort — 167
6. Diabetes Screening: Detection and Application of Saliva 1,5-Anhydroglucitol by Liquid Chromatography-mass Spectrometry — 168
7. Circulating Retinol-binding Protein 4 is Inversely Associated with Pancreatic β-cell Function Across the Spectrum of Glycemia — 170
8. Positioning Time in Range in Diabetes Management — 171
9. Neprilysin Inhibition: A New Therapeutic Option for Type 2 Diabetes? — 173
10. Early Pregnancy Prediction of Gestational Diabetes Mellitus Risk using Prenatal Screening Biomarkers in Nulliparous Women — 174
11. Six-month Randomized, Multicenter Trial of Closed-loop Control in Type 1 Diabetes — 176

Index — **179**

Section 1: BASIC SCIENCE

Soumik Goswami, Sreenivasa Murthy L, Rakesh Kumar Sahay, Vijay Viswanathan

1. Liver Iron Concentration is an Independent Risk Factor for the Prediabetic State in β-thalassemia Patients

Ref: Kosaryan M, Rahimi M, Zamanfar D, Darvishi-Khezri H. Liver iron concentration is an independent risk factor for the prediabetic state in β-thalassemia patients. Int J Diabetes Dev Ctries. 2020;4:227-34.

ABSTRACT

Background: Beta-thalassemia major (β-TM) comprises a group of inherited blood disorders characterized by the reduced synthesis of β-globin chains. Iron overload following blood transfusion can affect major tissues involved in glucose metabolism, leading to different glucose metabolic disorders in β-TM patients. The aim of this study was to compare glucose metabolism and iron overload indices in these patients with prediabetic and normoglycemic states.

Methods: This analytical study was performed on 49 patients with β-TM (age >18 years), receiving regular blood transfusions. The fasting plasma glucose (FPG) and glucose tolerance tests indicated 32 normoglycemic and 17 prediabetic cases. The serum levels of C-peptide, fructosamine, fasting serum insulin, and serum ferritin were measured. In addition, T2-weighted magnetic resonance imaging (MRI) of the heart and liver was carried out. Glycemic metabolism indices, including quantitative insulin sensitivity check index (QUICKI) and homeostatic model assessment for insulin resistance (HOMA-IR), were also calculated.

Results: The HOMA-IR score was significantly higher, while the QUICKI score was significantly lower in prediabetic patients, compared to normoglycemic patients [median (IR), 2.59 (2.19) vs. 1.46 (1.03), $p = 0.007$; mean ± SD, 0.34 ± 0.03 vs. 0.37 ± 0.04, $p = 0.01$]. On the other hand, β-cell function was not significantly different between the groups. The liver iron concentration (LIC) at a cutoff point of 5.82 mg/g dry weight showed 93% sensitivity and 70% specificity for differentiation of prediabetic and normoglycemic states [area under curve (AUC), 0.81 (95% CI 0.65–0.95); $p = 0.002$].

Conclusion: Based on the findings, HOMA-IR and QUICKI can be applied as useful glycemic metabolism indices for predicting prediabetic and normoglycemic states among β-TM patients. Also, LIC was an independent risk factor for the prediabetic state.

COMMENT

Beta-thalassemia major (β-TM) patients survive longer today, but frequent blood transfusions in them lead to iron overload and subsequent endocrine problems, such as abnormal glucose homeostasis (AGH), impaired fasting glucose (IFG) or prediabetes, and diabetes mellitus (DM). The incidence of impaired glucose tolerance (IGT) and DM in β-TM patients has been estimated at 4–30% and up to 26%, respectively. Iron overload is known to involve tissues related to glucose metabolism, including pancreatic β-cells, but the exact pathogenesis of AGH and the prediabetic state in β-TM patients remains unknown. There are several studies suggesting β-cell dysfunction and subsequent insulin deficiency secondary to iron overload as the pathogenic mechanism while there are several others which point to the presence of hyperinsulinemia and increased insulin resistance (IR) as the predominant mechanism. An increase in IR has been described in normoglycemic TM patients pointing to the occurrence of IR before the onset of glucose intolerance. An earlier study showed increased IR due to liver cell insult in patients with a history of blood transfusion associated with iron overload and severe hepatic injury compared to those without a history of blood transfusion and normal iron levels. This study compared glucose metabolism and iron overload indices in β-TM patients with prediabetic and normoglycemic states to shed further light on the pathophysiology of dysglycemia in TM and increase the objectivity and effectiveness of glucose metabolism and iron overload indices for differentiation of prediabetic and normoglycemic states in these patients.

This study showed that IGT was associated with hepatic and cardiac siderosis. AGH patients had higher HOMA-IR and lower QUICKI scores but similar β-cell function index compared to normoglycemic patients. This suggests that IR occurs first in TM followed by pancreatic β-cell dysfunction and decreased insulin secretion. This study also showed that increased LIC was related to an increased risk of prediabetes with a LIC cutoff of 5.82 mg/g dry weight showing 93% sensitivity and 70% specificity for differentiating prediabetic from normoglycemic state in TM. This LIC cutoff estimation is unique and adds to the existing literature which till date has only looked at serum ferritin levels in TM in relation to AGH.

The strength of this study lies in including AGH and normoglycemic patients with TM for comparison with regard to β-cell function and IR indices which provide an insight into the initial etiopathogenetic mechanisms that are operational in causing dysglycemia in TM. Most other studies have included either wholly normoglycemic patients or overt DM with TM. Use of MRI to estimate LIC and determine a cut-off for differentiation of dysglycemic state from normoglycemia is also a strength of this study as LIC has not been studied in such detail with regard to the glycemic state in previous studies. A limitation of this study is the small sample size of 49 patients and unequal distribution of them among the two groups. Additionally, this was a single center study from Iran which would not be entirely representative of glucose metabolic defects in TM in other ethnicities who might have a different background risk for AGH.

This study reiterates the importance of early, aggressive, and extensive iron chelation in TM patients. It also suggests monitoring and managing LIC as a risk marker for iron overload–related AGH. Additionally, the findings indicate the possible usefulness of insulin sensitizers in TM with early dysglycemia in preference to exogenous insulin and insulin secretagogues.

Studies with a larger number of participants of different ethnicities with a prespecified subgroup analysis would help confirm these findings. Future studies looking at muscle siderosis with use of additional markers such as hepcidin levels would further add to the existing knowledge in this field.

2. Nonalcoholic Fatty Liver Disease, Insulin Resistance, and Ceramides

Ref: Samuel TV, Shulman GI. Nonalcoholic fatty liver disease, insulin resistance, and ceramides. N Engl J Med. 2019;381(19): 1866-69.

ABSTRACT

Insulin resistance (IR) is found in majority of the obese as well as elderly patients; it is also present among some of the young and lean individuals. IR is precursor to and also accelerates coexisting conditions such as type 2 diabetes mellitus (T2DM), atherosclerosis, and nonalcoholic fatty liver disease

(NAFLD). There exists widespread consensus that IR is related to ectopic lipid deposition in skeletal muscle as well as liver. Several lipid species are involved, however, and the molecular mechanisms that impair insulin action are still being discussed. In this perspective, a large body of evidence suggests that ceramides play a role in promoting IR. Ceramides are bioactive lipid intermediates, similar to the diacylglycerols. Ceramides as well as their derivatives (such as sphingomyelin) are the structural membrane lipids; whereas diacylglycerols produce energy-storing triglycerides. Desaturases are the enzymes that convert dihydroceramides into ceramides, modifying the membrane biophysical properties. IR has been reported to be associated with ceramides as well as dihydroceramides. Changes in insulin signaling, mitochondrial function as well as inflammatory pathways have all been suggested as reasons for ceramide-associated IR. In the present article, Samuel and Shulman discussed the important role of ceramides in hepatic IR as well as in the pathogenesis of metabolically associated FLD.

COMMENT

Critical Appraisal

Insulin resistance (IR) is a precursor to an accelerant of coexisting conditions such as type 2 diabetes mellitus (T2DM), atherosclerosis, and nonalcoholic fatty liver disease (NAFLD). Although there is a broad consensus that IR is associated with ectopic lipid deposition in skeletal muscle and liver, the molecular mechanisms impairing the action of insulin are debated. A large body of evidence supports a role for ceramides in triggering IR.[1] Sphingolipids, e.g., ceramides and dihydroceramides, are products of fat and protein metabolism that have been shown to accumulate in humans with obesity and hyperlipidemia.[2] Unbiased lipidomic screens in large clinical cohorts have shown particularly strong associations between serum and tissue levels of ceramides and/or dihydroceramides and obesity-related comorbidities, including IR, T2DM, and major adverse cardiac events.[3]

In this article, Varman and Gerald discussed a recent study[4] that investigated the role of these sphingolipids as causative agents in the development of IR and hepatic steatosis. Authors (Chaurasia et al.) reported elegant mouse experiments targeting dihydroceramide desaturase-1 (Des1), a rate-limiting enzyme for de novo ceramide synthesis. Global Des1 deletion in both lean and obese (leptin-deficient) mice altered energy balance and reduced body weight and adiposity and led to the associated metabolic benefits: Reduced hepatic steatosis and increased insulin sensitivity and glucose tolerance, whereas depletion of Des1 specifically in adipose and/or liver tissue was linked to modest metabolic improvements without detectable changes in body weight or whole-body energy balance. Overall, depletion of Des1 improved insulin signaling and mitochondrial function and reduced lipogenesis and lipid uptake.[4] These observations suggest that lower ceramide levels improve the mitochondrial capacity for fatty acid oxidation and thereby reduce steatosis and lipid-mediated IR. Thus, inhibition of Des1 may provide a means of treating hepatic steatosis and metabolic disorders.

From an analytical point of view, these findings do not establish the necessity of ceramides for the development of IR. Chaurasia et al. did not find differences in the concentration of hepatic diacylglycerol in the Des1-deficient mice, although changes in the relatively small pool of bioactive diacylglycerols in the plasma membrane may be difficult to detect when the total diacylglycerol content is measured in whole cells. In this context, Varman and Gerald proposed that assaying specific species of diacylglycerol in distinct cellular compartments purified by cell fractionation would be interesting.[5] Models of ceramide- and diacylglycerol-mediated IR can be reconciled by considering how ceramides affect mitochondrial function as ceramide-mediated mitochondrial dysfunction may account for the observed association with metabolic diseases. Chaurasia et al. found that mice in which Des1 was systemically knocked out had a lower body weight than control mice, together with higher mitochondrial activity in isolated adipocytes, but differences in body-weight gain or energy balance were not evident in mice in which Des1 was knocked out specifically in adipose and/or liver tissue. Possibly enhanced mitochondrial function, brought about through suppression of Des1, improves whole-body glucose metabolism by reducing ectopic lipid and intracellular lipid metabolites independent of weight loss.[1]

In most clinical situations, IR ultimately reflects ectopic lipid accumulation in insulin-responsive organs. In certain patients, concurrent increases in intracellular ceramides may impair mitochondrial function and exacerbate lipid accumulation and IR. The findings of Chaurasia et al. are consistent with those of earlier studies that support the development of experimental medications that enhance mitochondrial oxidation in liver, perhaps by decreasing ceramide biosynthesis to treat patients with NAFLD and T2DM who are not able to achieve meaningful weight loss. In sum, current evidence indicates that ceramides contribute to metabolic disease and may offer an opportunity for clinical intervention.

3. Taking a Brown Adipose Tissue to the Chains of Diabetes

Ref: Arany Z. Taking a BAT to the chains of diabetes. N Engl J Med. 2019;381(23):2270-72.

ABSTRACT

Diabetes is generally understood to be a disease linked with sugars and fats. But extensive epidemiologic data long back have also demonstrated that plasma levels of the branched-chain amino acids (BCAAs; leucine, valine, and isoleucine) are frequently elevated in subjects with insulin resistance and diabetes. Robust support to the concept that these elevations actively contribute to the development of insulin resistance came from several additional studies based on human genetics, metabolomics, and animal models concept. In animal models of diabetes, pharmacologic lowering of BCAA levels has been found to improve insulin sensitivity. These observations give rise to a new theory that BCAAs synergize with excess fat and carbohydrates to cause insulin resistance. What causes increases in BCAA levels? And does BCAA metabolism present therapeutic opportunities? A recent study by Yoneshiro et al. on BCAA catabolism in brown adipose tissue (BAT) provides some answers.

COMMENT

Brown adipose tissue (BAT) is specialized fat tissue dedicated to thermogenesis and is different from white adipose tissue which serves mainly to store energy. Although BAT in humans was considered to be present only in newborns, recent studies have also shown its variable presence in adults. BAT is known to increase energy consumption and waste calories releasing heat in response to cold exposure which makes it an attractive therapeutic target for obesity management. Beyond its energy-dissipating effect, BAT may have a role to play in the metabolism of branched chain amino acids (BCAAs; leucine, valine, and isoleucine), which opens up another avenue of research into its relationship with diabetes causation. This is because studies have shown BCAA to be consistently elevated in patients with insulin resistance and diabetes and multimodal studies support the fact that these elevations actively contribute to the development of insulin resistance in synergy with excess fat and glucose. This study looks at the role of BAT in

BCAA metabolism and its relation to insulin resistance.

The investigators found cold exposure to significantly lower plasma BCAA levels in those with high BAT activity suggesting that cold exposure activates catabolism of BCAA in BAT and that BAT can be a primary site of BCAA breakdown. The study then used mouse models to show that absence of a BAT enzyme required for BCAA catabolism results in elevated BCAA levels and absence of thermogenesis in response to cold. This study thus unravels a previously unknown dependence of BAT thermogenesis on BCAA catabolism as well as a reciprocal dependence of BCAA homeostasis on BAT. Additionally, the authors also showed these mice to develop mild obesity, glucose intolerance, and insulin resistance, thereby showing that BCAA metabolism in BAT is a driver of glucose homeostasis. This study also pointed to the role of mitochondrial carrier protein SLC25A44 in shuttling BCAAs from the cytoplasm into the mitochondrial matrix, where all enzymatic steps of BCAA breakdown occur. The role of BAT in BCAA metabolism with subsequent effect on insulin resistance is the area where this study sheds light on. It also suggests low BAT activity to be responsible for elevated BCAA levels in metabolic syndrome patients.

The strength of this study lies in its stepwise multimodal approach, which not only shows an association between BCAA metabolism, BAT activity, and thermogenesis, but also points to its etiopathogenic role in the development of insulin resistance and diabetes. This study, however, does not delineate the exact mechanism by which BCAA causes insulin resistance. It does not indicate whether glycemic benefits of BCAA catabolism result primarily from reduction in BCAA levels or from activation of thermogenesis or a combination of both. Also, this study uses mouse models and the results might not always apply equally to humans.

In spite of minor limitations, this study points to BAT enzymes involved in BCAA catabolism as potential therapeutic targets to address insulin resistance. It suggests that activating BAT thermogenesis could be a unique way of reducing insulin resistance in addition to reducing obesity, thereby killing two birds with one stone.

Additional studies looking at the mechanisms linking elevated BCAA and decreased thermogenesis to insulin resistance are warranted. This study, though done in exquisite detail, needs to be replicated in humans before the fruits of its findings can be savored.

4. The *TCF7L2* Locus: A Genetic Window into the Pathogenesis of Type 1 and Type 2 Diabetes

Ref: Grant SFA. The TCF7L2 locus: A genetic window into the pathogenesis of type 1 and type 2 diabetes. Diabetes Care. 2019;42(9):1624-9.

ABSTRACT

Genome-wide association studies (GWAS) over the past approximately 15 years have enabled the researchers to develop better understanding of the genetics of both type 1 diabetes mellitus (T1DM) and type 2 diabetes mellitus (T2DM). Many distinct loci have now been reported for both traits, and *TCF7L2* locus for T2DM is one of them. This genetic signal has helped in exploring multiple aspects of disease risk, including developments in genetic risk scores, genetic commonalities with cancer, and for gaining insights into diabetes-related molecular pathways. Also, the genetics of both latent autoimmune diabetes in adults and various presentations of T1DM have been studied using *TCF7L2* locus. Here we review the knowledge gained so far from this locus and highlight how work with this locus leads the way in guiding how many other genetic loci could be similarly worked with to develop better understanding of the pathogenesis of diabetes.

COMMENT

Discovery of genes involved in disease causation may help develop novel therapies for the same. Since both type 1 diabetes mellitus (T1DM) and type 2 diabetes mellitus (T2DM) have a genetic component in their causation, genomic studies searching for relevant genes might help discover new pathophysiologic mechanisms and therapeutic targets. Although there is overwhelming evidence for a strong genetic component in T2DM, the genetic influence is stronger in T1DM, with it being most apparent within the major histocompatibility complex (MHC). Genome-wide association studies (GWAS) have helped unravel several genetic loci with both types of diabetes having strong polygenic traits. While >240 loci have been reported for T2DM, the most statistically significant association is with the *TCF7L2* locus which was first reported in 2006. *TCF7L2* is the most common locus most strongly associated with T2DM.

Studies looking at the causal variant have pinpointed the T allele of intronic single nucleotide polymorphism (SNP) rs7903146 situated within the fourth intron of the *TCF7L2* gene to be the likely ancestral allele across several populations and ethnicities. The exact mechanism by which *TCF7L2* contributes to diabetes pathogenesis remains undetermined although majority of evidence suggests that it regulates the proglucagon gene and influences glucagon-like peptide (GLP-1) production in the intestine. Studies have also shown its association with a decrease in insulin secretion due to a possible disruption in GLP-1 signaling in the pancreatic β cell. Additional mechanisms include its effect on adipose tissue and the liver.

Carriers of the rs7903146 T allele have impaired response to sulfonylureas but not to metformin. Studies have also shown that islet tissue harboring the risk variant has a reduced response to oral as well as intravenous glucose, arginine, and incretins. Interestingly, *TCF7L2* gene expression was shown to be five times higher in type T2DM islets leading to a decrease in insulin secretion.

Since the problem with *TCF7L2* lies in its intronic region, it very likely operates via an enhancer element. Its exact nature remains unknown with *PARP1*, *FOXA2*, and *HMGB1* being possible factors. Beyond these binders, *TCF7L2* functions as a transcription factor and functional studies with chromatin immunoprecipitation have shown *TCF7L2* to be a master regulator of genes associated with diabetes and its comorbidities. An additional hypothesis is that the *TCF7L2* variant could act through effector genes some distance away and a relationship was observed with *ACSL5* gene which influences fatty acid metabolism. However, later studies have not supported evidence for the same.

A large GWAS study has also implicated the *TCF7L2* locus in influencing risk for higher body mass index (BMI) although it is the nonrisk C allele which was involved rather than the T allele associated with diabetes. However, the authors noted the presence of a high degree of heterogeneity between cohorts and a later study showed it to be an index event bias resulting from improper stratification leading to a false-positive association with BMI.

Studies have also shown the association of *TCF7L2* locus with latent autoimmune diabetes in adults (LADA). Since LADA often mimics T2DM initially, this could lead to spurious genetic associations, especially when one is pursuing increasingly modest signals in larger and larger cohorts. *TCF7L2* is not associated with T1DM overall but shows a relationship with T1DM positive for a single autoantibody which reaffirms the LADA observation. Interestingly, autoantibody-positive individuals progress to T1DM less rapidly if they carry the T2DM incriminating allele. These observations could have significant implications in personalizing treatment with gene-based information helping in the management of diabetes subtypes.

Several studies have placed *TCF7L2* at the pinnacle of incriminating genes in the pathogenesis and causation of T2DM. However, the therapeutic opportunity that studies with *TCF7L2* have presented remains to be tapped and explored further.

5. Glycemic Index of Wheat and Rice are Similar when Consumed as Part of a North Indian Mixed Meal

Ref: Nayar S, Madhu SV. Glycemic index of wheat and rice are similar when consumed as part of a north Indian mixed meal. Indian J Endocrinol Metab. 2020;24(3):251-55.

ABSTRACT

Introduction: Wheat is preferable over rice due to its lower glycemic index (GI). It is not known if the same is true when these staples are a part of mixed meals; hence we compared the glycemic responses of wheat/rice-containing mixed meals.

Materials and methods: Glycemic responses of two mixed meals were compared with a reference meal (glucose) where each was designed to provide a total of 50 g of available carbohydrate (AvCHO) in 10 healthy adult volunteers as per recent recommendations. Test meal 1 comprised of a pulse preparation (green gram dal), a vegetable (ladyfingers), and two wheat chapattis. In test meal 2, these wheat chapattis were replaced by cooked rice supplying an equal amount of AvCHO. After an overnight fast of 10–14 hours, capillary blood glucose estimations were done subsequent to eating each test meal or glucose. The GI of test meals was calculated by comparing their area under curve (AUC) with AUC for glucose. The GI of test meals was compared using unpaired t-test.

Results: The study sample comprised of seven males and three females with mean age 30.9 ± 5.1 year. The GI of test meal 1 (85.5 ± 11.8%) and test meal 2 (83.6 ± 11.4%) was not significantly different ($p = 0.7095$).

Conclusion: This study found no differences in the GI of wheat chapatti and rice-based mixed meals with equivalent AvCHO content of the staple.

COMMENT

The glycemic index (GI) of a foodstuff determines its effect on postprandial glycemia and, therefore, several authorities recommend intake of low GI food in patients with diabetes. This has formed the basis for advising consumption of wheat in patients with diabetes in preference to rice due to the former's lower GI. However, in a multicultural country like India, it could affect compliance in those who have been brought up with rice as staple besides limiting the choice of cereal intake. Also, there could be an impact of greatly restricting food choices in those with concomitant coeliac disease. However, the GI of food which forms the basis of this recommendation is not the be-all and end-all determinant of post meal blood glucose response. The GI of an individual food may behave differently when consumed as a part of a mixed meal, and there is no robust long-term evidence that the intake of low GI food benefits patients with diabetes. Additionally, the concept of AvCHO has emerged which is defined as those carbohydrates that are digested and absorbed by the human small intestine and which are glucogenic. Earlier studies have used the total carbohydrate content of food rather than AvCHO which could have led to a possible overestimation of the CHO content. Keeping these factors in mind, this study used mixed North Indian meals with either wheat or rice with similar AvCHO to determine differences in glycemic responses and GI of these mixed meals.

This study found that when the total AvCHO consumed in healthy individuals was 50 g from a mixed meal containing either wheat or rice, the GI and postprandial glucose responses were similar. This finding of a similar GI of mixed meals containing either rice or wheat was a novel and unique one.

An important aspect of this study is the use of "available" CHO instead of the total CHO content for measurement of GI, which is both practically relevant and is as per the latest recommendations which mention the possibility of false overestimation with use of total CHO. Another strength of this study is the use of an everyday mixed meal rather than an individual foodstuff which makes the findings applicable to everyday practice. Also, the investigators ensured that all the mixed meals were prepared by a single person using standardized predefined methods to avoid any bias. However, this study was a pilot study with the obvious limitation of having a small sample size inclusion of only one type of mixed meal with green gram dal and ladyfingers.

These findings have implications for dietary recommendations for diabetes patients. The long-standing recommendation by some authorities of preferential consumption of wheat over rice has been debunked in this study which shows similar glycemic responses to both when the AvCHO is similar in a mixed meal. This also calls for making modifications in food exchange lists to include amount of foodstuff containing AvCHO rather than total CHO as has been a standard practice.

To clear the air on this issue once and for all, studies with a larger number of participants using different types of mixed meals (including nonvegetarian ones) are warranted.

6. *MACF1* Gene Variant rs2296172 is Associated with Type 2 Diabetes Susceptibility in Mizo Population from Northeast India

Ref: Lalrohlui F, Sharma V, Sharma I, Singh H, Kour G, Sharma S, et al. MACF1 gene variant rs2296172 is associated with T2D susceptibility in Mizo population from Northeast India. Int J Diabetes Dev Ctries. 2020;40(2):223-6.

ABSTRACT

Aim: Microtubule actin cross-linking factor 1 (*MACF1*) has been identified as a type 2 diabetes mellitus (T2DM) candidate gene, and variant rs2296172 of the gene was found associated with T2DM in multiple populations. However, it has never been explored in the Mizo population. The aim of this study was to replicate the association of variant rs2296172 of *MACF1* gene with T2DM in the Mizo population of Northeast India.

Methodology: The variation was genotyped using TaqMan allele discrimination assay in 755 individuals (425 cases and 330 healthy controls), belonging to the Mizo population.

Results: The variant rs2296172 MACF1 was found to be significantly associated with T2DM (p value = 0.001) in the Mizo population group with an observed odds ratio of 1.8 (1.3–2.8) at 95% confidence interval (CI) after correction with age, gender, and body mass index (BMI).

Conclusion: This study is the first replication report from Northeast India, showing variant rs2296172 of the MACF1 gene associated with T2DM in Mizo population. This independent study highlights *MACF1* as a candidate gene for T2DM in Asian Indian populations, suggesting that it is critical to evaluate the variant rs2296172 in other distinct endogamous Indian population cohorts.

COMMENT

Advances in genetics have changed the way we view several diseases with type 2 diabetes mellitus (T2DM) being one of the notable ones for which over 240 loci have been described till date, the most prominent of them being *TCF7L2*. Discovery of such loci helps develop insights into the pathogenetic mechanisms of disease as well as develop novel therapeutic modalities. However, in spite of there being a strong hereditary influence in developing T2DM, these loci explain <20% heritability. The likely reasons for the same include both ethnic disparity, as most of these studies were carried out in European populations, and possibly yet to be discovered genetic loci. Despite India being a land of great ethnic and genetic diversity and having the world's second largest population base, genetic studies in T2DM in Indians are lacking. Furthermore, India is home to nearly 7.7 million patients with diabetes which makes it even more pertinent to carry out gene discovery studies in this population. There is also lack of data of known genetic variants in different endogamous ethnic groups in India resulting in an unmet need of replication of data available for Caucasian population in these Indian population groups. One such locus is the variation rs2296172 (A > G) [p.(met2290val)] of *MACF1* which was discovered in an exome sequencing-based genome-wide association studies (GWAS) in European populations and was replicated in an independent Indo-European linguistic cohort in the Punjab region of the country.

This study replicated the *MACF1* variant rs2296172 in a distinct Mizo population group primarily speaking Tibeto-Burman languages and with a very highly reported prevalence of T2DM. The variant was significantly associated with T2DM with a dominant mode of inheritance although the population attributable risk (PAR) was only around 6%. The variant was further explored using established genetic portals and repositories which suggested possible implications on insulin secretion via effect on Poly (A) binding protein cytoplasmic 4 (PABPC4) and an effect on regulation of filamentous actin (F-actin) and microtubule cytoskeletal dynamics resulting in impaired glucose homeostasis. Genetic studies in the Mizo population are grossly lacking, with this study being the first replication study highlighting the association of variant rs2296172 and potential role of *MACF1* with T2DM susceptibility in Mizo population.

The major strength of this study lies in its uniqueness of generating data in a reasonably large-sized population cohort in which prior evidence was grossly lacking. However, although the study was sufficiently powered to begin with (based on the Punjab study), a post hoc analysis revealed a decrease in power to 74.4% due to reduced frequency of the allele in the Mizo population. This decrease could be on account of endogamy practices in Indian population and could also be the effect of gene admixture or founder gene effects or both in varying combination.

This study establishes *MACF1* as an ideal T2DM candidate gene in Indian population which might influence the development of disease and whose further characterization could help develop novel therapeutic options in our population.

Similar studies need to be conducted in other endogamous cohorts in India to establish the countrywide validity of these findings. Additionally, the small PAR in the Mizo population with this variant implies the need for searching for other genetic variants in this Northeast Indian population. Also, functional characterization of these genetic loci in future studies would help delineate its exact role in the development of T2DM.

7. Copeptin, a Surrogate Marker for Arginine Vasopressin Secretion, is Positively Associated with Glucagon

Ref: Lundegaard Asferg C, Bjørn Andersen U, Linneberg A, Goetze JP, Holst JJ, Jeppesen JL. Copeptin, a surrogate marker for arginine vasopressin secretion, is positively associated with glucagon. Diabet Med. 2019;36(11):1408-11.

ABSTRACT

Aim: To analyze the association of plasma copeptin and plasma glucagon in normal to obese men.

Methods: Fasting plasma concentrations of copeptin and glucagon were measured in 102 healthy obese men (mean ± SD age 49.4 ± 10.2 years). The control group had 27 normal weight healthy men (mean ± SD age 51.5 ± 8.4 years). Differences between groups were evaluated using t-tests. Calculation of unstandardized regression coefficients (β) with 95% confidence intervals (CIs) between copeptin and glucagon was done using multiple linear regression analysis, adjusted for age and weight status (normal weight vs. obese). Copeptin was (natural) log-transformed.

Results: Fasting plasma copeptin concentrations were higher in obese men [6.6 (4.6–9.5) vs. 4.9 (3.5–6.8) pmol/L; $p = 0.040$]. Also, the mean ± SD plasma glucagon concentrations (8.5 ± 3.8 vs. 5.3 ± 1.4 pmol/L; $p < 0.001$) were higher in this group. A significant association was observed between copeptin and glucagon ($\beta = 1.35$, 95% CI 0.13–2.57; $p = 0.031$).

Conclusions: Fasting plasma concentrations of copeptin and glucagon were higher in obese men than men of normal weight. There was a positive association between copeptin and glucagon. Increased arginine vasopressin-stimulated glucagon secretion might contribute to higher glucagon concentrations. So, the hyperglucagonemic state of obese men can get further worsened in case of increased arginine vasopressin (AVP) secretion.

COMMENT

Arginine vasopressin (AVP) has a well-established role in the control of body fluid homeostasis, but AVP also shown to play a role in carbohydrate metabolism and the endocrine stress response. AVP is difficult to measure on account of its lability and short half-life and therefore, studies commonly use copeptin, which is the stable, biologically inactive, C-terminal portion of pro-vasopressin, as a surrogate marker for AVP secretion. Studies using copeptin have suggested that a chronic increase in AVP secretion is involved in the development of glucose intolerance and insulin resistance although the underlying mechanism remains unclear. Individuals with insulin resistance have hyperinsulinemia and hyperglucagonemia at the same time which is interesting as in healthy individuals, the normal response of the glucagon-secreting pancreatic α cell to hyperinsulinemia is to reduce the secretion of glucagon. The reason behind this paradoxical hyperglucagonemia in such individuals is not known, but it is speculated that an increase in the activity of the AVP system could be involved as earlier studies have shown an increase in plasma glucagon in healthy volunteers following AVP infusion. This study tried to find this association in biobanked blood samples of obese and healthy volunteers.

The novel finding of this study was the evidence of chronic higher activity of the AVP system which reflected in its surrogate of copeptin concentration to be associated with higher plasma glucagon concentration in obese individuals with insulin resistance. Plasma glucagon levels were also associated with markers of insulin resistance in the study cohort. Both these associations were independent of body weight status.

The strength of this study lies in its novelty of measuring both glucagon and copeptin in the same sample to look at their possible association besides using strict inclusion criteria to avoid individuals with nighttime work and include only those with complete data sets. Limitations of this study include a small sample size which can lead to false-positive results and erroneous conclusions. In addition, this study being of a cross-sectional nature does not help draw conclusions on cause–effect relationships.

The relevance of this new finding is the knowledge that chronic increased AVP-stimulated glucagon secretion could contribute to the paradoxical hyperglucagonemia found in obese insulin-resistant individuals. This could form the basis of looking at therapeutic pathways with specific partial antagonists to AVP or its receptors to reverse the pathophysiology of diabetes. Another interesting area would be to note whether drinking adequate water to lower AVP levels could reduce glucagon levels and slow the pathogenesis of diabetes.

These results need confirmation in functional models as well as prospective studies with a larger number of participants in the future. This will help clarify the cause–effect relationship (if any) between AVP secretion and increased glucagon levels.

8. PAX Proteins and Their Role in Pancreas

Ref: Panneerselvam A, Kannan A, Mariajoseph-Antony LF, Prahalathan C. PAX proteins and their role in pancreas. Diabetes Res Clin Pract. 2019;155:107792.

ABSTRACT

Transcription factors are the proteins that alter cellular functions by binding to regions of specific genes and thereby modulating gene transcription. Paired box (PAX) transcription factors that exert their regulatory activity in many tissues are sequence-specific deoxyribonucleic acid (DNA)-binding proteins. The three members of the PAX family, namely PAX2, PAX4, and PAX6, are involved not only in the multiple steps of pancreatic development and differentiation, but also in the regulation of pancreatic islet hormones synthesis and secretion. Here, we provide a comprehensive review of these transcription factors and their role in the development of the pancreas and its associated disorders.

COMMENT

Understanding the molecular mechanisms involved in the development and function of the pancreas is necessary to improve our understanding of the pathogenesis of various forms of diabetes. Amongst the developmental regulators of the pancreas, paired box (PAX) proteins, a family of highly conserved transcriptional genes, play a key role in embryonic patterning and organogenesis. All PAX factors comprise a deoxyribonucleic acid (DNA)-binding domain, called bipartite paired domain (PD), with 128 amino acids and four of nine PAX factors (PAX3, PAX4, PAX6, and PAX7) contain additional helix-turn-helix homeodomain (HD) with 60 amino acids which play a part in DNA binding or transcriptional activation. In mammals, *PAX* genes are grouped under four subfamilies based on the presence or absence of octapeptide motif domain and complete or truncated homeodomain. The evidence till date indicates that *PAX2* and *PAX8* (subfamily II), as well as *PAX4* and *PAX6* (subfamily IV), are expressed in pancreas while PAX2, PAX4, and PAX6 have been primarily linked with pancreatic development and function. Small nucleotide polymorphism (SNP) or mutations in *PAX4*, *PAX6*, and *PAX8* genes have been shown to result in impaired glucose homeostasis and diabetes mellitus (DM).

PAX2 leads to dose-dependent transactivation of glucagon promoter and has also been found in human islets besides that of embryonic mice. PAX2 mutants have larger pancreatic volume composed predominantly of an increased number of large β-cell islets instead of alpha cells. PAX2 acts as a critical regulator in determining the endocrine–exocrine fate and its absence leads to expansion of the endocrine cells during embryonic development.

Genome-wide analysis has shown the expression of *PAX8* in islets of pregnant mice and in low levels in adult human islets. *PAX8* is also expressed in the thyroid and plays a key role in its development and the production of thyroxine (T4). Studies have linked low free T4 levels with gestational diabetes which suggest a link between altered *PAX8* expression and DM under specified metabolic conditions such as pregnancy. Studies have also confirmed the association of *PAX8* SNPs with type 2 diabetes mellitus (T2DM) in African-American families. The exact role of PAX8 in pancreatic endocrine physiology needs further investigation.

PAX4 plays an essential role in the development of all four types of pancreatic islets with a single copy of PAX4 being sufficient in heterozygous mutants to help in normal pancreatic β-cell development and function. *PAX4* overexpression has been shown to promote neogenesis of alpha cells followed by conversion into beta-like cells by *PAX4*-mediated downregulation of Arx. PAX8, therefore, has an important role in β-cell differentiation. Studies have also revealed PAX4 to decrease the expression of glucagon, ghrelin, and insulin by repressing islet hormone genes and inhibiting the expression of islet amyloid polypeptide and glucose transporter 2, thus highlighting the possible role of PAX4 in β-cell maturation. PAX8 may also play a role in β-cell proliferation and survival. Several studies have shown *PAX4* mutations to result in type1diabetes mellitus (T1DM), early onset T2DM, ketosis-prone DM, and maturity-onset diabetes of the young. *PAX4* is an important DM susceptibility gene and a valuable target for developing new therapeutic interventions. However, a lot remains to be unraveled regarding the *PAX4*-related mechanisms involved.

Functional studies have revealed PAX6 to directly mediate the expression of metabolic homeostasis genes such as insulin, glucagon, incretins, prohormone convertase, and somatostatin. PAX6 also regulates the transcription of different genes. It plays a particular role in transcriptional inhibition of glucagon gene expression during pancreatic development by direct DNA-binding competition with PAX4 and further protein–protein interaction with PAX4 through its PD. *PAX6* mutations result in deficiency of prohormone convertase and impaired conversion of proinsulin to insulin and glucose-challenged insulin secretion. Mice with *PAX6* mutation have deficient glucagon-like peptide (GLP-1) receptor expression with resultant diminution of glucose-stimulated insulin secretion. *PAX6* plays a prominent role in the regulation of islet function and glucose homeostasis and remains a key target for development of gene-based therapies for diabetes management.

PAX proteins hold considerable promise as a therapeutic tool in the management of DM. Studies with adenovirus-mediated *PAX4* expression and intrabile ductal injection of adenoviruses expressing human PAX4 have shown promising results in the laboratory. PAX4 through upregulation of galectin 9 and other pathways plays a role in reducing insulitis and β-cell apoptosis. PAX6 plays a crucial role in β-cell survival as well which might be suppressed by hyperglycemia. The overall evidence suggests that targeting PAX may help us better understand disease pathogenesis, develop prognostic aids, and use novel mechanism-based interventions to impede and cure DM.

9. What has Zinc Transporter 8 Autoimmunity Taught us About Type 1 Diabetes?

Ref: Williams CL, Long AE. What has zinc transporter 8 autoimmunity taught us about type 1 diabetes? Diabetologia. 2019;62(11):1969-76.

ABSTRACT

Zinc transporter 8 (ZnT8), a protein involved in the biosynthesis and secretion of insulin, is highly specific to β cells of pancreas that produce insulin. ZnT8 autoantibodies (ZnT8A) have been recently discovered that can help predict the risk of developing type 1 diabetes mellitus (T1DM). The fact that ZnT8A often appear late in the pathogenesis implies that the antigen probably is not a part of autoimmune reaction leading to T1DM. Based on the genotype of an individual for a polymorphic ZnT8 residue, the development of autoantibodies to different forms of ZnT8 occurs. This genetic variant is associated with susceptibility to type 2 diabetes mellitus (T2DM) but not T1DM. It has been observed that ZnT8A levels are often inconsistent and decrease rapidly after diagnosis in contrast to other islet autoantibodies that persist for longer duration. Here, we review our understanding of T1DM in relation to involvement of ZnT8 and prospects of further research.

COMMENT

Pancreatic islet autoantibodies play an important role in estimating the risk of development of type 1 diabetes mellitus (T1DM) as well as in its diagnosis. Zinc transporter 8 (ZnT8) autoantibodies (ZnT8A) were first described in 2007 and are one of the four major islet autoantibodies. ZnT8 encoded by SLC30A8 impacts insulin production and its polymorphism modulates the risk of developing type 2 diabetes mellitus (T2DM). ZnT8 is highly expressed in the pancreatic β cells in the insulin secretory granules and is important for β-cell function through its role in supplying zinc ions (Zn^{2+}) for insulin storage and biosynthesis. Less than half of ZnT8 protein structure is accessible to immune surveillance making it a target of autoimmune attack in T1DM. The whole protein or fragmented peptides are most likely to be accessible to the immune system upon β-cell death, although following granule exocytosis during insulin secretion, the luminal transmembrane domains are exposed extracellularly too.

ZnT8A have shown an association with some T1DM individuals and carry a high diabetes risk in first-degree relatives. T1DM patients have a higher frequency of proinflammatory ZnT8-specific CD4+ T cells than age- and HLA-matched nondiabetic individuals. Although the number and phenotype of ZnT8-specific T cells are not different in diabetes, greater ZnT8-stimulated IFN-γ secretion by isolated CD8+ T cells from people with diabetes has been reported. More ZnT8-specific CD8+ T cells are present in the pancreas of T1DM patients compared to T2DM patients or healthy individuals.

ZnT8A is rarely detected at seroconversion and more commonly appears later in the course of the disease and is more common in adolescents rather than younger children. ZnT8A mostly recognizes the C terminal of ZnT8 and often it is specific to amino acid 325 by the SLC30A8 polymorphism rs13266634. Therefore, individuals with the CC genotype (R325) rarely develop ZnT8 tryptophan specific autoantibodies (ZnT8WA) and individuals with the TT genotype (W325) rarely develop ZnT8 arginine-specific autoantibodies (ZnT8RA). So, individual response to endogenous ZnT8 protein is determined by the person's genome. This is a specific feature of ZnT8 as other antigens lack an amino acid polymorphism with such a specific influence on the autoantibody response. ZnT8A has been shown to cross-react with a viral protein from *Mycobacterium avium subspecies paratuberculosis* in several populations with around half of ZnT8A-positive individuals having antibodies recognizing epitopes independent of amino acid 325. Therefore, molecular mimicry could be a contributing factor in the initial response to ZnT8 although more research is warranted in this regard. A second SNP, rs16889462 (G/A) which encodes Q325, has also been identified which is present in <1% of Europeans. Identification of epitopes of ZnT8A associated with a higher risk of diabetes would aid prediction, but the pattern of prediagnosis epitope-specific responses has not proved useful for risk stratification till now.

ZnT8A identifies relatives who progress rapidly to disease in the most cost-effective way and in an age-dependent manner with the benefit of adding ZnT8A in single-islet-autoantibody-positive individuals seen when onset was after age 6 years. ZnT8A adds to risk prediction in relatives who are older or who are at a genetically lower risk. The added predictive value of ZnT8A in the general population is being assessed in an ongoing study.

About two thirds of children are ZnT8A positive at diagnosis and about one fourth of children who are negative for the other three antibodies have ZnT8A. ZnT8A has not been evaluated in details in adult disease but might still reduce the cost of discriminating monogenic diabetes. Studies over time have shown an increase in the prevalence of ZnT8 suggesting a shift toward more aggressive disease as it develops later in the pathogenesis.

ZnT8A is a potentially important marker for predicting β-cell loss as evidenced from studies using C peptide and in pancreatic transplant recipients.

The gold standard method for measuring ZnT8A is presently radioimmunoassay (RIA) although harmonization of this assay is still a work in progress. Alternatively, enzyme-linked immunosorbent assay (ELISA) or luciferase immunoprecipitation system (LIPS) can be used with LIPS requiring a smaller sample volume than RIA which would be an advantage in screening young infants and the general population with capillary bleeds.

The influence of variants in SLC30A8 on the rate of progression to clinical T1DM needs further studies which are also needed to answer why autoimmunity spreads to target ZnT8 later in the pathogenesis of the disease, why this response is lost rapidly after diagnosis, and whether these changes are related to β-cell function. Further research with ZnT8 and Znt8A will help improve our understanding of disease pathogenesis and provide better biomarkers of disease.

REFERENCES (Basic Science)

1. Samuel VT, Shulman GI. Nonalcoholic fatty liver disease as a nexus of metabolic and hepatic diseases. Cell Metab. 2018;27(1):22-41.
2. Chaurasia B, Summers SA. Ceramides—lipotoxic inducers of metabolic disorder. Trends Endocrinol Metab. 2015; 26(10):538-50.
3. Summers SA. Could ceramides become the new cholesterol? Cell Metab. 2018;27(2):276-80.
4. Chaurasia B, Tippetts TS, Mayoral Monibas R, Liu Jinqi, Li Y, Wang L, et al. Targeting a ceramide double bond improves insulin resistance and hepatic steatosis. Science. 2019;365(6451):386-92.
5. Samuel VT, Shulman GI. Nonalcoholic fatty liver disease, insulin resistance, and ceramides. N Engl J Med. 2019;381(19):1866-69.

Section 2: Epidemiology

Chitra Selvan, Jugal Kishor Sharma, Anand Moses, Vijay Kumar Panikar

1. Association of Maternal Lactation with Diabetes and Hypertension: A Systematic Review and Meta-analysis

Ref: Rameez RM, Sadana D, Kaur S, Ahmed T, Patel J, Khan MS, et al. Association of maternal lactation with diabetes and hypertension: A systematic review and meta-analysis. JAMA Netw Open. 2019;2(10):1913401.

ABSTRACT

Importance: In available literature, lactation has been reported to be associated with lower rates of maternal diabetes and hypertension. But these studies have been conducted in relatively small sample size and have shown varied range of strength of association.

Objective: To determine association of lactation with lower risk of diabetes and hypertension among mothers through a systematic review and meta-analysis.

Methodology: Manual search of the references in Ovid MEDLINE, Ovid Embase, Cochrane CENTRAL, and CINAHL databases from inception to July 2018. Studies conducted in adult women specifying at least 12 months of breastfeeding and assessing primary hypertension and diabetes in them were included in the review. The full-text articles in English reporting statistical outcomes as odds ratios were included. A standard spreadsheet template was used to extract the study characteristics independently and the data were pooled using the random-effects model. This review followed the Meta-analysis of Observational Studies in Epidemiology (MOOSE) guideline for reporting. The main outcomes included diabetes and hypertension.

Results: Out of 1,558 searched studies, six studies met inclusion criteria of association between lactation and diabetes and/or hypertension. The meta-analysis to explore the association between lactation and diabetes included four studies having a total of 206,204 participants. On the other hand, the meta-analysis to explore the association between lactation and hypertension included five studies having a total of 255,271 participants. This meta-analysis showed a relative risk reduction of 30% for diabetes in women reporting 12 months of lactation {pooled odds ratio, 0.70 [95% confidence interval (CI) 0.62–0.78]; $p < 0.001$} and a relative risk reduction of 13% for hypertension [pooled odds ratio, 0.87 (95% CI 0.78–0.97); $p = 0.01$].

Conclusion and relevance: This study demonstrated the benefits of breastfeeding in preventing maternal diabetes and hypertension that can be easily included in daily practice. The lactation may also have a positive impact on cardiovascular outcomes in mothers.

COMMENT

Cardiovascular disease is the most common cause of mortality in women. Diabetes and hypertension are the two important preventable risk factors of cardiovascular disease.

Women also have unique cardiovascular and metabolic stresses in the setting of pregnancy and the puerperium. Lactation has been known to decrease the risk of diabetes and hypertension, but the papers which have studied this association have all been relatively small with disparity in outcomes reported. This meta-analysis and systematic review has tried to study the relationship between maternal lactation and risk for diabetes and hypertension.

The four studies included in the meta-analysis for the association between lactation and diabetes had a total of 206,204 participants, and the five studies included in the meta-analysis for the association between lactation and hypertension had a total of 255,271 participants. Thus, one of the biggest advantages of the paper is the large number of participants studied.

Two independent investigators extracted information and were blinded. They included studies that looked at women who breastfed for at least 12 months and reported diabetes and hypertension as outcome.

Breastfeeding for more than 12 months was associated with a relative risk reduction of 30% for diabetes {pooled odds ratio, 0.70 [95% confidence interval (CI) 0.62–0.78]; $p < 0.001$} and a relative risk reduction of 13% for hypertension [pooled odds ratio, 0.87 (95% CI 0.78–0.97); $p = 0.01$].

Interestingly, one of the papers included did also note that exclusive breastfeeding was associated with a lower risk than nonexclusive breastfeeding.

Strength of the paper is the large sample size; they included papers that have looked at breastfeeding for at least 12 months and excluded studies which included gestational diabetes and preeclampsia/eclampsia.

Limitation of the meta-analysis is that none of the four studies which were included in the systematic review was randomized controlled trial. Second limitation of the paper is the fact that the history of lactation and breastfeeding duration were from self-reported questionnaires and interviews. The intervening years could have potentially brought in a recall bias. None of the studies included in the analyses reported blinding. The duration of follow-up was variable in the included studies. The authors included only those papers which reported the results of the association between lactation and diabetes and hypertension as odds ratio and excluded those papers which reported results in relative risk or hazard ratio but they went on to do a subanalysis of these papers whose findings corroborated with the papers included in the main analysis.

Breastfeeding for longer than 12 months was associated with a 30% lower risk of diabetes and a 13% lower risk of hypertension in mothers after adjusting for confounding variables. The prenatal and antenatal period is an important opportunity to educate women about lifestyle interventions that may protect their health in the future. Given the low-risk nature of this intervention, educating mothers about the potential benefits of breastfeeding for their cardiovascular health can be easily introduced into clinical practice when addressing prevention of cardiovascular outcomes in women.

Future research could be focused on a randomized controlled trial which provides a uniform protocol of lifestyle changes including exercise, eating, and weight management and after matching for factors such as family history, age, and body mass index (BMI), the risk reduction of lactation on diabetes and hypertension can be studied for longer period of follow-up and even beyond menopause.

2. Prevalence and Predictors of Osteopenia and Osteoporosis in Patients with Type 2 Diabetes Mellitus: A Cross-sectional Study From a Tertiary Care Institute in North India

Ref: Aleti S, Pal R, Dutta P, Dhibar DP, Prakash M, Khandelwal N, Dhiman V, et al. Prevalence and predictors of osteopenia and osteoporosis in patients with type 2 diabetes mellitus: a cross-sectional study from a tertiary care institute in North India. Int J Diabet Dev Ctries. 2020;40:262-8.

ABSTRACT

Background: Patients with type 2 diabetes mellitus (T2DM) have an increased risk of hip and vertebral fractures. The increased fracture risk has largely been attributed to poor bone quality and microarchitecture. The contribution of bone quantity, measured as areal bone mineral density (BMD), to the risk of fracture, is variable with most studies showing an increase in BMD in T2DM. The present study was undertaken to find out the prevalence of osteoporosis and osteopenia (based on BMD) in a cohort of patients with T2DM and delineate the possible modifiable and nonmodifiable risk factors.

Methods: In this cross-sectional observational study, 252 otherwise ostensibly healthy patients with T2DM underwent dual-energy X-ray absorptiometry (DEXA) scan. Osteoporosis and osteopenia were defined based on T-scores. The effects of modifiable and nonmodifiable risk factors on BMD and osteoporosis were assessed.

Results: The mean age of the cohort was 59.9 years with a male:female (M:F) ratio 2.9:3.4. The mean BMD at the lumbar spine and hip was 0.892 g/cm^2 and 0.715 g/cm^2, respectively. Males had significantly higher BMD at both the sites compared to females. The prevalence of osteoporosis and osteopenia was 33% and 40%, respectively. Female gender, increasing age, normal body mass index (BMI), low serum 25-hydroxyvitamin D, and use of pioglitazone were significantly associated with the risk of osteoporosis.

Conclusion: The prevalence of osteoporosis and osteopenia in patients with T2DM is high. Female gender, increasing age, normal BMI, low serum 25-hydroxyvitamin D, and pioglitazone use further increase the risk of osteoporosis.

COMMENT

Type 2 diabetes mellitus (T2DM), apart from contributing to micro- and macrovascular disease, also exerts a detrimental effect on bone health with moderately increased risk of hip and vertebral fractures. Hip and vertebral fractures not only contribute to significant morbidity but also independently predict mortality. The increased risk of fractures in T2DM is multifactorial with changes both in bone quality and microarchitecture. Bone quantity as measured by bone mineral density (BMD) in individuals with T2DM has been controversial with some studies showing increased BMD while others showing reduced BMD. The present study attempted to find out the prevalence of osteoporosis and osteopenia based on BMD in individuals with T2DM and to identify possible modifiable and nonmodifiable risk factors.

Individuals aged 50 years and above with T2DM for more than 5 years were included. Interestingly, individuals who are on calcium and vitamin D supplements were excluded. Hologic 6 machine was used to do the dual-energy X-ray absorptiometry (DEXA) scan to assess BMD and the World Health Organization (WHO) definition was used to diagnose osteoporosis and osteopenia.

Body mass index (BMI) had a positive correlation with both lumbar spine and hip BMD. Similarly, 25-hydroxy vitamin D had a positive correlation with lumbar and hip BMD. Normal BMI (18.5–22.9 kg/m^2) was associated with an odds ratio of 3.9 for having osteoporosis compared to obese subjects. Pioglitazone was significantly associated with osteoporosis with an odds ratio of 10.6 into confidence interval of 3.8–29.3 with p value being significant.

Diabetes duration, presence of nephropathy, or degree of glycemic control over the past 1 year did not have any significant effect on BMD or prevalence of osteoporosis. Female gender and increasing age were associated with risk of having osteoporosis.

The limitations of the study are the absence of an age and BMI-matched control group. It is also a cross-sectional study with no follow-up data on fracture incidence. Men and women both included in the study, which could have affected results. Lastly, attempts to study bone quality along with BMD with the use of trabecular bone score would have added value to the study, considering in T2DM, bone quality is affected more than mineral density.

In summary, the study demonstrates the high prevalence of osteoporosis and osteopenia (33% and 40 %) in patients with T2DM in India and reinforces the fact that BMD is actually decreased and not increased. Bone health must be added in all attempts made to provide comprehensive care for patients with T2DM.

3. Autoantibody Reversion: Changing Risk Categories in Multiple-autoantibody-positive Individuals

Ref: So M, O'Rourke C, Bahnson HT, Greenbaum CJ, Speake C. Autoantibody reversion: changing risk categories in multiple-antibody-positive individuals. Diabetes Care. 2020;43(4):913-17.

ABSTRACT

Objective: The majority of individuals with two or more islet autoantibodies progress to clinical type 1 diabetes mellitus (T1DM). Nevertheless, in certain individuals, autoantibodies are lost later on. Here, we aimed to determine the occurrence of autoantibody loss (reversion) in multiple-autoantibody-positive subjects and to determine the relationship between reversion and progression to clinical disease.

Research design and methods: Multiple-autoantibody-positive individuals participating in TrialNet Pathway to Prevention Study were analyzed for reversion and the effect of reversion on progression to clinical disease was determined using a Cox regression analysis.

Results: Out of 3,284 multiple-autoantibody-positive individuals, reversion occurred in 134 (4.1%) and was linked with decreased incidence of clinical T1DM. Reversion occurred more commonly with older age, lesser autoantibody titers, and fewer positive autoantibodies.

Conclusion: Even though reversion of multiple-autoantibody positivity is rare, when it happens, the risk of progression to clinical disease is decreased. This observation suggests unidentified mechanisms triggering immune remission in some individuals.

COMMENT

Islet autoantibodies are tested as a measure to distinguish type 1 diabetes mellitus (T1DM) from other forms of diabetes and to predict disease progression. Large scale prospective studies of relatives of individuals with T1DM revealed that nearly all individuals with two or more autoantibodies progressed to clinical diabetes. Some individuals noticed autoantibody titer levels dropping below threshold for positivity. The implication of this loss of multiple autoantibodies (reversion) on disease development is not known so this study was designed to evaluate the same.

Through TrialNet Pathway to Prevention Study, two lakh and more relatives of subjects with T1DM were screened for autoantibodies between 2004 and 2018. Multiple-autoantibody positivity was defined as two or more islet autoantibodies confirmed on two occasions within 12 months; the antibodies included are islet cell antibody (ICA) insulin antibody (IAA) GAD antibody (GAD) or zinc transporter.

Reverters were defined as an individual who demonstrated a loss of multiple-autoantibody positivity to one or zero autoantibodies on two consecutive encounters within 12 months.

Reverters were more likely to be older at the time of confirmed multiple-autoantibody positivity (19.4 vs. 13.1 years) with longer follow-up (5.2 vs. 2.1 years) and also had a lower number of autoantibodies (2.1 vs. 3.1). On the basis of univariate Cox model, each additional positive autoantibody decreases the risk of reversion by a factor of five. They also had a lower titer of autoantibodies as compared to maintainers.

Among reverters, ICAs were most likely to be lost, with 85 of the 87 (98%) who started with a positive ICA losing positivity. In contrast, reverters were unlikely to lose glutamic acid decarboxylase antibodies (GADAs), with only 19/129 (15%) reverters who had GADAs losing GADA positivity.

Estimated cumulative 5-year risk of T1DM was 42% for maintainers and 11% for the reporters with a confidence interval of 6–18%.

During follow-up, 41 of 134 (31%) reverters regained multiple-autoantibody status. There was no significant difference in diabetes incidence ($p = 0.99$) between the reverters who regained their multiple-autoantibody status (7/41, 17%) and those who did not (16/93, 17%). Nor was there a significant difference in distribution of autoantibody titers.

Strength of the study is to understand that there could be reversion of autoantibodies and this point might be relevant while recruiting individuals, especially for prevention trials.

Hide a group of individuals in home reversional multiple-autoantibodies and disease progression can be studied to find a mechanistic link of the pathophysiology of T1DM.

The limitation of the study is that it only looked at multiple-autoantibodies as against single autoantibodies or no antibodies.

4. Incidence and Associations of Chronic Kidney Disease in Community Participants with Diabetes: A 5-Year Prospective Analysis of the EXTEND45 Study

Ref: Sukkar L, Kang A, Hockham C, Young T, Jun M, Foote C, et al. Incidence and associations of chronic kidney disease in community participants with diabetes: a 5-year prospective analysis of the EXTEND45 study. Diabetes Care. 2020;43(5):982-90.

ABSTRACT

Objective: We intended to determine the incidence of and factors related with an estimated glomerular filtration rate (eGFR) <60 mL/min/1.73 m² in people with diabetes.

Research design and methods: We identified diabetic individuals in the EXTEND45 (EXamining ouTcomEs in chroNic Disease in the 45 and Up Study), a population-based cohort study (2006–2014) that connected the Sax Institute's 45 and Up Study cohort to community laboratory and administrative data in New South Wales, Australia. The outcome of the study was the first eGFR measurement <60 mL/min/1.73 m² documented during the follow-up period. Participants with eGFR <60 mL/min/1.73 m² at baseline were excluded. Poisson regression was used to calculate the incidence of eGFR <60 mL/min/1.73 m² and multivariable Cox regression was performed to examine factors associated with the outcome of the study.

Results: Out of 9,313 participants with diabetes, 2,106 (22.6%) developed incident eGFR <60 mL/min/1.73 m² over a median follow-up time of 5.7 years (interquartile range, 3.0–5.9 years). The incidence rate of eGFR <60 mL/min/1.73 m² per 100 person-years was 6.0 [95% confidence interval (CI) 5.7–6.3] overall, 1.5 (1.3–1.9) in individuals aged 45–54 years, 3.7 (3.4–4.0) for 55–64 year olds, 7.6 (7.1–8.1) for 65–74 year olds, 15.0 (13.0–16.0) for 75–84 year olds, and 26.0 (22.0–32.0) for those aged 85 years and above. A fully adjusted multivariable model showed an independent association of the incidence with age (hazard ratio 1.23 per 5-year increase; 95% CI 1.19–1.26), geography (outer regional and remote vs. major city: 1.36; 1.17–1.58), obesity (obese class III vs. normal: 1.44; 1.16–1.80), and the existence of hypertension (1.52; 1.33–1.73), coronary heart disease (1.13; 1.02–1.24), cancer (1.30; 1.14–1.50), and depression/anxiety (1.14; 1.01–1.27).

Conclusion: The incidence of an eGFR <60 mL/min/1.73 m^2 was high in people with diabetes. Older age, remoteness of residence, and the presence of various comorbidities were associated with greater incidence.

COMMENT

The leading cause of chronic kidney disease (CKD) worldwide is the presence of diabetes and CKD leads to increased risk of cardiovascular death and disease. Identifying individuals with diabetes who are at increased risk of developing CKD is a key step to develop preventive strategies for improving health outcomes in this high-risk population.

EXTEND45 (EXamining ouTcomEs in chroNic Disease in the 45 and Up Study) is a large population-based cohort built on Sax Institute's 45 and Up Study, a prospective cohort of residents aged 45 years or older in the state of New South Wales, Australia.

Follow-up data was collected from health and administrative databases. CKD-Epidemiology Collaboration (CKD-EPI) equation was used to calculate estimated glomerular filtration rate (eGFR). Among the 9,313 participants with diabetes, hypertension was present in 73.4% in hypercholesterolemia and 65.8%.

In this Australian population-based cohort of participants with diabetes aged 45 years and over, the age-adjusted incidence rates of eGFR <60 mL/min/1.73m^2 were six new cases per 100 person-years between 2006 and 2014, which is much higher than previously reported incidence rates. This high incidence could be explained by the fact that the cohort was 5–10 years older than other cohorts and also that this is real world clinical data from multiple sources.

Advancing age was found to be the strongest association of CKD in diabetes, followed by obesity and the presence of hypertension.

The social economic marker such as living remotely was an independent risk factor for greater incident CKD probably attributable to poorer access to health care. The study found no sex difference in the risk of CKD in those with diabetes.

History of cancer at baseline as well as baseline depression and anxiety predicted incident disease and these are interesting findings which have been observed before.

The strength of the study is the large number of the population in the real world set-up followed up for up to 5.7 years.

The first limitation of the study is the fact that the inclusion criteria only measured one creatinine in the 3 years prior to recruitment, the second important limitation is the fact that only eGFR was used to classify CKD and not albuminuria. The third limitation is the age of inclusion of individuals in this was only 45 years and higher. The type of diabetes was not specified. Yet the study is relevant in identifying factors which could potentially identify individuals with a higher risk of progression of eGFR decline and design interventions to mitigate the same.

5. Establishment and Validation of a Risk Prediction Model for Early Diabetic Kidney Disease Based on a Systematic Review and Meta-analysis of 20 Cohorts

Ref: Jiang W, Wang J, Shen X, Lu W, Wang Y, Li W, et al. Establishment and validation of a risk prediction model for early diabetic kidney disease based on a systematic review and meta-analysis of 20 Cohorts. Diabetes Care. 2020;43(4):925-33.

ABSTRACT

Background: Clinical outcome of diabetic kidney disease (DKD) can be improved by identifying patients at high risk.

Purpose: To establish a model for predicting DKD.

Data sources: The derivation cohort was from a meta-analysis. The validation cohort was from a Chinese cohort.

Study selection: We selected cohort studies that reported risk factors of DKD with their corresponding risk ratios (RRs) in patients with type 2 diabetes mellitus (T2DM). Their estimated baseline glomerular filtration rate (eGFR) was ≥60 mL/min/1.73 m^2 and urinary albumin-to-creatinine ratio (UACR) was <30 mg/g.

Data extraction: Only statistically significant risk factors were included in our DKD risk prediction model.

Data synthesis: Twenty cohorts including 41,271 patients with (T2DM) were included in our meta-analysis. Statistically significant risk factors were age, body mass index (BMI), smoking, diabetic retinopathy, hemoglobin A1c (HbA1c), systolic blood pressure (SBP), high-density lipoprotein (HDL) cholesterol, triglycerides (TGs), UACR, and eGFR. All, except eGFR, were included in the study because of the significant heterogeneity seen in eGFR among various studies. Risk factors were scored according to their weightage, with 37.0 being the highest score. Model validation was done in an external cohort with a median follow-up of 2.9 years. A cutoff value of 16 was selected with a sensitivity of 0.847 and a specificity of 0.677.

Limitations: A huge heterogeneity among studies involving eGFR was observed. So, more studies are needed to establish it as a risk factor of DKD.

Conclusion: High-risk patients of DKD can be easily predicted using this simple tool of DKD risk prediction model consisting of nine risk factors.

COMMENT

Diabetic kidney disease (DKD) is a major microvascular complication of diabetes with high prevalence, mortality, and treatment cost. Yet, there is low awareness and poor effective prevention and treatment strategy. Since most early predictive markers of DKD are difficult to promote in clinical practice due to high cost and/or stability, we have to rely on a comprehensive assessment of other risk factors which could potentially provide a window for intervention in high-risk individuals for preventing DKD.

The derivation cohort came from a systematic review and meta-analysis of 14 prospective cohorts and 6 retrospective cohorts. These 20 cohorts were identified by searching electronic databases. In total, 41,271 patients with type 2 diabetes mellitus (T2DM) from Europe, Asia, and America with an estimated glomerular filtration rate (eGFR) of

>60 mL/min/1.73 m² and urine albumin-to-creatinine ratio (UACR) <30 mg/g in baseline were included.

The validation cohort came from Tianjin Medical University Metabolic Disease Hospital and included 380 patients with T2DM who are followed up for at least 12 months.

The outcomes included were the occurrence of an eGFR <60 mL/min/1.73 m² or UACR ratio >30 mg/g for more than 3 months caused by diabetes.

The estimated incidence of DKD was approximately 29.1% in a derivation cohort and 25.8% in the validation cohort.

Of the 19 risk factors identified in the systematic review and meta-analysis, 10 risk factors were associated with the onset of DKD. These factors, followed by the respective pooled risk ratios (RRs), were age (1.09), body mass index (BMI) (1.07), diabetic retinopathy (DR) (1.72), smoking (1.49), HbA1c (1.17), systolic blood pressure (SBP) (1.03), high-density lipoprotein cholesterol (HDL-C) (0.75), triglycerides (TGs) (1.15), UACR (1.25), and eGFR (2.20). These factors are essentially consistent with the risk factors traditionally associated with DKD, further verifying that age and harmful lifestyle, together with poor glycemia, blood pressure, and plasma lipid control, initiate DKD. Except for age, most of these risk factors are modifiable, which is particularly important for DKD prevention.

Age, smoking, and TG were the most powerful baseline risk factors for detecting DKD in this systematic review and meta-analysis. With age incremented by 5–10 years, the risk for DKD was increased by 38%. The risk for DKD increased by 49% in patients with diabetes who smoked. TG increased by 1 mmol/L and the risk for DKD increased by 42%. With HDL-C increased by 1 mmol/L, the risk for DKD was reduced by 22%. For every 1% increase in HbA1c, the risk for DKD increased by 17%. With SBP increased by 10–20 mm Hg, the risk of DKD increased by 21%.

The risk of DKD increased by 16% when BMI increased by 5 kg/m² while patients with DR had their risk of DKD increased by 31%.

The limitations of the study are: First, the method of systematic review and meta-analysis was heterogeneous due to differences in research design and method as well as different race and sex compositions of the cohorts in included studies.

Second, the derivation cohort consisted of about 80% white patients and 20% Asian patients, leaving out some of the ethnicities with higher risk for DKD incidence (for instance, black and Hispanic patients). Third, amongst the Asians included, they were predominantly Chinese and the Chinese cutoffs for BMI were used in the risk prediction model making the model difficult to generalize to all Asians.

Fourth, a median follow-up period of 2.9 years may be insufficient follow-up for incidence of DKD validation cohort.

Yet, a simple DKD risk prediction model was developed using age, BMI, smoking, presence of diabetic retinopathy, HbA1c, SBP, TGs, HDL, and UACR which could identify individuals at risk for progression of kidney disease with high sensitivity and specificity, highlighting the importance of grouping use of risk prediction models.

6. Every Fifth Individual with Type 1 Diabetes Suffers from an Additional Autoimmune Disease: A Finnish Nationwide Study

Ref: Mäkimattila S, Harjutsalo V, Forsblom C, Groop PH, FinnDiane Study Group. Every fifth individual with type 1 diabetes suffers from an additional autoimmune disease: A Finnish nationwide study. Diabetes Care. 2020;43(5):1041-47.

ABSTRACT

Objective: To quantify the risk of coexisting autoimmune diseases (ADs) in type 1 diabetic adults of Finland.

Research design and methods: A total of 4,758 participants of Finnish Diabetic Nephropathy (FinnDiane) Study and 12,710 nondiabetic control individuals were enrolled for this study. Identification of the ADs like thyroid-related disorders, Addison disease, celiac disease, and atrophic gastritis was done with the help of Finnish nationwide health registries (1970–2015).

Results: The median duration of diabetes was 35.5 (26.5–44.0) years while the median age of the participants at the end of follow-up was 51.4 (interquartile range 42.6–60.1) years. 31.6% of women and 14.9% of men had at least one coexisting AD (overall 22.8%). The odds ratios (ORs) for hypothyroidism, hyperthyroidism, celiac disease, Addison disease, and atrophic gastritis were 3.43 [95% confidence interval (CI) 3.09–3.81], 2.98 (2.27–3.90), 4.64 (3.71–5.81), 24.13 (5.60–104.03), and 5.08 (3.15–8.18), respectively, in the participants compared to control group. The corresponding ORs for women compared with men were 2.96 (2.53–3.47), 2.83 (1.87–4.28), 1.52 (1.15–2.02), 2.22 (0.83–5.91), and 1.36 (0.77–2.39), respectively. Late onset of type 1 diabetes mellitus (T1DM) and ageing is associated with increased risk of hypothyroidism, while young age at onset of T1DM increased the risk of celiac disease.

Conclusion: The results of our study, which is one of the largest studies conducted in Finland, highlight the importance of screening of individuals with T1DM for risk of ADs.

COMMENT

Autoimmune disorders share common genetic factors and immunologic processes and hence, often coexist within the same individual and families. In individuals with type 1 diabetes mellitus (T1DM), celiac disease and hypothyroidism are the most frequently observed additional autoimmune disease (AD) amongst 80 different others. Although common genetic background is the main factor determining high prevalence of additional AD in individuals with T1DM, shared environmental or other pathological mechanisms cannot be ruled out. Finland has the highest incidence of T1DM in children (62.5 per 100,000) and is among the countries with the highest incidence of celiac disease in young adults (31 per 100,000) in the world.

This study aimed to quantify the excess risk of ADs in adult individuals with long-term T1DM compared with sex and age match control individuals without T1DM.

Autoimmune diseases were identified by linking the data with the Finnish nationwide health registry and prescription patterns of 4,758 individuals with T1DM in the Finnish Diabetic Nephropathy study cohort and 12,000 age and sex match control individuals without T1DM.

About 2,523 (53%) were diagnosed with T1DM under 15 years of age, and the median duration of diabetes was 35.5 (26.5–44.0) years. There were 1,245 additional ADs that were identified in 1,087 individuals with T1DM. The most prevalent AD on top of T1DM was hypothyroidism ($n = 859$, 18.1%) followed by celiac disease ($n = 207$, 4.4%), hyperthyroidism ($n = 112$, 2.4%), atrophic gastritis ($n = 49$, 1.0%), and Addison disease ($n = 18$, 0.4%).

There was a female preponderance for all ADs, although this was not significant for atrophic gastritis. It was most conspicuous for hyperthyroidism where the proportion of women reached 71.4%. Women were also more likely to develop multiple ADs with a prevalence of 31.6% compared with 14.9% in men ($p < 0.0001$). Individuals with hypothyroidism were older, had a longer duration of diabetes, and had a lower body weight but higher body mass index (BMI) (adjusted for sex) than those without any additional AD. Alongside female predominance, the individuals with hyperthyroidism more often had a history of smoking. Individuals with Addison disease had a worse lipid profile, lower high-density lipoprotein (HDL) cholesterol, and a tendency to higher triglyceride concentrations. Individuals with celiac disease had lower age at onset and longer duration of diabetes as well as lower body weight and BMI.

Of T1DM individuals, 937 (19.7%) had only one additional AD, 143 (3.0%) had two, 6 (0.13%) had three, and one patient (0.02%) had four ADs together with T1DM. The most prevalent combination was hypothyroidism and celiac disease. Although Addison disease was not a frequent AD, 16 out of 18 (89%) clustered with another AD and mostly with hypothyroidism (78%). Similarly, 53% of the cases of atrophic gastritis clustered with hypothyroidism.

The risk of hypothyroidism increased 1.7% [95% confidence interval (CI) 0.9–2.5%, $p < 0.0001$] by each increasing year of age at onset of diabetes. The risk increased 1.3% (0.7–2.0%, $p < 0.0001$) by year of age. Opposite to hypothyroidism, the risk of celiac disease was 1.5% (95% CI 0.1–3.0%, $p = 0.048$) higher for each decreasing year of age at onset of diabetes.

The highest risk was seen in those with an age at diagnosis of diabetes under 10 years compared with all other individuals with T1DM with an odds ratio (OR) of 1.38 (1.02–1.85, $p = 0.03$), but thereafter, the risk leveled off.

The main strength of the study is the large cohort of well-characterized patients with T1DM during a long diabetes duration with age and sex match controls. The limitations of the study are that it is a registry-based study with absence of clinical data and baseline, and also the fact that the age of onset of ADs is not determined.

In conclusion, this nationwide study showed that 22.8% of individuals with T1DM have an additional AD. Hypothyroidism, celiac disease, and hyperthyroidism are the most prevalent ADs. Late onset of T1DM and ageing increases the risk of hypothyroidism. Screening for celiac disease is important during childhood, since age 10 years at onset of T1DM but not ageing, per se, increases the risk of celiac disease. ADs should be screened throughout life equally for both sexes and more often in those with a family history of T1DM.

7. Absence of Islet Autoantibodies and Modestly Raised Glucose Values at Diabetes Diagnosis Should Lead to Testing for MODY: Lessons from a 5-year Pediatric Swedish National Cohort Study

Ref: Carlsson A, Shepherd M, Ellard S, Weedon M, Lernmark Å, Forsander G, et al. Absence of Islet Autoantibodies and Modestly Raised Glucose Values at Diabetes Diagnosis Should Lead to Testing for MODY: Lessons From a 5-Year Pediatric Swedish National Cohort Study. Diabetes Care. 2020;43(1):82-9.

ABSTRACT

Objective: To identify the discriminatory factors for maturity onset diabetes of the young (MODY) in the pediatric population at the time of diagnosis of diabetes.

Research design and methods: A total of 3,933 Swedish patients, aged 1–18 years, from a national consecutive prospective cohort were enrolled for the study. Clinical data and other information related to islet autoantibodies [glutamic acid decarboxylase (GAD) insulinoma antigen-2 (IA-2), zinc transporter-8 (ZnT8), and insulin autoantibodies (IAAs)], human leukocyte antigens (HLAs) type, and C-peptide were collected at diagnosis. Confirmation for MODY was done by glucokinase (GCK), hepatocyte nuclear factor-1A (HNF1A), and HNF4A sequencing.

Results: Discriminatory factors for MODY at diagnosis included four islet autoantibody negativity (100% vs. 11% not-known MODY; $p = 2 \times 10^{-44}$), hemoglobin A1c (HbA1c) [7.0% vs. 10.7% (53 vs. 93 mmol/mol); $p = 1 \times 10^{-20}$], plasma glucose (11.7 vs. 26.7 mmol/L; $p = 3 \times 10^{-19}$), parental diabetes (63% vs. 12%; $p = 1 \times 10^{-15}$), and diabetic ketoacidosis (0% vs. 15%; $p = 0.001$). Detection rate for MODY was 15% in islet autoantibody-negative patients, and 49% in islet autoantibody-negative patients having HbA1c <7.5% (58 mmol/mol) at diagnosis. On follow-up, the 46 patients with MODY showed good glycemic control, having an HbA1c level of 6.4% (47 mmol/mol).

Conclusion: Absence of all islet autoantibodies and modest hyperglycemia [HbA1c <7.5% (58 mmol/mol)], at the diagnosis of pediatric diabetes, should prompt the clinician to test for GCK, HNF1A, and HNF4A MODY. Testing all patients negative for four islet autoantibodies is an effective strategy for not missing MODY but will result in a lower detection rate.

COMMENT

Maturity onset diabetes of the young (MODY) is noninsulin dependent, dominantly inherited monogenic variant of diabetes which is diagnosed in young age typically. It has been recognized that management of MODY is different from type 1 diabetes mellitus (T1DM) and type 2 diabetes mellitus (T2DM). MODY is found to be accountable for 1–2% of pediatric diabetes but misdiagnosis results in unnecessary treatment of many young people with insulin resulting in delay in diagnosis of MODY. The most common subtypes of MODY or glucose kinase MODY does not require any treatment whereas other two subtypes, i.e., hepatocyte nuclear factor-1A (HNF1A) MODY and HNF4A MODY are optimally treated with low-dose sulfonylureas in case therapy is needed.

Islet autoantiantibodies can be useful in diagnosis of MODY, non-T1DM. These antibodies are detected in 90% of pediatric cases of T1DM but are rarely detected in MODY, i.e., only 1% of cases which are similar to healthy population. In routine clinical practice, comprehensive islet autoantibody testing of all four subtypes—antibodies against glutamic acid decarboxylase (GAD), insulinoma antigen-2 (IA-2A), zinc transporter-8 (ZNT8A), and insulin autoantibodies (IAA)—is not performed. The present study was carried out in a pediatric national cohort with the aim to characterize discriminatory clinical features of the most common types of MODY in diagnosis of diabetes.

This study, i.e., better diabetes diagnosis study (BOD), was carried out from May 2005 to December 2010 in 42 hospital pediatric clinics in Sweden. Total 3,933 eligible pediatric patients were included in the study cohort with the mean age of 10.1 years at the time of diagnosis and 45% being female.

The study reported 88% of patients to be positive for at least one islet autoantibody. Anti-glutamic acid decarboxylase antibody (GADA) alone were reported negative in 49% patients. 17% of patients were reported to be negative for GADA and IA-2A; 13% for GADA, IA-2A, and ZNT8A; and 12% with all the four autoantibodies.

It was found that MODY was not identified in any autoantibody-positive patient.

The characteristic clinical feature of MODY and diagnosis was found to be absence of islet autoantibodies. Additionally, lower HbA1c (7% vs. 10.7%), parental diabetes (63% vs. 12%), and not having DKA (0 out of 46 vs. 601 out of 3,887) $p < 0.001$ were other keys discriminating features.

Maturity onset diabetes of the young was detected in 45% of the islet autoantibodies-negative patients who were tested on clinicians request. Whereas it was detected in 5% of the autoantibody-negative patients who were tested genetically as part of this research project.

Glucokinase (GCK) MODY subtype was detected in 63%, HNF1A MODY subtype in 22%, and HNF4A MODY subtype in 15%.

The detection rate of MODY was found to be 33% with 96% of case subjects with MODY detected in patients with HbA1c <7.5% or an affected parent. It shows that glycemic index at the time of diagnosis and family history helps in identification of autoantibody-negative patients for further testing, but HbA1c <7.5% is both more sensitive and more specific than family history.

Excellent glycemic control with a mean HbA1c of 6.4% has been seen in the patients with genetic diagnosis of MODY after a mean of 5.9 years of initial diabetes diagnosis and 91% of patients were not on insulin.

The present study is the first large prospective national study to provide clear support to identify characteristic discriminatory clinical features in pediatric patients for MODY testing by excluding T1DM. This is the first study which was carried out at the time of diabetes diagnosis with a large cohort and also considers clinical features in addition to detection of all the four subtypes of islet autoantibody in diagnosis of MODY. But this study was limited to testing for three most common subtypes of MODY only and the other rare subtypes were not tested.

In conclusion, MODY had a prevalence of 1.2% in pediatric diabetes and a comprehensive approach of islet autoantibody testing, glycemic index, and key clinical features of MODY at the time of diagnosis of pediatric diabetes allows its differentiation from T1DM.

8. Effect of Age at Menarche on Microvascular Complications Among Women with Type 1 Diabetes

Ref: Y Yi, Denic-Roberts H, Rubinstein D, Orchard TJ, Costacou T. Effect of age at menarche on microvascular complications among women with Type 1 diabetes. Diabet Med. 2019;36(10):1287-93.

ABSTRACT

Aim: To test the hypothesis that type 1 diabetic women with delayed menarche are at an increased risk of microvascular complications.

Methods: Data of 315 out of 325 women who were enrolled in a prospective study of childhood-onset type 1 diabetes diagnosed during 1950–1980, were included in our study. These 315 women who had menarche during 1986–1988 could report their age at that time. For assessment of the relationship of age at menarche with microvascular complications, that included overt nephropathy, proliferative retinopathy, and confirmed distal symmetric polyneuropathy (DSP), cross-sectional and prospective analyses over the 25-year follow-up were conducted.

Results: The odds of overt nephropathy increased 1.24 times ($p = 0.02$) and the cumulative incidence of overt nephropathy increased 1.16 times ($p = 0.01$) with annual delay in menarche onset. Also, women with delayed menarche were twice at increased risk of overt nephropathy (hazard ratio 2.30, $p = 0.001$) compared to women with no delay in menarche. However, there was no significant association between age at menarche and proliferative retinopathy or confirmed DSP.

Conclusion: A significant association was observed between age at menarche and prevalence and cumulative incidence of overt nephropathy in type 1 diabetic women. However, this was not seen with proliferative retinopathy or confirmed DSP. Hence, targeting women with delayed menarche for early screening along with appropriate interventions can prevent the development of nephropathy.

COMMENT

Delayed menarche has been found commonly in type 1 diabetic women especially if the diagnosis of diabetes precedes menarche. The National Health and Nutrition Examination Survey (NHANES), a population-based survey conducted from 1988-1994 to 2001-2006, has suggested the persistence of the delay in the age of menarche over time. As the delay in menarche has been seen among type 1 diabetic girls in spite of intensive diabetes treatment and good glycemic control, there is conflict in the association of delayed menarche and glycemic control.

A 2-fold increase in the prevalence of retinopathy and nephropathy has been reported in women with delayed menarche (after 15 years) as compared to women with a normal menarche timing (11-15 years) by the Finnish Diabetic Nephropathy study (Finn Diane group) independent of covariates.

The two possible hypotheses for delayed menarche in type 1 diabetic women include insulin deficiency along with elevated hemoglobin A1c (HbA1c) or appearance of hyperandrogenism. But evidences also suggest delayed menarche in spite of adequate diabetes treatment and good glycemic control.

The Pittsburgh Epidemiology of Diabetes Complication (EDC study), an ongoing prospective study of childhood onset type 1 diabetes mellitus (T1DM), included patients with T1DM diagnosed between 1950 and 1980. Biennial surveys were carried out for their follow-up for up to 25 years with clinical examinations at 10 years and again at 18 and 25 years. The age at menarche was self-reported by the girls at baseline. The age at menarche was categorized into early age of menarche (before 11.5 years of age), normal (11.5-15 years of age), and delayed (after 15 years of age).

The median age of menarche was reported to be 13 years (9-23 years) in the study cohort. The age of menarche was found to be normal in 78%, delayed in 13%, and early in 9% of the participants. Approximately 77.8% of the study participants achieved menarche after more 1 year after the onset of diabetes.

Increase in prevalence of hypertension, overt nephropathy, and proliferative retinopathy was found from early to delayed menarche group.

Approximately 1.24 times increase in the odds of overt nephropathy was reported with each year increase in age at menarche ($p = 0.02$) after adjusting for the variables, i.e., age at diabetes onset, baseline diabetes duration, HbA1c, total insulin units per weight, hypertension, and estimated glomerular filtration rate (GFR). Delayed menarche was found to be associated with 3.2 times greater odds of overt nephropathy as compared to the normal age at menarche ($p = 0.009$) when menarche group was taken as the main exposure variable whereas no such association was found between the early and normal menarche categories after adjustment. Delayed menarche was not found to be associated with the prevalence of either proliferative retinopathy or polyneuropathy.

This study reflected the more severe latent microvascular damage by delayed menarche reflects caused by poor glycemic control earlier in life. Another possibility for the observation of greater risk of kidney damage could be due to delay in exposure to higher estrogen level in view of delayed menarche. The renoprotective effects of estrogen have been reported by numerous studies in both general and diabetes population. Additionally a few randomized controlled trials also reported a reduction in albumin creatinine ratio and even improve creatinine clearance with the use of hormone replacement therapy.

The data related to age and duration of diabetes at the onset of microvascular complications were lacking prior to the study date. Small number of cases with the incidence of complications and lack of data of HbA1c over the follow-up period of 25 years were other limitations of the present study.

More studies are required to be conducted to confirm the role of age of menarche in type 1 diabetic women in subsequent microvascular complications so that early screening and timely interventions can be done in women with a delayed menarche to prevent development of advanced microvascular disease.

9. Geographic Variation and Associated Covariates of Diabetes Prevalence in India

Ref: Hernandez AM, Jia P, Kim HY, Cuadros DF. Geographic variation and associated covariates of diabetes prevalence in India. JAMA Netw Open. 2020;3(5):e203865.

ABSTRACT

Importance: In modern era, diabetes is emerging as a severe metabolic disorder worldwide with higher prevalence in low- and middle-income countries and affecting human health. There is gap in the knowledge regarding risk factors for diabetes and due to lack of large-scale dual testing and appropriate evaluation methods; it is still found to be associated with tuberculosis (TB) endemicity at the national scale.

Objectives: To identify the hotspots of diabetes with concentrated prevalence, to explore the association of diabetes with sociodemographic and behavioral covariates, and to locate the high regional TB endemicity areas overlapping with diabetes.

Design, setting, and participants: A total of 803,164 men in the age group of 15–54 years and women in the age group of 15–49 years who reported their diabetic status were enrolled in this cross-sectional study. The participants had also participated in the Demographic Health Survey (2015–2016) carried out by the Indian Ministry of Health and Family Welfare using a two-stage clustered sampling, including a diabetes estimation component. The data were collected from January 2015 to December 2016 and analyzed from July 2018 to January 2019.

Main outcomes and measures: The association of prevalence of self-reported diabetes was estimated with covariates including educational level, sex, age, religion, marital status, alcohol use, tobacco use, obesity status, and socioeconomic level. Additionally, the estimated regional TB endemicity level according to the India TB report for 2014 from the Revised National TB Control Program was used to assess the national extent of the spatial overlap of diabetes and TB.

Results: A total of 803,164 individuals were sampled with the mean age of 30.09 ± 9.97 years and 691,982 (86.2%) women. A significant geographic variation was found in diabetes prevalence in India. A concentrated burden was reported at the southern coastline. The prevalence of 3.01% (1,864 of 61,948 individuals) was found in cluster 1 in Andhra Pradesh and Telangana, prevalence of 4.32% (3,429 of 79,435 individuals) in cluster 2 in Tamil Nadu and Kerala, prevalence of 2.81% (330 of 11,758 individuals) in cluster 3 in east Odisha, and prevalence of 4.43% (83 of 1,883 individuals) in cluster 4 in Goa. The presence of obesity and overweight [odds ratio (OR) 2.44; 95% confidence interval (CI) 2.18–2.73; $p < 0.001$; OR 1.66; 95% CI 1.52–1.82; $p < 0.001$, respectively], tobacco smoking (OR 3.04; 95% CI 1.66–5.56; $p < 0.001$), and consumption of alcohol (OR 2.01; 95% CI 1.37–2.95; $p < 0.001$) were found to be associated with increased odds of diabetes. A lack of consistent geographical overlap between TB and diabetes were shown with regional TB endemicity and diabetes spatial distributions, e.g., TB cluster 4 with 60,213 TB cases and 0.93% diabetes prevalence, i.e., 186.79 diabetes cases in 20,183.88 individuals; TB cluster 8 with 47,381 TB cases and 0.80% diabetes prevalence, i.e., 180.53 diabetes cases in 22,449.18 individuals; TB cluster 9 with 37,620 TB cases, 4.67% diabetes prevalence, i.e., 601.45 diabetes cases in 12,879.36 individuals.

Conclusion and relevance: The identification of spatial clusters of diabetes on the basis of a nationally representative survey suggested that India faces different levels of disease severity. Each region might need to implement appropriate control strategies according to its unique epidemiologic context.

COMMENT

Diabetes has been identified by the World Health Organization as an important public health issue. The estimated global burden of diabetes in 2014 was 422 million adults and it is expected to increase to 552 million by 2030. Interest regarding the biological and epidemiological interactions between diabetes and other diseases has recently grown. For example, tuberculosis (TB) has been considered part of the spectrum of diabetes-associated diseases. Possible causes of diabetes–TB interaction include impaired glucose tolerance associated with TB treatment with potential increases the risk of diabetes. However, the mechanisms underlying glucose intolerance in diabetes in individuals with TB infections are not completely understood.

India, the second most populous country in the world with 1.3 billion residents, has the largest number of diabetes cases with a prevalence of 7.8%. Tuberculosis also severely affects the Indian population with an incidence of 2.79 million in 2016.

Such high burdens of both TB and diabetes might increase the likelihood of disease interactions that could worsen mortality from both diseases.

Lack of information regarding the interaction between diabetes and TB exist particularly in India. First, previous studies have overlooked the roles of behavioral risk factors in the prevalence of diabetes at a large scale. Second, little attention has been paid to the spatial structures of diabetes. Third, few studies have examined questions regarding the association between regional TB endemicity and diabetes mainly because of lack of affordable large-scale dual testing for TB or diabetes. Moreover, spatial variation in the association between diabetes and TB and the behavioral and environmental risk factors for diabetes-TB concurrence have not been assessed.

Against this background, data from a national survey of more than eight lakh individuals were obtained by the Indian Demographic Health Survey (DHS) 2015–2016 and the Revised National TB Control Program (RNTCP) data from 2014 in India were obtained to identify the location where the burden of diabetes is clustered and the areas where the burden of diabetes TB exist.

The study aimed to assess the association of diabetes with regional TB endemicity after controlling for important covariance and to examine sociodemographic and behavioral factors associated with diabetes in India. The hypothesis was that individuals living in areas with high TB exposure would have an increased likelihood of developing diabetes.

Self-reported diabetes status was used as the outcome variable for the study so the question which was asked was "Has a doctor or other health professional ever told you that you had diabetes?" As a measure for diabetes, only individuals answering yes or no were included in the analysis.

A total of seven covariance were included in the final model which were sex, age, religion, marital status, alcohol consumption, smoking tobacco, and body mass index (BMI). Control variables were added to control for confounding including educational level rural or urban residents, wealth index, and land travel friction.

Body mass index classification was according to the World Health Organization standards defining normal weight as a BMI 18.5 to <25 kg/m^2.

Data from RNTCP was used for reclassification of TB exposure areas and was conducted using the following quantiles: level 1, <210 cases per 100,000 inhabitants; level 2, 210–311 cases per 100,000 inhabitants; level 3, 312–411 per 100,000 inhabitants; and level 4, >411 cases per 100,000 inhabitants.

A scan statistical analysis was implemented in the SaTscan software to identify locations where diabetes cases were clustered. The spatial scan statistic is a cluster detection test able to identify geography clusters.

About 86.2% of individuals were women with the mean age of the cohort 30 years. The prevalence of self-reported diabetes was 1.76%. Four special clusters of diabetes cases were identified comprising 40.4% of total cases compared with 1.3% in noncluster areas.

The clusters of diabetes were cluster 1, Andhra Pradesh and Telangana with prevalence 3.01%; cluster 2, Tamil Nadu and Kerala with prevalence 4.32%; cluster 3, Odisha with prevalence 2.8%; and cluster 4, Goa with prevalence 4.43%. Having obesity and overweight, smoking tobacco, and consuming alcohol were associated with increase of diabetes.

Fourteen TB clusters were identified mainly distributed across northern states: Jammu, Himachal Pradesh, Punjab, Uttar Pradesh, Delhi, Haryana, Gujarat, and Madhya Pradesh; northeastern states Sikkim and Assam.

Regional TB endemicity and diabetes special distributions showed that there is a lack of consistent geographical overlap between these two diseases.

The highly dense areas of self-reported diabetes in southern India are consistent with other studies, whereas TB clustering indicates a high burden in North India where diabetes prevalence was lower compared with southern regions. The analysis of covariance association for diabetes clusters and nonclusters showed increase odds of diabetes in areas with higher levels of TB exposure only within diabetes hotspots. Furthermore, regional TB density exposure did not increase the likelihood of reporting diabetes after controlling for important confounders consistently.

The strength of the study is that this was one of the first studies to implement spatial analysis to investigate geographic structures of diabetes and to identify if locations with high prevalence of diabetes and TB coexist.

The limitation of the study was that the diabetes was self-reported and will exclude individuals who have undetected diabetes, and in a country like India we should not be surprised if individuals were on medication for diabetes and did not know that they had diabetes. Second limitation is it included only individuals aged 15–54 years excluding older individuals who have a much higher prevalence of diabetes.

In conclusion, the spatial variation of diabetes highlighted the existence of clusters of diabetes at different scales of disease severity as were clusters of TB and each region might need to implement control strategies unique to their epidemiological context.

10. Sex Differences in the Burden of Type 2 Diabetes and Cardiovascular Risk Across the Life Course

Ref: Huebschmann AG, Huxley RR, Kohrt WM, Zeitler P, Regensteiner JG, Reusch JEB, et al. Sex differences in the burden of type 2 diabetes and cardiovascular risk across the life course. Diabetologia. 2019;62(10):1761-72.

ABSTRACT

It is estimated that approximately 90–95% of 425 million people affected globally with diabetes mellitus (DM), have type 2 diabetes mellitus (T2DM) (in 2017). In this review, we have highlighted the differences in prevalence and incidence of T2DM, and in the associated cardiovascular risk in both sexes. Even though the absolute rates of cardiovascular disease (CVD) between men and women though decreases in the presence of T2DM, it remains higher in men. There is 25–50% higher risk of CVD in type 2 diabetic women compared with men, as suggested by large-scale observational studies. In this review, we will discuss the probable physiological and behavioral mechanisms responsible for the observed differences and also the differences in sociobehavioral norms and disparities in provider-level treatment patterns in both sexes. Further investigations are needed to fill the gaps found in our study.

COMMENT

The rates of type 2 diabetes mellitus (T2DM) and its impact on cardiovascular disease (CVD) outcomes across the life span have been identified different according to sex and gender. The burden of future cancer, dementia, and renal disease in individuals with T2DM is also influenced by the same features. Slightly higher prevalence of T2DM among men as compared to females has been suggested by the data from the Western European or Asian descent which may be region specific.

The sex difference in T2DM may be due to higher insulin resistance from late puberty into adult life among men as compared to women. Although the incidence of T2DM is approximately equal among men and women in older age which could be attributed to hormonal transition during menopause around age of 50 years leading to visceral fat deposition promoting insulin resistance and elevated incidence of the metabolic syndrome in older women.

The absolute rates of CVD are reported to be higher among men as compared to women at all ages without diabetes, the prevalence of stroke is found to be higher in women as compared to men irrespective of diabetic status. However, the female advantage concerning cardiovascular outcomes in type 2 diabetic women is negated by diabetes although not fully eliminated but it is substantially reduced.

There is need of clinical trials to be conducted in type 2 diabetic young population with prespecified evaluation by sex and gender to identify optimal lifestyle/medication interventions for risk reduction of CVDs and also to optimize treatment and prevention strategies for prevention of diabetes. There is also need to assess prospectively and identify mechanisms contributing to sex/gender differences in diabetes prevalence and the relatively worse CVD risk among type 2 diabetic women than men including biological as well as behavioral factors. More studies need to be carried out to identify approaches, i.e., education and point-of-care risk-recognition protocols, medication adherence surveillance, and equitable revascularization for acute coronary syndrome to improve risk factor control of CVDs.

Offspring born as intrauterine growth restriction (IUGR), parental obesity or high-fat diet, or mothers with diabetes in pregnancy are at high risk for developing obesity, diabetes, and CVDs. Hence, there is need to implement their early screening for CVDs risk and their parents should be counseled on lifestyle.

Patients should be counseled to adopt lifestyle with healthy diet/physical activity by the clinicians and they should also assist patients to implement the lifestyle changes. Men and women should be prescribed gender equitable and guideline concordant screening and therapy and the reasons for nonadherence with the therapy, i.e., depression, medication intolerance, and access to healthcare need to be uncovered and addressed by the clinicians.

11. Incidence of New-onset Diabetes and Post-transplant Metabolic Syndrome after Liver Transplantation - A Prospective Study from South India

Ref: Oommen T, Arun CS, Kumar H, Nair V, Jayakumar RV, Sudhindran S, et al. Incidence of new-onset posttransplant metabolic syndrome after transplantation - a prospective study from South India. Indian J Endocrinol Metab. 2020;24(2):165-9.

ABSTRACT

Background and aims: Liver transplantation has become an effective therapy for patients with end-stage liver disease. The risk of new-onset diabetes after transplantation (NODAT) and post-transplant metabolic syndrome (PTMS) is high among patients after liver transplantation. These are thought to be associated with increased risks of graft rejection, infection, cardiovascular disease, and death. Our study aimed to document the incidence of NODAT and PTMS and analyze pre- and post-transplant predictive factors for their development in patients undergoing a liver transplant.

Methods: This was a prospective comparative study on 51 patients who underwent live donor liver transplantation. They were evaluated at baseline, 3 and 6 months after transplantation with fasting glucose, lipids, serum insulin levels, C-peptide, and hemoglobin A1c (HbA1c). They were followed up at 5 years to document any cardiovascular events or rejection.

Results: The incidence of preoperative diabetes mellitus (DM) in the study group was 25/51 (49%). The incidence of NODAT was 38.5% (10/26 patients) and PTMS 29% (10/35), respectively. Age (47.7 ± 5.4 vs. 41.5 ± 12.7 years), homeostatic model assessment - insulin resistance (HOMA2-IR) (2.3 ± 1.8 vs. 2.1 ± 1.6), serum insulin (16.1 ± 12.0 vs. 17.9 ± 14.5), and C-peptide (4.6 ± 0.5 vs. 4.8 ± 0.7) were similar at baseline in the NODAT group compared to those who did not develop it. Mean tacrolimus levels were higher in PTMS group (6.8 ± 2.9 vs. 5.0. ± 2.0, p value = 0.042). By the end of 5 years, 7 patients expired; 6 due to rejection and 1 due to cardiovascular disease. Moreover, two of these patients had preexisting DM and two had NODAT.

Conclusion: None of the baseline metabolic factors in patients undergoing liver transplant were predictive of the development of NODAT or PTMS. Mean tacrolimus levels were significantly higher in the PTMS group. A 5-year follow-up showed no excess risk of cardiovascular events or rejection in those with preexisting DM or in those who developed NODAT.

COMMENT

Diabetes mellitus (DM) occurring after organ transplantation in a previously nondiabetic person is termed as new-onset diabetes after transplantation (NODAT). A number of retrospective studies have reported the prevalence of the individual components of metabolic syndrome (MS), which include DM, hypertension, dyslipidemia, and obesity, among patients who have undergone liver transplantation.

The incidence rates of NODAT vary depending upon the organ transplanted and post-transplant interval and are estimated to be around 9–30% for liver transplant patients.

The estimated prevalence rates of post-transplant metabolic syndrome (PTMS) range around 44–58% according to previous studies. Knowledge about these metabolic parameters is important as NODAT is associated with increased cardiovascular morbidity and mortality, more severe infections, higher incidence of rejection, and poorer graft survival though the overall survival rates are still debatable.

The present study aimed at studying the incidence of NODAT and PTMS following living donor liver transplantation and identifies pre- and postoperative risk factors for the development of NODAT.

There was a high incidence of preoperative DM in the study which was around 49% compared to 9% in a study done by Harada et al. in Japanese population. And the incidence of NODAT was 38.5% compared to 9–30% in the western population. Metabolic syndrome was seen in 31% before transplantation and further 29% developed it post-transplant.

In the present study, there was no difference in preoperative or postoperative variables in the groups with or without PTMS and also there was no significant association between complications and NODAT or PTMS.

The limitations of the study include small sample size and short duration, which could have influenced the correlation of preoperative and postoperative variables and incidence of NODAT and PTMS. Presence of ascites might have influenced the anthropometric parameters like body mass index (BMI) and waist-to-hip ratio (WHR).

Large-scale prospective studies with longer duration of follow-up are required to further clarify the pathogenesis of NODAT and PTMS and also to assess their effects on the long-term outcome in the Indian population.

Future studies should focus on better follow-up protocols and usage of metabolic parameters with less confounding effect which could help us to arrive at better conclusion. Planning a large scale study with uniform protocol and treatment regimes may be needed.

12. Use of Antihyperglycemic Medications in U.S. Adults: An Analysis of the National Health and Nutrition Examination Survey

Ref: Le P, Chaitoff A, Misra-Hebert AD, Ye W, Herman WH, Rothberg MB. Use of antihyperglycemic medication in U.S. adults: an analysis of the nation health and nutrition examination survey. Diabetes Care. 2020;43(6):1227-33.

ABSTRACT

Objective: To analyze the trend of antidiabetic agents' usage and approach of the physicians toward recommendations of American Diabetes Association (ADA).

Research design and methods: Individuals of ≥18 years age with history of diabetes at any point of time, hemoglobin A1c (HbA1c) >6.4%, or a fasting plasma glucose >125 mg/dL, during 2003–2016, were selected from National Health and Nutrition Examination Survey (NHANES) data. Trend of use of seven classes of ADAs, namely sulfonylureas, thiazolidinediones (TZDs), insulin, meglitinides, canagliflozin, empagliflozin, and liraglutide was analyzed. Use by hypoglycemia risk, weight effect, cardiovascular benefit, and cost were also assessed.

Results: The proportion of antidiabetic agent use increased by 9% from 2003–2004 to 2015–2016 ($p < 0.001$). The choice of drug did not change significantly based on age, weight, or presence of cardiovascular disease (CVD), irrespective of 2012 recommendations by American Diabetes Association. Older patients with comorbidities were more likely to receive hypoglycemia-inducing drugs. The use of higher-cost medications was associated with insurance, and not income.

Conclusion: ADA recommendations did not change the treatment approach of physicians in relation to individualization as per patients' characteristics.

COMMENT

Type 2 diabetes mellitus (T2DM) is associated with serious complications, higher mortality, and enormous costs. Management of diabetes requires multidisciplinary approach, which includes lifestyle measures and pharmacologic therapies. Appropriate management of glycemia is important to prevent complications. Glycemic control is best achieved by oral antihyperglycemic drugs and insulin. Among the available drugs, metformin, sulfonylureas, and thiazolidinediones (TZDs) were the most commonly available drugs to which newer drugs like dipeptidyl peptidase-4 (DPP-4) inhibitors, glucagon-like peptide-1 (GLP-1) analogs, and sodium-glucose cotransporter-2 (SGLT-2) inhibitors have added with advantage of lesser hypoglycemia chances and better weight control. Among these drugs, at least two classes of drugs have shown to reduce all-cause mortality and also cardiovascular events.

However, the latest class of drugs is 50- and 200-fold more expensive than older medications.

Latest in the group of drugs are SGLT-2 inhibitors and GLP-1 receptor agonists (GLP-1 RA) for patients with cardiovascular disease (CVD) in conjunction with lifestyle management and metformin based on cardiovascular outcome trials.

Prescribing trends of these drugs are not uniform in view of higher cost and multiple choices of available drugs. The aim of the study is to examine temporal trends in pharmacologic management for T2DM overall and by drug class. And also to know if the diabetes treatment was individualized by assessing the patient risk factors to avoid hypoglycemia and for better cardiovascular health.

Present study helps to understand how pharmacologic treatment for T2DM increased from 2003 to 2016. And the use of sulfonylureas and TZD decreased with metformin being the most frequently prescribed first-line therapy in accordance with the ADA's standards of care. Usage of insulin increased throughout the study period, with insulin analogs displacing human insulin almost entirely.

More than 50% of patients aged >65 still received drugs that cause hypoglycemia, and there was little evidence that doctors tailored treatment for patients with obesity or CVD as recommended by the ADA. The study identified the current baseline to which new guidelines will be applied and demonstrated a substantial opportunity for improvement.

Limitations of the study: Exact number of patients using generic versions was not known. The study did not distinguish between type 1 diabetes mellitus (T1DM) and T2DM. NHANES prescription medication data were available only through 2015–2016; thus ADA's most recent recommendation regarding patients with chronic kidney disease could not be assessed. Data being cross-sectional, the information regarding the initial drug combination or switching of drugs is not available.

Thus, translating recommendation into clinical practice is a challenge and identifying the extent of the scenario is a reasonable place to begin improvement.

13. Why are South Asians Prone to Type 2 Diabetes? A Hypothesis Based on Underexplored Pathways

Ref: Venkat Narayan KM, Kanaya AM. Why are South Asians prone to type 2 diabetes? A hypothesis based on underexplored pathways. Diabetologia. 2020;63(6):1103-9.

ABSTRACT

Type 2 diabetes mellitus (T2DM) is highly prevalent in South Asian population, even at a lower body mass index (BMI). This can be attributed to lower ability to secrete insulin resulting in poor compensation in presence of unhealthy lifestyles, as suggested by emerging data from epidemiological studies. So, resistance to insulin may not be the prime reason for development of T2DM in this population. Also, with lower average muscle mass, accumulation of ectopic hepatic fat and intramyocellular fat deposition occur that further inhibits insulin action. We assume that these two mechanisms increase the susceptibility to diabetes: Decrease in function of beta cell and impairment of insulin action due to low lean mass that leads to ectopic fat accumulation.

COMMENT

South Asians are at increased risk of diabetes even with lesser body weight. Change in the environmental factors, lifestyle, and epidemiological transition has been proposed to play important role in the causation. Visceral adiposity which drives insulin resistance is the most important reason for increased diabetes risk in these ethnic people. On an average, low lean mass is found in South Asians which could be a reason of specific susceptibility for diabetes. The long-term intergenerational influences attributable by major changes in the nutrition status especially affecting adversely maternal and/or early childhood during the first 3 years of life. These nutritional changes affect the metabolic capacity of the people resulting in shorter stature, lower lean muscle mass, inadequate organ development, and increased susceptibility to diabetes. Several metabolic pathways (e.g., poor insulin secretion, ectopic fat deposition, and low lean mass) have been linked to early malnourishment with diabetes risk.

South Asians even at lower body mass index (BMI) are having higher risk of developing type 2 diabetes mellitus (T2DM) than other ethnic groups. Additionally higher risk of T2DM is also found in South Asians with normal weight as compared to normal weight people of other ethnic groups like whites, black, and pima Indians.

There is evidence of lowest secretion of insulin among South Asians in every age group followed by Chinese Americans in a review comparing nondiabetic South Asian adults with Chinese Americans, Hispanics, African Americans, and whites in the USA. The potential role of deficient insulin secretion has been reported in the early natural history of T2DM in South Asians by studies carried out among adults in India; youth-onset diabetes populations in India and South Asian adults in the USA, thus making a strong case of reduced beta cell mass as an important contributor to the increased risk of diabetes in South Asians.

Understanding about the metabolic pathways of the disease process helps us in deciding the treatment strategies. Insulin sensitizers like glitazones which target insulin sensitivity and other drugs which target the insulin resistance are less useful here in these ethnic populations. Strategies to preserve or help recover beta cell function during early normoglycemic periods in these people needs to be researched. Other interventions like high intensity interval training or specific pharmacological approaches can be tried.

A dual mechanism has been postulated by the authors for the significant susceptibility of South Asians to T2DM endowed by their evolutionary history. This susceptibility is hypothesized to be driven primarily by poor metabolic capacity, i.e., reduced beta cell mass and/or function leading to impaired insulin secretion. Impaired insulin secretion coupled with low lean muscle mass could be responsible for reduced insulin action. The insulin action is further impaired by the ectopic fat deposition in the liver and muscle. There is need to consider these unique evolutionary features of South Asians compared to other ethnic groups to formulate an innovative research agenda for solving the problem. There is need to carry out interdisciplinary research, basic/translational sciences, longitudinal epidemiology, and intervention studies taking into consideration the intensive measures of insulin secretion, lean mass, hepatic fat, and glucose patterns. There is also need to study the biological mechanisms leading to poor insulin secretion, low lean mass, hepatic steatosis, myosteatosis, and mitochondrial metabolism in detail.

Parallel research into clinical and public health interventions to address the increased propensity of diabetes in these individuals needs to be done. Treatment strategies improving the beta cell mass and lean muscle mass have to be developed. Methods to reduce ectopic fat deposition need to be focused.

14. Prevalence and Clinical Characteristics of Individuals with Newly Detected Lean Diabetes in Tamil Nadu, South India: A Community-based Cross-sectional Study

Ref: Oommen AM, Kapoor N, Thomas N, George K. Prevalence and clinical characteristics of individuals with newly detected lean diabetes in Tamil Nadu, South India: a community-based cross-sectional study. Int J Diabetes Dev Ctries. 2019;39:680-4.

ABSTRACT

Background and objectives: Lean diabetes is an entity that has been observed to be higher in Asian populations. The estimates of the burden of lean diabetes in India are mainly from hospital-based studies. This study reports the prevalence of lean diabetes among individuals with newly detected diabetes, from Vellore, Tamil Nadu, South India.

Methods: A cross-sectional World Health Organization (WHO) STEPwise approach to surveillance (STEPS) survey was conducted among adults aged 30–64 years, in one rural block and 48 urban wards, in Vellore. Physical and anthropometric parameters were assessed in addition to fasting lipid profile and plasma glucose. Newly detected diabetes was defined as fasting plasma glucose ≥126 mg/dL and lean diabetes as nonketotic diabetes mellitus, without clinical features to suggest pancreatic diabetes, with a body mass index (BMI) <18.5 kg/m^2.

Results: Among 3,445 rural and 2,019 urban subjects, the proportion of lean diabetes among 280 subjects (146 rural, 134 urban) with newly detected diabetes was 5.5%, 95% confidence interval (CI) 1.7–9.3% (eight subjects) and 1.5%, 95% CI 0–3.6% (two subjects), in the rural and urban areas respectively. The proportion of those with a normal BMI (18.5–22.9 kg/m^2) was 25.3% and 18.7% in the rural and urban populations, while 69.2% and 79.9% had a BMI ≥23 kg/m^2. Those with lean diabetes were more likely to be older, illiterate, and involved in manual labor, than those with nonlean diabetes ($p < 0.05$).

Conclusion: The prevalence of lean diabetes was low (5.5% of newly detected rural diabetes, 1.5% of newly detected urban diabetes) in Vellore, South India. Further documentation of the burden of this condition across India is needed to assess the public health implications for prevention and control.

COMMENT

Type 2 diabetes mellitus (T2DM) is emerging as a major public health problem in the low- and middle-income countries in the recent past. The reasons being unhealthy lifestyle and obesity which are well studied. Lean T2DM is suspected to be higher in Asian and African populations as compared with others, in whom obesity is a more common risk factor. Definition of lean diabetes is described as body mass index (BMI) <18.5 kg/m^2 or as Ketosis Resistant Diabetes of the Young (KRDY) as BMI <18.0 kg/m^2, while high-income countries the cutoff values are ranging from 18.0 to 24.9 kg/m^2.

Genome-wide association studies have shown that diabetes in lean individuals may be related to genetic factors irrespective of obesity and lifestyle factors.

Studies from India are hospital based rather than population level based for patients with lean T2DM. This information adds on to the current understanding of the disease burden and helps to judge the public health importance of the condition. There is dearth of data regarding the lean diabetes from South India and hence A World Health Organization (WHO) STEPwise approach to surveillance (STEPS) cross-sectional survey was carried out in Vellore, in 2011-2012, among adults aged 30-64 years.

The present study demonstrates the epidemiological transition in the diabetic individuals in a rural place of Tamil Nadu from India.

Among the newly detected diabetes lean diabetes accounted for around 5.5% in rural areas compared to 1.5% in the urban areas. And also lean individuals with diabetes were older and seen more common in lower socioeconomic population. Other important features are higher total cholesterol and hypertension and were reported in lean diabetics as compared to lean nondiabetics which indicated the independence of risk factors from body weight among the lean group.

Strength of the study is that it is a community-based survey and both previously and newly diagnosed diabetic patients were identified giving better estimation of the burden of the disease as compared to hospital-based surveys.

Limitations include lack of body fat measurement and being community-based study a low power to assess risk factors for lean diabetes is obtained. Detailed evaluation for the type of diabetes using GAD (glutamic acid decarboxylase) antibodies and ultrasonography (USG) of abdomen were not done. Fasting plasma glucose alone was used to diagnose diabetes where a considerable number of patients would be missed when only this parameter is used.

The proportion of lean individuals is decreasing as the prevalence of obesity is being doubled or tripled in the last two decades. Consensus is not clear about the causal relationship between leanness and diabetes, i.e., whether the leanness is the cause or effect of T2DM. This causal relationship is important to understand the future estimate, i.e., if leanness is a causal factor for diabetes, the burden of lean diabetes will decrease but if it is the effect of T2DM, the burden of T2DM might remain same or increase in the future, possibly mediated by genetic factors.

There is need to report the prevalence of lean diabetes in addition to overall burden of T2DM by future WHO STEPS surveys which are being conducted in the region for surveillance of noncommunicable diseases to explore its public health significance and need for interventions for the better detection of diabetes in lean patients whose risk is mostly under-recognized.

15. Prevalence of Diabetes Mellitus in 2019 Novel Coronavirus: A Meta-analysis

Ref: Wang X, Wang S, Sun L, Qin G. Prevalence of diabetes mellitus in 2019 novel coronavirus: A meta-analysis. Diabetes Res Clin Pract. 2020;164:108200.

ABSTRACT

Background: The prevalence of diabetes mellitus (DM), a major public health concern, has been increasing over the past 10 years with the most recent being 2019 novel coronavirus (2019-nCoV). This research aimed to systematically assess the prevalence of DM among those infected with 2019-nCoV.

Methods: Observational studies up to February 25, 2020 were searched on PubMed, Embase, Web of Science, and Medline with application of random effects model or fixed effects model for evaluation of the pooled prevalence of DM in patients infected with 2019-nCoV.

Findings: We selected nine papers meeting the eligibility criteria. The pooled prevalence of DM was 9% [95% confidence interval (CI) 6–12%] with obvious heterogeneity (I^2 65%, $p = 0.004$). The prevalence of DM in patients with moderate symptoms and severe symptoms of 2019-nCoV infection was 7% (95% CI 4–10%) and 17% (95% CI 13–21%), respectively.

Interpretation: This is probably the first paper showing the prevalence of DM in 2019-nCoV infected patients which can be beneficial in preventing the spread of 2019-nCoV in the future.

COMMENT

Diabetes mellitus (DM) is a noncommunicable disease which is also a pandemic leading to severe morbidity and mortality. There have been predictions of increase in number of diabetic patients to 439 million in 2030 by the International Diabetes Federation. Increased risk of infectious diseases hospitalization is reported to be linked with DM. Higher incidence of postoperative pneumonia has been demonstrated among type 2 diabetic patients than nondiabetics in the previous studies. Similarly, the long-term mortality in community-acquired pneumonia has been indicated to be higher among patients with undiagnosed DM as compared to patients without diabetes in another study. Diabetic patients are also reported to be admitted to hospital with infection more likely as compared to the nondiabetic patients.

This meta-analysis has demonstrated the pooled prevalence of DM to be 9% [95% confidence interval (CI) 6–12%)] in coronavirus disease 2019 (COVID-19)—infected individuals with obvious heterogeneous prevalence of DM (I^2 65%, $p = 0.004$) in the studies. Among 2019 novel coronavirus (2019-nCoV) patients, the prevalence of DM was found to be 7% (95% CI 4–10%) in moderate patients and 17% (95% CI 13–21%) in severe patients demonstrating the significantly higher prevalence of DM in severe patients with 2019-nCoV than that in moderate patients with 2019-nCoV (OR 2.49, 95% CI 1.70–3.64).

No subgroup analysis could be done in this meta-analysis as many of the included studies did not categorize the participants into different groups for outcome analysis. Secondly, this meta-analysis included retrospective studies with obvious heterogeneity. Thirdly, it is hard to determine the causality as the present study is the single-arm meta-analysis without a control group. Fourth, age adjustment analysis could not be performed because this meta-analysis included retrospective studies and most of them did not mention age groups.

This study concluded that diabetes is prevalent in patients with 2019-nCoV, specifically among severe patients. The demonstrated prevalence of DM in patients with 2019-nCoV will be beneficial to inhibit the spread of 2019-nCoV in the future.

16. Vitamin D Supplementation and Prevention of Type 2 Diabetes

Ref: Pittas AG, Dawson-Hughes B, Sheehan P, Ware JH, Knowler WC, Aroda VR, et al. Vitamin D supplementation and prevention of type 2 diabetes. N Engl J Med. 2019;381(6):520-30.

ABSTRACT

Introduction: In some of the previous observational studies, an association has been reported between low blood 25-hydroxyvitamin D level and the risk of type 2 diabetes mellitus (T2DM). However, it is still not known if vitamin D supplementation reduces the risk of diabetes.

Methods: The study population included adults who fulfilled minimum two of three glycemic criteria for prediabetes (fasting plasma glucose level, 100–125 mg/dL; plasma glucose level 2 hours following a 75-g oral glucose load, 140–199 mg/dL; and glycated hemoglobin level, 5.7–6.4%) and no diagnostic criteria for diabetes. Participants were randomly assigned to receive either 4,000 IU/day of vitamin D3 or placebo, irrespective of the baseline level of serum 25-hydroxyvitamin D. New-onset diabetes was considered as the primary outcome in this time-to-event analysis. The design of the trial was event-driven, with a target number of diabetes events of 508.

Results: Study included 2,423 participants, who were randomized to either vitamin D group ($n = 1,211$) or placebo group ($n = 1,212$). By month 24, in the vitamin D group, the mean serum 25-hydroxyvitamin D level was 54.3 ng/mL (from 27.7 ng/mL at baseline), in comparison to 28.8 ng/mL placebo group (from 28.2 ng/mL at baseline). At the median follow-up of 2.5 years, in the vitamin D group and the placebo group, the primary outcome of diabetes was observed in 293 and 323 participants, respectively (9.39 and 10.66 events per 100 person-years, respectively). The hazard ratio for vitamin D in comparison to placebo was 0.88 [95% confidence interval (CI) 0.75–1.04; $p = 0.12$]. There was no significant difference in the incidence of adverse events between the vitamin D and placebo groups.

Conclusion: As compared to placebo, individuals who are at high risk for T2DM and not selected for vitamin D insufficiency, supplementation of vitamin D3 at a dose of 4,000 IU/day did not significantly reduce the risk of diabetes. (Funded by the National Institute of Diabetes and Digestive and Kidney Diseases and others; D2d ClinicalTrials.gov number, NCT01942694).

COMMENT

25-hydroxyvitamin D level has emerged as a treatment for many illnesses in the recent past. Hence vitamin D deficiency is linked to diabetes as well. Vitamin D supplementation has been proposed as a potential intervention to lower diabetes risk. The cause for diabetes is hypothesized as both impaired pancreatic beta cell function and insulin resistance. Many observational studies have shown an association between a low blood 25-hydroxyvitamin D level and the risk of diabetes.

In few studies, vitamin D supplementation improved disposition index, a measure of pancreatic beta cell function by 40% but whether vitamin D supplementation lowers the risk of diabetes is unclear. In a trial, Tromso Vitamin D and type 2 diabetes mellitus (T2DM) trial (Norway), which randomly assigned 511 white adults with prediabetes to 20,000 IU per week (approximately 2,900 IU/day) of vitamin D3 or placebo, the risk of diabetes was numerically lower in the vitamin D group than in the placebo group, but the difference was not significant (hazard ratio 0.90; 95% CI 0.69–1.18). In the Diabetes Prevention with Active Vitamin D study (Japan), which randomly assigned 1,256 adults with prediabetes to an active form of vitamin D analog (eldecalcitol) or placebo, the risk of diabetes was also lower in the vitamin D group than in the placebo group, but the difference was again not significant (hazard ratio 0.87; 95% CI 0.68–1.09).

This is a randomized, double-blind, placebo-controlled clinical trial which evaluated the safety and efficacy of oral administration of vitamin D3 (cholecalciferol; 4,000 IU/day) for diabetes prevention in adults at high risk for T2DM. The mean age of the participants was 60 years; mean body mass index (BMI) was 32.1 kg/m^2; and mean HbA1c was 5.9%; the total follow-up was 2.5 years in both groups.

The mean baseline level of serum 25-hydroxyvitamin D was 28 ng/mL with no significant difference between the two groups. By the end of the trial, diabetes had developed in 616 patients. New-onset diabetes occurred in 293 participants in the vitamin D group and 323 participants in the placebo group. The hazard ratio in the vitamin D group was 0.8 (CI 0.75–1.04) $p = 0.12$.

Strengths of the study are glycemic criteria used to diagnose diabetes were closely matching the standard clinical practice, the dose of vitamin D used was decided based on the safety and efficacy, i.e., 4,000 IU/day, and follow-up was better to reduce the confounding effect of seasonal variation and adherence was high.

Limitations: There were a high percentage of patients with adequate levels of vitamin D, which would have limited the ability of the drug to have an impact on outcome. 24-hour urine calcium level was not measured, which is a parameter to monitor when a patient is on vitamin D supplementation.

Vitamin D supplementation at a dose of 4,000 IU/day in patients with high risk for T2DM not selected for vitamin D insufficiency, did not significantly reduce the risk of diabetes compared to placebo.

Dose of vitamin D and duration required for the impact to occur are still not clear. Supplementation of vitamin D to vitamin D sufficient people, the benefits are not understood.

17. Prognostic Significance of Long-term HbA1c Variability for All-cause Mortality in the ACCORD Trial

Ref: Sheng CS, Tian J, Miao Y, Cheng Y, Yang Y, Reaven PD, et al. Prognostic Significance of Long-term HbA1c Variability for All-Cause Mortality in the ACCORD Trial. Diabetes Care. 2020;43(6):1185-90.

ABSTRACT

Objective: High glycemic variability and all-cause mortality have been invariably associated in various epidemiological studies but rarely validated in glucose-lowering clinical trials. Our aim was to identify the prognostic significance of hemoglobin A1c (HbA1c) variability in treated patients in the Action to Control Cardiovascular Risk in Diabetes (ACCORD) trial population.

Research design and methods: The risk of all-cause mortality was assessed in relation to long-term visit-to-visit HbA1c variability, and expressed as coefficient of variation (CV), variability independent of the mean (VIM), and average real variability (ARV), from the 8th month to the transition. Estimation of adjusted hazard ratio (HR) and 95% confidence interval (CI) was done using multivariable Cox proportional hazards model.

Results: The mean HbA1c was lower in the intensive therapy group ($n = 4,755$) when compared with the standard therapy group ($n = 4,728$) [6.6% (49 mmol/mol) vs. 7.7% (61 mmol/mol), $p < 0.0001$]. So were the values of CV, VIM, and ARV ($p < 0.0001$). In multivariate adjusted analysis, all three HbA1c variability indices were significantly associated with total mortality in all patients as well as in the standard- and intensive-therapy groups analyzed separately. The hazard ratios for a 1 standard deviation (1-SD) increase in HbA1c variability indices for the all-cause mortality were 1.19 and 1.23 in intensive and standard therapy, respectively. Cross-tabulation analysis showed the third tertile of HbA1c mean and VIM had significantly higher all-cause mortality (HR 2.05; 95% CI 1.17–3.61; $p < 0.01$) only in the intensive-therapy group.

Conclusion: Long-term HbA1c variability has a strong association with all-cause mortality.

COMMENT

Type 2 diabetes mellitus (T2DM) is a potent risk factor for cardiovascular disease (CVD) events. Prior several studies have shown the association between the degree of hyperglycemia and the risk of these outcomes.

Hemoglobin A1c (HbA1c) and plasma blood glucose have been considered as the markers to measure glycemic control, which has been proved in the previous clinical trials.

Glycemic variability is a recent marker added to the armamentarium of diabetes management. Previous trials have shown the relation between glycemic variability and microvascular and macrovascular complications. Glycemic variability can have both short-term and long-term components to measure. Long-term glycemic variability can be calculated by visit-to-visit fluctuations of HbA1c over periods of follow-up lasting months to years.

In previous studies, there was increased mortality and hospitalization in patients with T2DM, which was not explained by average HbA1c but could be associated with HbA1c variability. Systematic ascertainment of glycemic variability may provide additional value in the prediction of future complications among diabetes, both in clinical practice and in large clinical trials.

Large clinical trials showed increased all-cause mortality in the intensive-treatment group compared to those receiving conventional treatment among patients with diabetes.

In this study, data from the ACCORD (Action to Control Cardiovascular Risk in Diabetes) trial were used to investigate associations of the long-term visit-to-visit HbA1c variability with outcomes among participants with type two diabetes and tested the hypothesis that HbA1c variability white plays an important role in outcomes of treated type two diabetes. Long-term visit-to-visit HbA1c variability was evaluated using three or more HbA1c measures from the eighth month to the transition calculating individual participant coefficient of variation, variation independent of the mean, and average real variability.

The hazard ratios for a 1 standard deviation (1-SD) increase in HbA1c variability indices for the all-cause mortality were 1.19–1.50 in the intensive-therapy group and 1.23–1.28 in the standard-therapy group. Present study confirmed that in patients with diabetes, long-term visit-to-visit variability in HbA1c was a strong predictor of a variety of all-cause mortality in these patients. HbA1c variability combined with HbA1c mean conferred an increased risk for all-cause mortality in the intensive therapy group in the ACCORD trial. These findings emphasize that visit-to-visit glycemic variability as well as higher levels of glycemia might be important risk factors for all-cause mortality and should be considered in the management of diabetes.

Strengths of our study include a large number of high-risk patients and a large number of HbA1c measures, which enable us to accurately calculate HbA1c variability. They used three variability indices, which enabled them to study HbA1c variability more comprehensively. The variability index, VIM, can diminish the tight correlation between the coefficient of variation (CV) and mean and was more suitable for the mean and variability cross-tabulation analysis. Study being a post-hoc analysis which included high risk CVD patients, the results can be extended to real-world studies including patients with T2DM having a variety of risk characteristics.

Limitations of the analysis were, in this study HbA1c was used rather than glucose as the target.

Evaluation indices and glucose were not recorded at every visit, so in this study we only focused on HbA1c.

Glycemic variability has to be considered as a most important parameter for the intensive therapy of diabetes. But variables which have to be used to measure glycemic variability is a matter of debate and of clinical interest. Hence research has to be based on measuring this glycemic variability and variables used to measure this entity.

18. Evaluating the Performance of the Indian Diabetes Risk Score in Different Ethnic Groups

Ref: Nugawela MD, Sivaprasad S, Mohan V, Rajalakshmi R, Netuveli G. Evaluating the performance of the indian diabetes risk score in different ethnic groups. Diabetes Technol Ther. 2020;22(4):285-300.

ABSTRACT

Aim: This study aimed to assess the effectiveness of MDRF-IDRS (Madras Diabetes Research Foundation-Indian Diabetes Risk Score) in different ethnic groups (consisting of Indians, Hispanic, non-Hispanic blacks, non-Hispanic whites, and other Americans).

Methods: Calculation of the MDRF-IDRS is done on the basis of risk equation including age, waist circumference, physical activity, and family history of diabetes. In the study, the National Health and Nutrition Examination Survey (NHANES) data on American and CURES (Chennai Urban Rural Epidemiology Study) data on Indians were included. Study population included individuals of ≥20 years with and without type 2 diabetes mellitus (T2DM). Evaluation of the performance of the MDRF-IDRS was done by analyzing sensitivity, specificity, positive predictive value, negative predictive value, and the area under the receiver operating characteristic curve [area under curve (AUC)] measures in each ethnic group. Performance of IDRS was compared with available noninvasive American diabetes risk scores.

Results: Total 11,035 participants were included; out of which 8,743 were Americans and 2,292 were Indians. Performance of MDRF-IDRS (cutoff ≥60) was good in Indians with an AUC of 0.73, sensitivity 80.2%, and specificity of 57.3%. In Hispanic, non-Hispanic whites, and non-Hispanic blacks, the highest discriminative performance was shown by MDRF-IDRS cutoff ≥70 with sensitivity in the range of 70.1% to 86.9% and specificity between 61.2% and 72.2%. The AUC for American was 0.77–0.81; highest AUC in non-Hispanic blacks and lowest AUC in non-Hispanic whites was observed. In comparison with the available noninvasive American diabetes risk score, with a smaller number of variables, IDRS demonstrated nearly the same performance in prediction of diabetes.

Conclusion: In Indians as well as Americans (comprising Hispanic, non-Hispanic blacks, non-Hispanic whites, and other American), performance of the MDRF-IDRS is good. This is beneficial in early diagnosis, management as well as optimal control of diabetes mostly in mass screening programs conducted in India and America.

COMMENT

Indian Diabetes Risk Score (IDRS) has good performance not only among Indians but also in other ethnic groups including Hispanic, Non-Hispanic whites, Non-Hispanic blacks, and other Americans. IDRS can be used in mass screening programs by nonmedically trained healthcare workers and as a self-administered tool among public to help in early diagnosis, management, and optimal control of diabetes in India and America. This was derived from the noninvasive risk factors identified in the CURES (Chennai Urban Rural Epidemiology Study), which include waist circumference, family history of diabetes, age, and level of physical activity. Compared with other noninvasive diabetes risk scores developed for Indians, IDRS is the most commonly externally validated tool in a large number of studies across India. It has been identified as a cost-effective, simple, and easy-to-use tool mainly in resource restricted settings.

Indian Diabetes Risk Score is a noninvasive cost-effective tool diabetes risk score derived from risk factors identified in the CURES. The validity of the score is not only established for Indians but also for other races like Hispanic, non-Hispanic whites, non-Hispanic blacks, and other Americans. It has been identified as a simple, cost-effective tool mainly in resource restricted settings as it includes only four variables age, family history of diabetes, level of physical activity, and waist circumference.

The Madras Diabetes Research Foundation (MDRF)-IDRS performs well not only among Indians but also among other ethnic groups like Hispanic, non-Hispanic whites, non-Hispanic blacks, and other Americans. Hence, it can be used in mass screening programs in India and America as a screening tool for early diagnosis of diabetes.

In this study, was DMDRF-IDRS course performance among Indian and American ethnic groups tested? The National Health and Nutrition Examination Survey (NHANES) and CURES were used to assess the score performance in different ethnic groups. About 11,035 study participants were included in the study.

With a smaller number of variables IDRS score showed almost the same performance in predicting diabetes amongst Americans compared with the existing noninvasive American diabetes risk score.

Strength of the study is involvement of different ethnic backgrounds and it includes very few parameters for assessment. This score can be used by even nonmedical personnel easily as it is simple. This risk score has a high negative predictive value for all ethnicities and therefore it is suitable as a triage tool to rule out those with a negative test result. IDRS performs well in different settings and in different population characteristics such as age distribution, physical activity levels, and family history.

The MDRF-IDRS score slightly overestimates the risk scores among Indians as same Indian dataset that was used to develop IDRS was used here also. Physical activity was measured using an estimate for 24-hour energy expenditure, which may not be accurate enough.

The MDRF-IDRS score performed well among Indians and Americans. The IDRS score cutoff ≥60 had the highest performance among Indians with sensitivity and specificity of 80.2% and 57.3%, respectively. MDRF-IDRS score cutoff ≥70 had the highest discriminative performance among Hispanic, non-Hispanic whites and non-Hispanic blacks ethnic groups with sensitivity and specificity ranging between 70.1–86.9% and 61.2–72.2%, respectively. For other Americans, IDRS score ≥60 was identified as the highest performing cutoff with sensitivity and specificity of 94.8% and 48.9%, respectively. So these cutoffs can be used among these ethnic groups to diagnose diabetes.

Performance of IDRS in low- and middle-income countries is limited and also the validity of this score in different population subgroups is not available. According to the MDRF-IDRS model development study by Mohan et al., the sensitivity and specificity of IDRS is only 72.5% and 60.1%, respectively. Hence the applicability of this score on large scale basis is questionable. In future, development of tools which contains proper objective methods of assessing the parameters should be used, like in this study the physical activity is recorded by patient's feedback.

Section 3: Comorbidities

Amritava Ghosh, Shalini Jaggi, Mithun Bhartia, Bikash Bhattacharjee

1. Usefulness of Routine Fractional Flow Reserve for Clinical Management of Coronary Artery Disease in Patients with Diabetes

Ref: Van Belle E, Cosenza A, Baptista SB, Vincent F, Henderson J, Santos L, et al. Usefulness of Routine Fractional Flow Reserve for Clinical Management of Coronary Artery Disease in Patients With Diabetes. JAMA Cardiol. 2020;5:272-81.

ABSTRACT

Importance: Diabetes has been reported to be a major determinant for the choice of revascularization strategy and the clinical outcome among the patients considered for coronary revascularization is diabetes. Diabetes has been seen in approximately one-third of these patients. There is lack of studies showing the usefulness of fractional flow reserve (FFR) to guide treatment in these patients.

Objective: To explore the usefulness and rate of major adverse cardiovascular events (MACE) of integrating FFR in management decisions for diabetic patients undergoing coronary angiography.

Design, setting, and participants: The data from two prospective multicenter registries sharing a common design; the PRIME-FFR study derived from the merger of the POST-IT study (Portuguese Study on the Evaluation of FFR-Guided Treatment of Coronary Disease) conducted from March, 2012 to November, 2013 and R3F study (French Study of FFR Integrated Multicenter Registries Implementation of FFR in Routine Practice) conducted from October, 2008 to June, 2010 were used in this cross-sectional study. Both diabetic and nondiabetic patients in whom angiography revealed ambiguous lesions were analyzed for rates, patterns, and outcomes associated with management reclassification including revascularization deferral. Data were analyzed from June to August, 2018.

Main outcomes and measures: This study measured incidence of death from any cause, myocardial infarction or unplanned revascularization (MACE) at 1 year.

Results: Total 1,983 patients were enrolled in this study with the mean age of 65 ± 10 years and 1,503 (77%) males. Of recruited 1,983 participants, 701 had diabetes. FFR was carried out for 1.4 lesions per patient. 58.2% of the lesions were found in the left anterior descending artery with the mean stenosis of 56% ± 11% and mean FFR of 0.81 ± 0.01. Although reclassification by FFR was found to be high and similar in both diabetic and nondiabetic patients (41.2% vs. 37.5%, $p = 0.13$) but reclassification from medical treatment to revascularization was more frequent in diabetic patients [142 of 342 (41.5%) vs. 230 of 730 (31.5%), $p = 0.001$]. There was no statistical significant difference between the 1-year rates of MACE in reclassified and nonreclassified patients (9.7% vs. 12.0%) ($p = 0.37$). Lower risk of MACE at 12 months was found in FFR-based deferral identified patients [25 of 296 (8.4%)] compared with those undergoing revascularization (13.1%, $p = 0.04$) among diabetic patients whereas the same magnitude of the observed rate among deferred patients was found in nondiabetic patients (7.9%, $p = 0.87$). The outcomes were not found to be associated with the status of insulin treatment. FFR was disregarded in 6.6% patients and they had the highest MACE rates irrespective of their diabetes status.

Conclusion and relevance: Among diabetic patients, routine integration of FFR for the management of coronary artery disease (CAD) resulted in a high rate of treatment reclassification. Management strategies guided by FFR including revascularization deferral may be useful for diabetic patients.

COMMENT

Critical Appraisal
What was Known Prior to this Study?

Fractional flow reserve (FFR) is the ratio of maximum blood flow in the poststenotic region of the coronary artery to the maximum blood flow that would have occurred in the same artery if the stenosis was not there. It is measured by the ratio of coronary pressure to aortic pressure at maximum blood flow. Pressure is measured using a coronary artery guidewire with a pressure sensor located at the tip, while hyperemia is achieved by continuous intravenous infusion or intracoronary bolus injection of adenosine. The normal value of FFR in a normal coronary artery is expected to be 1.0. An FFR value of <0.8 indicates a hemodynamically significant stenosis. It has been proposed as a method to guide treatment decisions and revascularization in coronary artery disease (CAD). A number of studies—including DEFER study, FAME (Fractional Flow Reserve Versus Angiography for Multivessel Evaluation) study, and FAME2 study—have demonstrated reduction in major adverse cardiovascular events (MACE) with use of FFR in guiding revascularization strategy in participants with CAD. Although, FFR has received class 1A recommendation in recent guidelines as a physiology-based guidance to revascularization in CAD, it has found limited utilization in actual practice. One of the issues which have been flagged include use of adenosine to achieve hyperemia which makes the procedure more prolonged and complex and exposes the patient to adverse effects. Also true bifurcations and/or tandem lesions are difficult to interrogate, which limits the use of this strategy in these settings. Certain studies have also raised concern about the safety of this approach, e.g., the Functional Testing Underlying Coronary Revascularization study was halted prematurely on account of doubled risk of death observed among participants with multivessel disease receiving an FFR-guided percutaneous coronary intervention.[1]

What this Study Adds?

Diabetes mellitus (DM) is associated with an increased risk of CAD. However, there is limited data on the utility of FFR in guiding revascularization among CAD patients with DM. Concerns regarding impaired microvascular responsiveness to hyperemia, and accelerated atherosclerosis among people with DM (resulting in the possibility that FFR may underestimate the severity of lesions in presence of DM) has cast doubts on the utility of FFR in this population. This study assessed the utility of routine use of FFR among participants with DM having intermediate stenosis on diagnostic angiography. The parameters assessed were rate of reclassification of the patient management strategy, comparison of such change among participants with DM with those without DM, rate of revascularization deferral, and the rates of MACE at 1 year in deferred patients with DM compared with those without DM. The main findings of the study were as follows: (1) DM was associated with significantly lower FFR values for a given stenosis severity; (2) the rate of FFR-based reclassification of treatment strategy was similar in those with and without DM (41.2% vs. 37.5%), although the pattern of reclassification was different, those with DM were more likely to be reclassified from medical management to revascularization strategy; (3) the clinical outcome was similar among participants with DM in whom treatment strategy was reclassified based on FFR, as compared to those in whom the treatment strategy was not reclassified (1-year MACE rates of 9.7% and 12.0% respectively); (4) disregarding the information derived from FFR was associated with a worse outcome regardless of diabetes status.

Major Strengths of the Study

This study used data from a large PRIME-FFR [Insights From the POST-IT and R3F (French FFR Registry) Integrated Multicenter

Registries Implementation of FFR in Routine Practice] population ($n = 1,983$), which resulted from the merger of two nationwide multicenter prospective cohorts—(1) R3F and (2) POST-IT. The major strengths of the study were its large sample size and prospective nature.

Limitations of the Study

- The study population was derived from the merger of two separate cohorts and some unaccounted for differences between the two cohorts may have influenced the results.
- The study included patients with mostly intermediate results. Thus, the results of the study may not be generalizable to more severe multivessel disease and tight lesions.
- Fractional flow reserve was disregarded in a very small proportion of the study population with diabetes. The study was inadequately powered to detect difference between outcomes between those in whom FFR was disregarded compared to those in whom FFR was included in management strategy.

Implications of the Findings for the Clinicians

The findings of this study suggest that FFR may be useful in guiding treatment decisions and revascularization in people with DM and CAD.

Knowledge Gaps Identified and Scope for Future Research

The results of this cross-sectional study need to be confirmed by randomized controlled trials comparing FFR-based management strategy with angiography-based approach, powered for clinical outcomes.

2. The Long-term Effects of Metformin on Patients with Type 2 Diabetic Kidney Disease

Ref: Kwon S, Kim YC, Park JY, Lee J, An JN, Kim CT, et al. The long-term effects of metformin on patients with type 2 diabetic kidney disease. Diabetes Care. 2020;43:948-55.

ABSTRACT

Objective: The type 2 diabetic population having a deranged kidney function are predisposed to the risk of developing lactic acidosis with the use of metformin. Here, we intend to observe the long-term effects of metformin in type 2 diabetic kidney disease (DKD).

Research design and methods: A total of 10,426 patients with type 2 DKD from two tertiary care centers were included in this retrospective observational cohort study. All-cause mortality and progress to end-stage renal disease (ESRD) were the primary outcomes while metformin-associated lactic acidosis was the secondary outcome. Propensity score matching (PSM) was done as only those with less severe DKD were probably advised metformin.

Results: The multivariate Cox analysis showed that the all-cause mortality and progression to ESRD were lower in the group that received metformin. As the two groups differed significantly in their baseline characteristics, PSM was performed. Metformin usage still had lower all-cause mortality [adjusted hazard ratio (aHR) 0.65; 95% confidence interval (CI) 0.57–0.73; $p < 0.001$] and progression to ESRD (aHR 0.67; 95% CI 0.58–0.77; $p < 0.001$). Metformin-associated lactic acidosis was observed only in one case. No increased risk of lactic acidosis events from all causes was observed with metformin in both the original and PSM groups (aHR 0.92; 95% CI 0.668–1.276; $p = 0.629$).

Conclusion: It was concluded that metformin decreased the risk of all-cause mortality and incident ESRD in advanced chronic kidney disease (CKD) patients, especially those with CKD 3B, with no increase in the risk of developing lactic acidosis. However, more randomized controlled trials, which are less biased, are required to establish the same.

COMMENT

Critical Appraisal

What was Known Prior to this Study?

Metformin has been widely accepted as first-line drug in management of diabetes mellitus. However, concerns regarding risks of lactic acidosis have led to caution in use of this agent in patients with chronic kidney disease (CKD). Current guidelines recommend that metformin can be used when estimated glomerular filtration rate (eGFR) is ≥45 mL/min/1.73 m^2; when eGFR is 30–44 mL/min/1.73 m^2, metformin treatment should not be started, however, if metformin is already in use, daily dose should be limited to ≤1,000 mg, while metformin contraindicated when the eGFR is <30 mL/min/1.73 m^2.[2] Increasing evidence suggests low incidence of lactic acidosis associated with use of metformin. A recent Cochrane review reported that metformin does not increase incidence of lactic acidosis compared to other antidiabetic agents.[3] A limited number of observational studies have reported on beneficial effects of metformin use on long-term mortality and progression of renal disease among patients with diabetic kidney disease (DKD). In an observational study (2 years follow-up) by Roussel et al. (2010), on participants with type 2 diabetes mellitus (T2DM) with established atherothrombosis, metformin use was associated with reduced all-cause mortality in patients with eGFR 30–60 mL/min/1.73 m^2.[4] In an analysis of Swedish National Diabetes Register (4 years mean follow-up) by Ekstrom et al. (2012), use of metformin was associated with lower all-cause mortality in patients with eGFR 45–60 mL/min/1.73 m^2.[5] In another retrospective study (4 years follow-up) by Charytan et al. (2019), use of metformin lead to a reduction in the risk of all-cause mortality, cardiovascular death, cardiovascular composite, and kidney disease composite [defined as end-stage renal disease (ESRD) or death] in patients with CKD stage ≥4.[6]

What this Study Adds?

This study demonstrated the safety of metformin and its benefits on mortality and progression of kidney disease in Asian population with DKD. This study offers the advantage of longer term follow-up and also evaluated the utility of use of metformin in subgroup with eGFR <30 mL/min/1.73 m^2, a population excluded in a number of studies. The main findings of the study were as follows: (1) metformin use was associated with reduction in all-cause mortality in CKD patients across all strata of eGFR, (2) use of metformin was associated with reduction in progression to ESRD particularly in those with eGFR >30 mL/min/1.73 m^2, and (3) metformin use was not associated with increased risk of lactic acidosis.

Major Strengths of the Study

The major strengths of the study were its large sample size and long follow-up period.

Limitations of the Study

- The study was a retrospective cohort study. Thus, this study was dependent on the accuracy of medical records. Additionally, the difference between prescription and actual adherence to drugs could not be ascertained. Concerns have also been raised about the influence of immortal time bias on the outcome.
- Although, the authors tried to balance baseline characters of patients with propensity score matching (PSM), unmeasured characteristics and confounders could have affected the results.
- The effect of cumulative metformin dose on outcome was not calculated.

Implications of the Findings for the Clinicians

Metformin is well-recognized for its efficacy, low cost, weight neutrality, and benefits regarding cardiovascular outcomes and is a preferred drug for treatment of T2DM. This study provides additional evidence regarding the safety and benefits of this agent even among individuals with DKD.

Knowledge Gaps Identified and Scope for Future Research

The findings of this study need to be confirmed with randomized controlled trials assessing the effect of metformin on outcome among patients with DKD with reduced eGFR.

---

3. Impact of Treating Oral Disease on Preventing Vascular Diseases: A Model-based Cost-effectiveness Analysis of Periodontal Treatment Among Patients with Type 2 Diabetes

Ref: Choi SE, Sima C, Pandya A. Impact of treating oral disease on preventing vascular diseases: a model-based cost-effectiveness analysis of periodontal treatment among patients with type 2 diabetes. Diabetes Care. 2020;43:563-71.

ABSTRACT

Objective: The treatment of periodontitis in type 2 diabetic patients improved glycemic control in previous randomized trials, and thus it has potential to lower the risk of developing type 2 diabetes mellitus (T2DM)-related microvascular diseases and cardiovascular disease (CVD). This has prompted some payers in the United States to expand coverage to nonsurgical treatment modalities for periodontitis in people suffering from chronic diseases such as diabetes. We aim to analyze the cost-effectiveness of covering nonsurgical periodontal treatment among patients with T2DM.

Research design and methods: We conducted a cost-effectiveness analysis to estimate lifetime costs and health gains using a stochastic microsimulation model of oral health conditions, T2DM, T2DM-related microvascular diseases, and CVD.

Population: Model parameters were obtained from the nationally representative National Health and Nutrition Examination Survey (NHANES) (2009–2014) and randomized trials of periodontal treatment among patients with T2DM.

Results: It was observed that expanding periodontal treatment coverage among patients with T2DM and periodontitis can reduce the incidence of tooth loss by 34.1% [95% confidence interval (CI) –39.9, –26.5], microvascular diseases by 20.5% (95% CI –31.2, –9.1) for nephropathy, 17.7% (95% CI –32.7, –4.7) neuropathy, and 18.4% (95% CI –34.5, –3.5) for retinopathy. This will have a total net savings of $5,904 (95% CI –6,039, –5,769), and an estimated gain of 0.6 quality-adjusted life years (QALYs) per capita (95% CI 0.5, 0.6).

Conclusion: Expanding treatment coverage to nonsurgical modalities for periodontitis can significantly bring down the rate of tooth loss or any microvascular diseases in T2DM patients. So, such patients need to be encouraged to receive periodontal treatment when needed as it would not only improve health outcomes, but is also cost-effective.

COMMENT

Critical Appraisal

What was Known Prior to this Study?

Periodontitis is a chronic inflammatory condition of the gums and supporting bone. Diabetes mellitus (DM) is associated with 3-fold increased risk of periodontitis. Conversely, presence of periodontitis contributes to poor glycemic control in DM and is associated with increased risk of vascular complications. Treatment of periodontitis has been shown to improve glycemic control and reduce risk cardiovascular disease (CVD). However, periodontal care is often neglected in people with DM. Studies based on insurance claims data have shown that treatment of periodontitis among people with DM is associated with reduction in medical costs and hospitalization. Additionally, cost-effectiveness of the approach has also been demonstrated in a cohort-based simulation modeling study from the UK.[7]

What this Study Adds?

This study used a mathematical model-based analysis to demonstrate the cost-effectiveness of periodontal treatment among people with type 2 diabetes mellitus (T2DM) in the US. The benefits would be expected to accrue from long-term reductions in tooth loss, reduction in risk of T2DM complications (microvascular diseases, CVDs), cost savings, and gain of quality-adjusted life years (QALYs).

Major Strengths of the Study

The study took into account a wide range of key model parameters.

Limitations of the Study

- The modeling was based on secondary sources. Most trials of periodontal treatment are of short duration.
- The study only included effects of periodontal treatment on diabetes and its vascular complications; suggested associations between periodontal treatment and other conditions such as respiratory diseases, CKD, and cognitive impairment were not considered.
- The study used data from National Health and Nutrition Examination Survey (NHANES) which are subject to limitations of survey studies including recall bias, acceptability bias, and under-reporting.
- The results are subject to the assumptions inherent in modeling.

Implications of the Findings for the Clinicians

The results of this study should encourage clinicians to integrate periodontal treatment with routine diabetes care.

Knowledge Gaps Identified and Scope for Future Research

Large trials on periodontal treatment in DM, involving larger sample sizes and longer follow-up periods, are an important need for future research.

4. Risk of Rapid Kidney Function Decline, All-cause Mortality, and Major Cardiovascular Events in Nonalbuminuric Chronic Kidney Disease in Type 2 Diabetes

Ref: Buyadaa O, Magliano DJ, Salim A, Koye DN, Shaw JE. Risk of rapid kidney function decline, all-cause mortality, and major cardiovascular events in nonalbuminuric chronic kidney disease in type 2 diabetes. Diabetes Care. 2020;43:122-9.

ABSTRACT

Objective: We intended to investigate the rate of progression of nonalbuminuric chronic kidney disease (CKD) to end-stage kidney disease (ESKD) or death or major adverse cardiovascular events (MACE) compared with albuminuric and nonalbuminuric phenotypes.

Research design and methods: A total of 10,185 participants with type 2 diabetes mellitus (T2DM) were enrolled in the Action to Control Cardiovascular Risk in Diabetes (ACCORD) study. Participants were classified as having no kidney disease (no CKD), albuminuria only (albuminuric non-CKD), reduced estimated glomerular filtration rate (eGFR) only (nonalbuminuric CKD), or both albuminuria and reduced eGFR (albuminuric CKD) based on baseline albuminuria and eGFR. The rate of decline of eGFR and hazard ratios (HRs) for ESKD or death or MACE was calculated.

Results: For subjects with absent CKD and those with nonalbuminuric CKD, the rates of eGFR decline were −1.31 and −0.60 mL/min/year, respectively ($p < 0.001$). In competing risk analysis (no CKD as the reference), HRs for ESKD indicated no elevated risk for nonalbuminuric CKD [0.76 (95% CI 0.34, 1.70)] and highest risk for albuminuric CKD [4.52 (2.91, 7.01)]. In adjusted Cox models, HRs for death and MACE were greatest for albuminuric CKD [2.38 (1.92, 2.90) and 2.37 (1.89, 2.97), respectively] and were greater for albuminuric non-CKD [1.82 (1.59, 2.08) and 1.88 (1.63, 2.16), respectively] than for those with nonalbuminuric CKD [1.42 (1.14, 1.78) and 1.44 (1.13, 1.84), respectively].

Conclusion: Individuals with nonalbuminuric CKD showed a slower rate of eGFR decline than did any other group; however, these patients still carry a higher risk for death and MACE than do those without CKD.

COMMENT

Critical Appraisal

What was Known Prior to this Study?

Diabetes is the leading cause of chronic kidney disease (CKD). Clinical course of diabetic kidney disease (DKD) is classically characterized by appearance of albuminuria followed by a decline in glomerular filtration rate (GFR). However, nonalbuminuric CKD is an emerging pattern of renal impairment in diabetes. Several factors, including, use of renin–angiotensin system blockers, advances in antihypertensive antidiabetic and hypolipidemic agents, and smoking cessation have been implicated in rising prevalence of nonalbuminuric DKD. The natural history and outcome of nonalbuminuric DKD appear significantly different from that of albuminuric DKD, only a few studies have addressed the same. In the Finnish Diabetic Nephropathy (FinnDiane) study among participants with type 1 diabetes mellitus (T1DM), presence of nonalbuminuric CKD was not associated with increase in the risk of end-stage renal disease (ESRD). During the 13-year follow-up, ESRD developed in 1.3% of participants with nonalbuminuric CKD, as compared to 0.3% of patients with normal albumin excretion rate (AER) and GFR at baseline, 13.9% of patients with isolated albuminuria, and in 63% of patients with a combination of albuminuria and reduced GFR. However, nonalbuminuric CKD was associated with an increased risk of cardiovascular events and all-cause mortality. Similarly, in the Chronic Renal Insufficiency Cohort (CRIC) Study, nonalbuminuric CKD was associated with much lower incidence of CKD progression and ESRD compared with albuminuric CKD.[8]

What this Study Adds?

This study adds to the limited knowledge about the natural history and outcome of nonalbuminuric DKD. The main findings of the study were as follows: (1) The rate of decline in estimated GFR (eGFR) among those with nonalbuminuric CKD was lower than in other groups (including those with no CKD), (2) nonalbuminuric CKD was not associated with an increased risk of progression to ESRD, and (3) nonalbuminuric CKD was associated with a greater risk of all-cause mortality and major adverse cardiovascular events (MACE) as compared to those with no CKD.

Major Strengths of the Study

The study included participants with type 2 diabetes mellitus (T2DM) who were enrolled in the Action to Control Cardiovascular Risk in Diabetes (ACCORD) study and followed up further in the ACCORD Follow-on (ACCORDION) study with a sample size of 10,185 participants and a combined duration of follow-up of 9 years. The strengths of the study were the large sample size, long follow-up period and availability of records of frequent serum creatinine sampling.

Limitations of the Study

- The study may have limitations in generalizability as the participants were drawn from a clinical trial which included those with DM with either established cardiovascular disease or additional cardiovascular risk factors.
- Follow-up data on urine albumin creatinine ratio was lacking.

Implications of the Findings for the Clinicians

The study gives a better understanding of the outcomes associated with nonalbuminuric DKD.

Knowledge Gaps Identified and Scope for Future Research

With increasing prevalence of nonalbuminuric CKD in diabetes, more studies are required to clarify its pathogenesis and underlying mechanisms. Researches investigating molecular pathways that determine the different patterns of DKD are warranted. Differences in the patterns of DKD and their outcomes in different ethnic populations need to be explored. Search should also be made for early diagnostic markers of nonalbuminuric DKD and renal function decline.

5. Performance of Plasma Biomarkers and Diagnostic Panels for Nonalcoholic Steatohepatitis and Advanced Fibrosis in Patients with Type 2 Diabetes

Ref: Bril F, McPhaul MJ, Caulfield MP, Clark VC, Soldevilla-Pico C, Firpi-Morell RJ, et al. Performance of plasma biomarkers and diagnostic panels for nonalcoholic steatohepatitis and advanced fibrosis in patients with type 2 diabetes. Diabetes Care. 2020;43:290-7.

ABSTRACT

Objective: To assess the performance of noninvasive diagnostic panels and plasma biomarkers for the diagnosis of nonalcoholic steatohepatitis (NASH) and advanced fibrosis in patients with type 2 diabetes mellitus (T2DM).

Research design and methods: A total of 213 patients who underwent liver magnetic resonance spectroscopy (MRS) were included in this cross-sectional study. Several noninvasive clinical models/scores and plasma biomarkers were measured to identify NASH and advanced fibrosis [NASH: alanine aminotransferase (ALT), cytokeratin-18, NashTest 2, HAIR, BARD, and OWLiver; advanced fibrosis: aspartate aminotransferase (AST), fragments of propeptide of type III procollagen (PRO-C3), fibrosis-4 (FIB-4), aspartate aminotransferase-to-platelet ratio index (APRI), nonalcoholic fatty liver disease (NAFLD) fibrosis score, and FibroTest].

Results: We could not find any of the noninvasive tools having an optimum performance for the diagnosis of NASH in patients with T2DM [all areas under the curve (AUCs) <0.80]. Plasma ALT [AUC 0.78 (95% CI 0.71–0.84)] performed better than any other panel or biomarker. Plasma PRO-C3, AST, and APRI performed better in diagnosing advanced fibrosis, than the other approaches [AUC 0.90 (0.85–0.95); 0.85 (0.80–0.91); and 0.86 (0.80–0.91) respectively]. Plasma AST was better than any other approach.

Conclusion: Noninvasive clinical models/scores and plasma biomarkers were found suboptimal for the diagnosis of NASH or advanced fibrosis in patients with T2DM. However, need for liver biopsies may be limited by the sequential use of plasma AST and other noninvasive tests to detect patients with advanced fibrosis.

COMMENT

Critical Appraisal

What was Known Prior to this Study?

Nonalcoholic fatty liver disease (NAFLD) occurs in up to 70% of people with type 2 diabetes mellitus (T2DM), with 20–30% having more severe morphology—nonalcoholic steatohepatitis (NASH) and can progress to advanced fibrosis or cirrhosis. Liver biopsy is the gold standard for diagnosis of NASH/advanced fibrosis/cirrhosis. However, because of its invasive nature, it is often not preferred by patients and clinicians alike. Other available clinical tools also have significant limitations. Although aminotransferases are widely used as screening tool, they have limited sensitivity in diagnosing NASH/advanced fibrosis. The other commonly prescribed tool—ultrasonography has only modest sensitivity and specificity. More advanced diagnostic tools, transient elastography, and magnetic resonance elastography have limited availability. Additionally, several other clinical models/scores and plasma biomarkers have been tested in recent years as tools to diagnose NASH/advanced fibrosis. Some of the tools to diagnose NASH include: (1) Alanine aminotransferase (ALT); (2) plasma cytokeratin 18 (CK-18); (3) BARD score (sum of: BMI ≥28 = 1 point, aspartate aminotransferase (AST)/ALT ratio ≥0.80 = 2 points, and diabetes = 1 point); (4) NashTest 2 [a proprietary score based on serum α_2-macroglobulin, apolipoprotein A1, haptoglobin, total bilirubin, γ-glutamyl transpeptidase (GGT), AST, cholesterol, and triglycerides]; (5) OWLiver (a proprietary, BMI-dependent logistic regression algorithm based on serum levels of a panel of 20 triglycerides); (6) HAIR score [sum of: hypertension = 1 point; ALT >40 units/L = 1 point; and insulin resistance index (log fasting insulin + log fasting glucose) >5.0 = 1 point]. Some of the tools to diagnose advanced fibrosis include: (i) AST; (ii) APRI [defined as (AST)/(upper limit of normal)/(platelets in 10^9/L)]; (iii) FibroTest (a proprietary score based on serum α_2-macroglobulin, apolipoprotein A1, haptoglobin, total bilirubin, and GGT); (iv) FIB-4 [(age × AST)/(platelets × $\sqrt{ALT}$)]; (v) NAFLD fibrosis score [−1.675 + 0.037 × (age in years) + 0.094 × (BMI in kg/m^2) + 1.13 (for diabetes) + 0.99 × (AST/ALT) − 0.013 × (platelets in 10^9/L) − 0.66 × (albumin in g/dL)]; (vi) plasma PRO-C3.[9]

What this Study Adds?

This study assessed the performance of various available noninvasive clinical models/scores, plasma biomarkers and their combinations in the diagnosis of biopsy proven NASH or advanced fibrosis in patients with T2DM. The main findings of the study were as follows: (1) None of the tested clinical models/plasma biomarkers performed better than ALT and AST in the diagnosis of NASH and advanced fibrosis respectively; and (2) A combination of the tools did not significantly improve their performance or discriminatory capacity.

Major Strengths of the Study

- The study evaluated a wide range of clinical models/biomarkers and their combinations.
- Comparison was made against the gold standard method of diagnosis (liver biopsy).
- The study included a wide range of liver disease (from absence of NAFLD to severe NASH with advanced fibrosis).

Limitations of the Study

- The study included a multiethnic cohort, which could have influenced the results.
- The study participants were recruited from different sources to ensure that all stages of the disease were well represented, and there was possibility of a selection bias.
- Liver biopsy was not performed in controls (those without evidence of NAFLD on H-MRS).

Implications of the Findings for the Clinicians

Although a number of clinical models/plasma biomarkers have been proposed as tools for diagnosis of NASH/advanced liver fibrosis, they should be used with caution in people with DM, taking into account their clinical characteristics. As none of the other tested clinical models/biomarkers performed better than ALT or AST, these less costly and widely available tests should be preferred as stand-alone tools to guide clinicians in selecting cases to be biopsied.

Knowledge Gaps Identified and Scope for Future Research

The results of this study highlight the need for continued search for new, noninvasive and affordable tools with greater accuracy to diagnose NASH, and advanced fibrosis.

6. Time in Range is Associated with Carotid Intima-media Thickness in Type 2 Diabetes

Ref: Lu J, Ma X, Shen Y, Wu Q, Wang R, Zhang L, et al. Time in range is associated with carotid intima-media thickness in type 2 diabetes. Diabetes Technol Ther. 2020;22:72-8.

ABSTRACT

Introduction: Time in range (TIR), an evolving metric of glycemic control, is associated with microvascular complications of diabetes. This study aimed at evaluating the association of TIR [achieved from continuous glucose monitoring (CGM)] with carotid intima-media thickness test (CIMT) as a surrogate marker of cardiovascular disease (CVD).

Methods: This was across-sectional study including 2,215 patients with type 2 diabetes mellitus (T2DM). Evaluation of TIR of 3.9–10.0 mmol/L was done with CGM. High-resolution B-mode ultrasonography was used for measuring CIMT. Abnormal CIMT was defined as a mean CIMT 1.0 mm or more. For examining the independent association of TIR with CIMT, logistic regression models were utilized.

Results: Participants with abnormal CIMT were found to have significantly lower TIR ($p < 0.001$) than patients with normal CIMT. A progressive reduction was observed in the prevalence of abnormal CIMT across the categories of increasing TIR ($p < 0.001$). In a fully adjusted model controlling for traditional risk factor of CVD, each 10% increase in TIR was found to be associated with 6.4% lower risk of abnormal

CIMT. On stratification of the data by sex, there was a significantly association between TIR with CIMT in males but not in females. In 612 patients with complete data on diabetic retinopathy and albuminuria, the association between TIR and CIMT was significant, irrespective of the status of microvascular complications.

Conclusion: In patients with T2DM, TIR was associated with CIMT indicating a relation between TIR and macrovascular disease.

COMMENT

Critical Appraisal

What was Known Prior to this Study?

Although glycated hemoglobin (HbA1c) is a widely accepted criterion to assess adequacy of glycemic control, and HbA1c is strongly associated with vascular complications of diabetes mellitus (DM), it has its limitations, e.g., it is affected by pregnancy, anemia, hemoglobinopathies, ethnicity. Additionally, it cannot detect glycemic variability or acute events such as hypoglycemia. Continuous glucose monitoring (CGM) tracks glucose profile over days/weeks. Time in range (TIR) is one of the glycemic metrics obtained from CGM readings which has been found to have strong correlation with HbA1c. Additionally, it has also been shown to be independently associated with diabetic retinopathy and albuminuria.[10,11] However, there is no data demonstrating association of TIR with cardiovascular disease (CVD).

What this Study Adds?

This study investigated the association between TIR and carotid intima-media thickness test (CIMT) in participants with type 2 diabetes mellitus (T2DM). CIMT is an ultrasound-based marker of subclinical atherosclerosis and can serve as a surrogate marker of CVDs. In the study, TIR was found to be inversely associated with CIMT. However, the association was found to be significant only in males and not in females.

Major Strengths of the Study

The major strengths of the study were its large sample size and well-characterized study population.

Limitations of the Study

- Cross-sectional study design
- Continuous glucose monitoring was conducted only for 3 days for each participant. Longer duration of CGM, up to 14 days, may be required to optimally assess glycemic control.
- Carotid intima-media thickness test was analyzed only in the common carotid artery. Carotid bulb and internal carotid artery were not assessed.

Implications of the Findings for the Clinicians

The association between TIR and CIMT (a predictor of future cardiovascular events) found in this study highlight the importance of TIR as an additional parameter (in addition to HbA1c) for assessing glycemic control.

Knowledge Gaps Identified and Scope for Future Research

Further prospective studies and clinical trials are required to establish the relationship between TIR and CIMT/CVDs.

REFERENCES (Comorbidities)

1. Moscarella E, Gragnano F, Cesaro A, Ielasi A, Diana V, Conte M, et al. Coronary Physiology Assessment for the Diagnosis and Treatment of Coronary Artery Disease. Cardiol Clin. 2020;38(4):575-588.
2. Tuttle Kr, Bakris GL, Bilous RW, Chiang JL, de Boer IH, Goldstein-Fuchs J, et al. Diabetic kidney disease: a report from an ADA Consensus Conference. Diabetes Care. 2014;37(10):2864-83.
3. Salpeter SR, Greyber E, Pasternak GA, Salpeter EE. Risk of fatal and nonfatal lactic acidosis with metformin use in type 2 diabetes mellitus. Cochrane Database Syst Rev 2010;(4):CD002967.
4. Roussel R, Travert F, Pasquet B, Wilson PWF, Smith Jr SC, Goto S, et al. Metformin use and mortality among patients with diabetes and atherothrombosis. Arch Intern Med. 2010;170(21):1892-9.
5. Ekström N, Schiöler L, Svensson AM, et al. Effectiveness and safety of metformin in 51,675 patients with type 2 diabetes and different levels of renal function: a cohort study from the Swedish National Diabetes Register. BMJ Open. 2012;2:e001076.
6. Charytan DM, Solomon SD, Ivanovich P, et al. Metformin use and cardiovascular events in patients with type 2 diabetes and chronic kidney disease. Diabetes Obes Metab 2019; 21:1199-1208.
7. Solowiej-Wedderburn J, Ide M, Pennington M. Cost-effectiveness of non-surgical periodontal therapy for patients with type 2 diabetes in the UK. J Clin Periodontol 2017;44:700-707.
8. Klimontov VV, Korbut AI. Albuminuric and non-albuminuric patterns of chronic kidney disease in type 2 diabetes. Diabetes Metab Syndr. 2019;13(1):474-9.
9. Bril F, Cusi K. Nonalcoholic Fatty Liver Disease: The New Complication of Type 2 Diabetes Mellitus. Endocrinol Metab Clin North Am. 2016;45(4):765-81.
10. Lu J, Ma X, Zhou J, et al. Association of Time in Range, as Assessed by Continuous Glucose Monitoring, With Diabetic Retinopathy in Type 2 Diabetes. Diabetes Care. 2018;41(11):2370-6.
11. Beck RW, Bergenstal RM, Riddlesworth TD, et al. Validation of Time in Range as an Outcome Measure for Diabetes Clinical Trials. Diabetes Care. 2019;42(3):400-5.

Section 4: Complications

Indira Maisnam, Amit Gupta, Neeta Deshpande, Brij Mohan Makkar

1. Reduced Pancreatic Polypeptide Response is Associated with Early Alteration of Glycemic Control in Chronic Pancreatitis

Ref: Aslam M, Vijayasarathy K, Talukdar R, Sasikala M, Reddy DN. Reduced pancreatic polypeptide response is associated with early alteration of glycemic control in chronic pancreatitis. Diabetes Res Clin Pract. 2020;160:107993.

ABSTRACT

Aim: To study the incidence of glucose intolerance in nondiabetic patients of chronic pancreatitis (CP) based on oral glucose tolerance test (OGTT).

Methods: Consecutive Indian CP patients without diabetes over 6 months were screened by performing OGTT, and correlation with physical characteristics and glycated hemoglobin (HbA1c) was established. Comparison of c-peptide and pancreatic polypeptide (PP) response across different groups based on OGTT was done. $p < 0.05$ was considered significant.

Results: Mean duration of CP among 171 screened patients was 5.03 ± 4.32 years. OGTT detected diabetes in 40, while 55 were detected to have prediabetes. A significant dilatation of pancreatic duct was observed in CP patients with diabetes and prediabetes compared to nondiabetic CP (4.2 ± 2.7 mm, 3.6 ± 2.7 mm, 2.84 ± 2.25 mm; $p = 0.018$). Fasting blood glucose (FBS) and 2 hour OGTT were 109.35 ± 19.06, 97.47 ± 11.94, 85.24 ± 9.95 and 236.13 ± 31.42, 154.65 ± 19.53, 112.89 ± 16.32 in patients with diabetes mellitus (DM), prediabetes, and CP patients without diabetes ($p < 0.0001$). CP patients showed good c-peptide response ($p = 0.001$) and reduced PP response ($p = 0.003$) in CP patients compared to controls.

Conclusion: We concluded that reduced PP response in the presence of good c-peptide response may result in development of DM, in the early course of disease.

COMMENT

What was Known Prior to this Study?

Diabetes that develops in patients with pre-existing exocrine pancreatic disorder is known as type 3c diabetes. The condition is often undiagnosed or misdiagnosed. Type 3c is a disease of heterogenous etiology, including but not limited to tropical calcific pancreatitis, alcoholic pancreatitis, cystic fibrosis, postpancreatectomy, etc. The proposed mechanisms of diabetogenic are not fully known but have been linked to genetic factors, loss of β-cell mass and function, and disruption of incretin axis. The prevalence of diabetes mellitus (DM) in chronic pancreatitis (CP) ranges from 25 to 80%.[1,2] Diabetes development has been linked to the duration of CP while the age of presentation varies in different studies.[2,3] Presence of pancreatic calcification was a determinant of diabetes in some studies.[1,2] β-cell dysfunction and apoptosis due to local and systemic inflammatory response, and β-cell dedifferentiation has been linked to development of diabetes in CP.[4,5] The effect of CP on glucagon secretion is mixed. While most studies suggest impaired α-cell function and glucagon secretion due to generalized inflammation, other studies have shown increased α-cell response and glucagon secretion.[6] Pancreatic polypeptide (PP) cells which are proposed to protect β-cells are also reported to be diminished in CP. PP has been reported to improve hepatic insulin sensitivity.[7] Systemic insulin resistance and alteration in gut microbiota are increasingly being realized to be involved in the pathogenesis of diabetes in CP.

What Does this Study Add?

This study included 171 CP without a known diagnosis of diabetes and 20 healthy controls. Specifically, the study excluded acute on CP, cystic fibrosis, postpancreatectomy CP, pre-existing DM, pancreatic malignancy, hypertriglyceridemia, or hypercalcemia induced pancreatitis, alcoholics, and smokers.

About 23.39%, 32.16%, and 44.45% of the patients were found to have diabetes, prediabetes, and normoglycemia (nondiabetes) based on the American Diabetes Association Criteria. Thus, a significant number of patients with CP (55.55%) had hyperglycemia that was asymptomatic or undiagnosed.

Diabetes was seen more frequently in those with longer duration of CP, but was not statistically significant. Compared to other studies, diabetes was diagnosed at a younger age in the study population, possibly due to presentation of CP at a younger age. The presence of dilated pancreatic ducts rather than pancreatic atrophy and calcification was significantly more in diabetes with CP compared to prediabetes and normoglycemic with CP.

The c-peptide response to mixed meal was increased in CP compared to controls ($p = 0.001$); with no difference in c-peptide response among diabetes, prediabetes, and nondiabetes with CP. HOMA2-β% (marker of β-cell function) was reduced in diabetes and prediabetes with CP, compared to nondiabetes with CP and controls, but was not statistically significant. Insulin sensitivity was decreased and HOMA-IR (marker of insulin resistance) was increased in CP compared to controls though not statistically significant. PP response was significantly lower in patients with CP compared to controls ($p = 0.001$). PP response was significantly lower in CP with diabetes compared to non-DM with CP ($p = 0.003$).

The major information which the study adds is that in the studied population, there is a high prevalence of hyperglycemia in CP that is undiagnosed and/or asymptomatic; the age of DM in CP is younger; low PP response and decreased insulin sensitivity are seen in CP compared to controls; PP response is worse in CP with DM compared to CP with prediabetes; and the c-peptide response is increased in CP compared to controls suggesting presence of viable islet cells for quite sometime, even in those with diabetes.

Major Strengths of the Study

The study represents patients with tropical pancreatitis, as other secondary causes of pancreatitis were excluded. It highlights the importance of screening in such patients for diabetes as many are asymptomatic/undiagnosed. Reduced PP response is an important finding and reduction in PP is known to contribute to hepatic insulin resistance, but a viable islet cell response is still present even in those with diabetes. Insulin resistance rather than the loss of islet cell response was identified as an important determinant of hyperglycemia. This finding of greater role of diminished PP response and insulin resistance in diabetes pathogenesis, if confirmed in larger studies, could shift focus to improving PP response and systemic/hepatic insulin sensitivity in the management of similar patients with CP.

Limitations of the Study

The limitations are single-center and cross-sectional nature of the study. The cross-sectional nature of the study cannot determine the natural history of the disease. From the study, it is not possible to determine the frequency of screening for DM. Other pancreatic hormones like glucagon were not studied. The study cannot explain the mechanism of increased c-peptide response, diminished PP response, impaired insulin sensitivity, and pancreatic duct dilatation in the pathogenesis of diabetes as it was not designed to do so.

Implications of the Findings for the Clinicians

Diabetes should be screened for in patients with CP. Diminished PP response and insulin resistance plays an important role in its pathogenesis and measures to improve insulin resistance like physical activity and avoidance of truncal obesity (even if lean) may help in improving glycemic outcomes.

Knowledge Gaps Identified and Scope for Future Research

Research is needed to identify the factors responsible for early appearance of CP and therefore of DM. Studies need to be performed on heterogenous population groups including those with other causes of CP.

2. Young-Onset Type 2 Diabetes and Younger Current Age: Increased Susceptibility to Retinopathy in Contrast to other Complications

Ref: Middleton TL, Constantino MI, Molyneaux L, D'Souza M, Twigg SM, Wu T, et al. Young-onset type 2 diabetes and younger current age: Increased susceptibility to retinopathy in contrast to other complications. Diabet Med. 2020;37(6):991-9.

ABSTRACT

Aim: To determine if people with young-onset type 2 diabetes mellitus (T2DM) are more susceptible to long-term complications like retinopathy than those diagnosed later.

Methods: We analyzed the prospective data from 3,322 individuals with T2DM, who had onset during 15–70 years and collected up to 10–25 years after diabetes diagnosis. Logistic regression models were used to analyze the associations between age at diagnosis and long-term complications, after adjusting for duration of diabetes and metabolic risk factors.

Results: Retinopathy was observed in highest frequency in those with onset between 15 and 40 years, with the odds being higher for longer duration of exposure to diabetes. After 10–15 years' diabetes duration, the adjusted odds ratio for retinopathy in this population was 2.8 (95% CI 1.9–4.1; reference group those diagnosed at 60 to <70 years of age). For other complications, no such pattern was observed.

Conclusion: In our study, people with young-onset T2DM appeared to be more susceptible to retinopathy after accounting for disease duration and other important confounders.

COMMENT

What was Known Prior to this Study?

The past few decades have seen an exponential rise in young-onset type 2 diabetes mellitus (T2DM). Young-onset T2DM is known to have a more aggressive course of vascular complications compared to type 1 diabetes mellitus (T1DM) and T2DM with onset in older people. Young-onset T2DM was associated with greater risk of death, after a shorter duration of diabetes, and at a younger age compared to T1DM.[8] The same study found that despite similar glycemic control and shorter duration of disease, the chances of albuminuria, cardiovascular risk factors, cardiovascular disease, neuropathy, and cardiovascular deaths were higher in young-onset T2DM. A study from India also concluded that young-onset T2DM was more aggressive than T1DM.[9]

The Restoring Insulin Secretion (RISE) consortium suggest that young-onset T2DM has a different pathophysiological basis compared to older-onset T2DM.[10] The increased complications in young-onset T2DM compared to older-onset T2DM have been linked to longer exposure to the cardiovascular risk, poorer glycemic control, and pharmacotherapy failure.[11,12] However, what is not clear is whether or which complication risk persists after accounting for the above-mentioned factors in young-onset T2DM.

What Does this Study Add?

The study describes the data from 1996 to 2016 of a single-center database of 3,322 individuals of people with T2DM. Age at diagnosis was categorized as 15 to <40 years (young-onset T2DM), 40 to <50 years, 50 to <60 years, and 60 to <70 years. Complications status was considered during three distinct diabetes exposure bands (10 to <15 years, 15 to <20 years, and 20 to <25 years after diagnosis).

Within the duration band of 10 to <15 years, young-onset T2DM had significantly higher updated mean glycated hemoglobin (HbA1c), low-density lipoprotein (LDL) cholesterol, and triglyceride levels, significantly higher body mass index (BMI) and smoking rates, and lower blood pressure (BP), and HDL cholesterol than those diagnosed at older ages. Similar patterns were seen for the duration bands 15 to <20 years and 20 to <25 years.

Using logistic regression models, the cross-sectional associations between age at diagnosis and microvascular and macrovascular complications were analyzed after adjusting for duration of diabetes exposure and metabolic risk factors including BP, cholesterol, and updated mean HbA1c. The following findings were seen after adjusted modeling.

For each diabetes duration band, the prevalence of diabetic retinopathy was highest in the young-onset T2DM subgroup. Differences in the prevalence of diabetic retinopathy were observed across the age-at-diagnosis spectrum for each duration band ($p \leq 0.001$ for all). Higher odds of retinopathy were seen in the younger age-at-onset group in each of the three models of retinopathy. The odds of retinopathy across the age-at-diagnosis spectrum for the 0 to <5 years exposure band were not significantly different, but the pattern of increased risk of retinopathy in the young-onset group emerged after 5 to <10 years of diabetes exposure.

Within each diabetes duration band, the prevalence of albuminuria and chronic kidney disease was highest in the subgroup of people diagnosed at 60 to <70 years of age, which was statistically significant. After 10 to <15 years of diabetes exposure, the odds of albuminuria or chronic kidney disease were significantly lower in each of the younger age of diagnosis subgroups. However, after 20 to <25 years of diabetes exposure, no significant differences in albuminuria were observed across the age of diagnosis spectrum. Age of diagnosis was not consistently associated with peripheral neuropathy across the duration of diabetes exposure bands. Younger age at diagnosis was associated with lower odds of macrovascular disease.

The information that is available from the study is that young-onset T2DM had higher cardiometabolic risk like BMI, HbA1c, LDL, triglyceride, and smoking across all duration bands. However, after adjustment modeling for duration, BP, cholesterol, and updated mean HbA1c, the study found that the odds ratio of retinopathy (but not for albuminuria, peripheral neuropathy, and macrovascular disease) was higher in young-onset T2DM compared to older-onset T2DM. Earlier studies have suggested that the increased incidence of retinopathy in younger people and young-onset diabetes could be due to a robust vascular endothelial response or growth hormone and insulin-like growth factor 1 effects.[13,14] The novel finding in this study is that retinopathy is a risk specifically seen in young-onset T2DM after adjustment for other confounders.

Major Strengths of the Study

Relatively large data with comprehensive information and prolonged follow-up.

Limitations of the Study

Single-center data from a referral hospital, which may not reflect the general population. Survival bias cannot be completely ruled out.

Implications of the Findings for the Clinicians

The risk of retinopathy is high in young-onset T2DM and therefore more frequent retinopathy screening should be offered to this group of patients. Even if the risk of peripheral neuropathy, albuminuria, and macrovascular disease was not found to be higher after adjustment for duration of diabetes, BP, updated mean HbA1c, and cholesterol; it needs to be remembered that these were findings after adjustments of important risks. The purpose of adjustment was to identify the specific contribution of age to diabetes complications. The fact remains and was also found in the study that there is higher BMI, LDL cholesterol, triglyceride, HbA1c, and smoking in young-onset T2DM. Therefore, the risk of both macrovascular and microvascular disease continues to remain high in young-onset T2DM.

Knowledge Gaps Identified and Scope for Future Research

It is quite evident that T2DM in young is different from older-onset diabetes mellitus. More research is needed to exactly identify the pathogenesis of T2DM and its complications in the young. Data needs to be available from a diverse range of individuals across population and ethnic groups as we know T2DM to be an extremely heterogeneous disease.

3. Dipeptidyl Peptidase 4 Inhibitors and the Risk of Bullous Pemphigoid among Patients with Type 2 Diabetes

Ref: Douros A, Rouette J, Yin H, Yu OHY, Filion KB, Azoulay L. Dipeptidyl peptidase 4 inhibitors and the risk of bullous pemphigoid among patients with type 2 diabetes. Diabetes Care. 2019;42(8):1496-1503.

ABSTRACT

Objective: Bullous pemphigoid (BP), a potentially severe autoimmune skin disease can have an association with dipeptidyl peptidase-4 (DPP-4) inhibitors as suggested by some literature. Here, we aim to assess if there is an increased risk of BP in type 2 diabetic patients, when compared with other second- to third-line antidiabetic drugs.

Research design and methods: A cohort study that included 168,774 patients who initiated antidiabetic drugs between January 2007 and March 2018, was conducted using the U.K. Clinical Practice Research Datalink. Estimation of adjusted hazard ratios (HRs) with 95% CIs of incident BP associated with current use of DPP-4 inhibitors, was done using time-dependent Cox proportional hazards models, and compared with other antidiabetic drugs. To assess the impact of residual confounding, a propensity score-matched analysis was done.

Results: Total of 150 patients were newly diagnosed with BP during 711,311 person-years of follow-up. An increased risk of BP [HR 2.21 (95% CI 1.45–3.38)] was observed with the current use of DPP-4 inhibitors. HRs gradually increased with longer durations of use, with a peak after 20 months [HR 3.60 (95% CI 2.11–6.16)]. The propensity score-matched analysis [HR 2.40 (95% CI 1.13–4.66)] showed similar results.

Conclusion: Although the absolute risk of BP in patients with type 2 diabetes mellitus (T2DM) was low, the use of DPP-4 inhibitors can double the risk.

COMMENT

What was Known Prior to this Study?

Bullous pemphigoid (BP) is an autoantibody-mediated blistering skin disease. The incidence of BP has been increasing over the past few decades. The independent risk factors of BP are advanced age, dementia, parkinsonism, multiple sclerosis, and medications. The list of drugs that can cause BP is extensive and includes antibiotics, antihypertensives, diuretics, anti-TNF, and vaccines.[15] Increasingly, there are reports of dipeptidyl peptidase-4 (DPP-4) inhibitors induced/associated BP in case reports and pharmacovigilance studies.

Dipeptidyl peptidase-4 protein is expressed in numerous cells including T lymphocytes with increased expression in skin diseases like T-cell lymphomas, psoriasis, lichen planus, and atopic dermatitis.[16,17] Besides antihyperglycemic effects, gliptins effect on cells and tissues include tissue modeling, e.g., myocardial regeneration and regulation of inflammatory cells such as T lymphocytes.[18,19]

Skandalis et al., were the first researchers to report DPP-4 inhibitor associated BP when they reported five cases of BP following exposure to metformin and gliptins.[20] Following this there has been a number of case reports. The European, French, Finnish, and Korean pharmacovigilance studies reported increased incidence of BP with gliptins.[21-24] Other case-controlled studies also reported increased incidence of BP with gliptins.[25]

What Does this Study Add?

This study assessed a huge database, the U.K. Clinical Practice Research Datalink, and conducted a cohort study among 168,774 patients initiating antidiabetic drugs between January 2007 and March 2018.

Time-dependent Cox proportional hazards models were used to estimate hazard ratios (HRs) and 95% CIs of BP associated with use of DPP-4 inhibitors, when compared with use of other second- to third-line treatments. The models were adjusted for age, sex, year of cohort entry, alcohol related disorders, smoking status, BMI category, HbA1c and duration of treated diabetes, macrovascular and microvascular complications, cancer, dementia, parkinsonism, multiple sclerosis and depression. Secondary analyses performed were whether there was a duration-response relation according to the current use of DPP-4 inhibitor on the incidence of BP; and assessed the association between BP and use of individual DPP-4 inhibitors. Propensity score-matched analysis to assess the impact of residual confounding was also done.

In the 711,311 person-years of follow-up, 150 patients developed BP (21.1 per 100,000 person-years). Current use of DPP-4 inhibitors increased the risk of BP [(47.3 vs. 20.0 per 100,000 person-years; HR 2.21 (95% CI 1.45–3.38)]. The risk was increased with increased duration of use, with a peak after 20 months. The highest point estimate was for linagliptin and vildagliptin. In the propensity score-matched analysis, DPP-4 inhibitors use was associated with doubling of the risk of BP, compared with the use of other second- to third-line antidiabetic drugs, however, the absolute risk was low.

The important addition from this study is that it aggressively addressed shortcomings in previous case reports, case series, and pharmacovigilance studies. The study addressed potential time-window bias, lack of adjustment for potentially important confounders, and duration response relations.

Major Strengths of the Study

Data was derived from a very large cohort with >700,000 patient years of follow-up with adjustments for numerous potential confounders thereby addressing the shortcomings of previous reports.

Limitations of the Study

There is no mention of adjustment for some important confounders especially, other medications that can cause BP. BP diagnosis was made on the basis of drugs used and/or dermatologist referral, and not by histology.

Implications of the Findings for the Clinicians

There is an increased risk of BP with gliptin use compared to nonusers, however, the absolute risk is low. Physicians need to be alert too, but not alarmed to the possibility of gliptin induced BP.

Knowledge Gaps Identified and Scope for Future Research

Research into the mechanism of gliptin induced BP is required. There is a need to identify diabetes specific factors and comorbidities that increase gliptin-induced BP risk.

4. Seroprevalence and Risk Factors Associated with HBV and HCV Infection among Subjects with Type 2 Diabetes from South India

Ref: Juttada U, Smina TP, Kumpatla S, Viswanathan V. Seroprevalence and risk factors associated with HBV and HCV infection among subjects with type 2 diabetes from South India. Diabetes Res Clin Prac. 2019;153:133-7.

ABSTRACT

We intend to summarize the seroprevalence data of hepatitis C virus (HCV) and hepatitis B virus (HBV) viral infections and associated risk factors in type 2 diabetic patients from South India. Among the 388 screened subjects, prevalence of HBV (9%) was higher as compared to HCV (2%) infection. These infections were independent of the liver damage. The importance of hepatitis vaccination once the subject is diagnosed with diabetes has been emphasized by the fact that longer duration of diabetes, hospital admission, history of jaundice, and history of surgeries are prominent risk factors for HBV and HCV infections.

COMMENT

What was Known Prior to this Study?

Chronic viral hepatitis has been reported to coexist with type 2 diabetes mellitus (T2DM). Studies have shown an increased risk of chronic hepatitis C virus (HCV) infection in people with diabetes.[26,27] At the same time, chronic HCV is a risk factor for T2DM.[1] The data on the prevalence of HBV infection in diabetes mellitus (DM) is mixed. While some studies showed no increase in prevalence compared to background population,[28-31] some studies showed increased prevalence of both HCV and hepatitis B virus (HBV) infection.[32]

The liver plays a vital role in glucose metabolism and therefore chronic diseases of the liver like chronic viral hepatitis may adversely affect body glucose handling. HCV can also disturb the insulin signaling pathway, cause insulin resistance and induce autoimmunity.[33,34] HBV outbreaks and infection have been reported in diabetes patients.[35,36] The increased risk of chronic viral hepatitis has been linked to factors like impaired immunity in DM, the greater chances of parenteral and surgical procedures in patients with diabetes and other unknown factors.

India has a huge prevalence of both DM and chronic HBV and HCV infection. However, there is scarce data on the chronic viral hepatitis seroprevalence in people with diabetes.

What Does this Study Add?

This was a single hospital-based cross-sectional study of 388 patients with T2DM. They were divided into Group-I T2DM with abnormal liver function, Group-II T2DM with normal liver function test, and Group-III control with normal liver function and without T2DM.

The prevalence of HBV (9.3%) was more prevalent compared to HCV (2.8%) among subjects. HCV in Group I, Group II, and Group III were 3.3%, 4.3%, and 0.8%, respectively. HBV prevalence in Group I, Group II, and Group III were 5.8%, 20.3%, and 0.8%, respectively.

Thus, most of the patients with chronic HBV and HCV infection, and diabetes had normal liver function tests. HBV infection was seen more frequently in those with longer duration of diabetes, history of hospital admission, history of jaundice, and history of surgeries, which was all statistically significant. The only statistically significant risk factor for a chronic HCV infection was a history of surgery.

Higher number of positive cases was observed in group II as compared to group I. Group II showed the higher prevalence rates of both the hepatitis infections, which may mean that deranged liver function was not provoking the chronic viral hepatitis infections.

The study added some interesting observations. One, the prevalence of chronic HBV was much higher than chronic HCV in the study population, the major contribution being from patients with diabetes rather than controls. Two, the most patients with chronic HCV and HBV infection have normal liver function tests implying that most may be asymptomatic despite the presence of infection. This highlights the importance of screening and prevention of infection. Three, a number of factors were noted to be significantly associated with the development of HBV infection, but only past history of surgery was found to be associated with development of HCV. This re-emphasizes the current understanding that the acquisition of HCV infection is often occult and asymptomatic in the acute phase.

Major Strengths of the Study

The study provides data about the prevalence of chronic HBV and HCV infection in patients with diabetes from a hospital in India. The prevalence is significant and the major contribution is from HBV rather than HCV. It also provided information that majority of the patients with chronic viral hepatitis have normal liver function tests, highlighting the importance of screening and prevention. HBV, the more prevalent of the two chronic viral hepatitis can be prevented by vaccination and both the types of chronic hepatitis can be prevented by healthy practices.

Limitations of the Study

It was a single-center study performed in a short period of time. It therefore cannot reflect the general prevalence in the region or the country. Some patients with chronic liver disease, namely, compensated cirrhosis can have an apparently normal liver function test, and therefore, anatomical evaluation (ultrasonography and upper gastrointestinal endoscopy) could have added more information.

Implications of the Findings for the Clinicians

There is a huge prevalence of chronic hepatitis, especially, HBV in patients with T2DM. In most of these patients the liver function test is normal. Therefore, prevention of chronic hepatitis in DM by healthy practices and of HBV by vaccination is vital.

Knowledge Gaps Identified and Scope for Future Research

There is need to explore the mechanisms linking diabetes to chronic viral hepatitis.

5. Prevalence and Patterns of Cardiac Autonomic Dysfunction in Male Patients with Type 2 Diabetes Mellitus and Chronic Charcot's Neuroarthropathy: A Cross-sectional Study from South India

Ref: Naik D, Singh HS, Gupta RD, Jebasingh F, Paul TV, Thomas N. Prevalence and patterns of cardiac autonomic dysfunction in male patients with type 2 diabetes mellitus and chronic Charcot's neuroarthropathy: A cross-sectional study from South India. Int J Diabetes Dev Ctries. 2019;39:633-40.

ABSTRACT

Aim: Our study aimed to look at the prevalence and patterns of cardiac autonomic neuropathy (CAN) related dysfunction in male patients of type 2 diabetes mellitus (T2DM) with chronic Charcot's foot.

Methods: A total of 74 male patients with T2DM were included in this study. Three groups of patients were selected: Group 1 included patients with chronic Charcot's foot (n = 24), group 2 included patients with diabetic peripheral neuropathy without chronic Charcot's foot (n = 22), and group 3 included patients without peripheral neuropathy or chronic Charcot's foot (n = 28). The autonomic functions were tested using a personal computer-based cardiac autonomic neuropathy system (CANS-504) analyzer.

Results: The combined sympathetic nervous system (SNS) and parasympathetic autonomic function [parasympathetic nervous system (PNS)] abnormalities were detected in about 70.8% in the chronic Charcot's group, 55.6% in the peripheral neuropathy group, and 35.7% in the non-neuropathic group. In patients with chronic Charcot's foot (n = 24), 29.2% had normal, 20.8% had borderline, and 50% had abnormal PNS functions, while 4.2% had normal, 16.7% had borderline, and 79.2% had abnormal SNS functions. The Meary's angle (183.18 ± 73.83 vs. 157.98 ± 14.11; $p < 0.196$) and calcaneal pitch (7.07 ± 3.30 vs. 8.5 ± 1.88; $p < 0.219$) were greater in the subjects with combined autonomic neuropathy, suggesting more structural deformity in them.

Conclusion: Cardiac autonomic neuropathy-related dysfunction was found to be more common in type 2 diabetic patients with chronic Charcot's foot. This study has highlighted that patients with diabetic mellitus and chronic Charcot's foot should be screened comprehensively in order to prevent complications related to cardiac autonomic dysfunction.

COMMENT

What was Known Prior to this Study?

Charcot's neuroarthropathy (Charcot's foot) is a lower extremity complication of diabetes arising from a complex interplay of sensorimotor and autonomic neuropathy, metabolic abnormalities of the bone, trauma, and infection. The condition begins with inflammation of bones, joints, and soft tissues of the ankle and foot; followed by varying degree of deformities arising out of destruction, subluxation, and dislocation of the bones, joints, and soft tissues of the foot and ankle.

Neuropathy plays a significant role in the pathogenesis of the condition. Both sensory and motor neuropathy predispose to trauma, by loss of sensation and foot deformity, respectively. Autonomic neuropathy can cause localized increase in blood flow through arteriovenous shunting, contributing to the pathogenesis of Charcot's neuroarthropathy.[37,38]

Cardiac autonomic neuropathy (CAN) is an often ignored serious complication of diabetes, symptomatic CAN at 5 years of diabetes was a predictor of mortality at 10 years, even after adjusting for conventional cardiovascular disease (CVD) risk factors.[39] CAN has been linked to longer duration of diabetes in some studies but not all.[40-43] Some earlier studies have found association of CAN with Charcot foot, while some studies did not find any such association.[44,45] These discrepancies are mostly due to the differences in methodology used and the lack of standardization in the diagnosis of CAN. Data on the prevalence of CAN in patients with Charcot's neuroarthropathy in Indian population is scarce.

What Does this Study Add?

This was a single-center study which took 74 male patients with type 2 diabetes mellitus (T2DM) and divided them into three groups. Group 1: Chronic Charcot's foot (n = 24), group 2: Peripheral neuropathy without chronic Charcot's foot (n = 22), and group 3: Without peripheral neuropathy or chronic Charcot's foot (n = 28). The tests for sympathetic nervous system (SNS) and parasympathetic nervous system (PNS) were done using a personal computer-based CANS-504 analyzer. The results were categorized as normal, borderline, and abnormal based on Ewing's criteria.[46,47] Meary's angle and calcaneal pitch were calculated to assess extent of structural deformity.

The important highlights of the study were, there is a high prevalence (71%) of CAN in Charcot's foot, Charcot's foot was diagnosed in a mean shorter duration of diabetes in the study population compared to earlier studies.[39-41] Charcot's foot occurred at a higher mean body mass index (BMI) which was comparable to earlier studies.[48] The Meary's angle and calcaneal pitch were greater in the subjects with combined autonomic neuropathy, suggesting more structural deformity in them. Other chronic diabetic complications like diabetic retinopathy and urinary microalbuminuria were significantly higher in those with Charcot's foot.

Major Strengths of the Study

The study assessed CAN in patients with Charcot's neuroarthropathy and found the prevalence to be high. CAN is an often neglected but an extremely important condition in diabetes. Standardized criteria for diagnosing CAN were used.

Limitations of the Study

Major limitations were single-center study in a small population. There were no controls without diabetes.

Implications of the Findings for the Clinicians

Since Charcot's neuroarthropathy presents in Indian population with a shorter duration of disease, one should be alert to the possibility of its existence at an earlier stage of diabetes. Appropriate footwear, avoidance of barefoot walking, and neuropathy testing are essential to prevent the condition. Besides specifically addressing and managing the foot in a patient presenting with a Charcot's neuroarthropathy; the search for CAN should be made. This is because there is a high prevalence of CAN in Charcot's foot and CAN is an important cause of morbidity and mortality.

Knowledge Gaps Identified and Scope for Future Research

A comprehensive understanding of the risk, associations, and pathogenesis of Charcot's foot is needed. Larger prospective data on evolution of Charcot's foot, CAN, and studying their association is needed.

6. Longitudinal Associations between Depression and Diabetes Complications: A Systematic Review and Meta-analysis

Ref: Nouwen A, Adriaanse MC, van Dam K, Iversen MM, Viechtbauer W, Peyrot M, et al. Longitudinal associations between depression and diabetes complications: a systematic review and meta-analysis. Diabet Med. 2019;36(12):1562-72.

ABSTRACT

We conducted a systematic review and meta-analysis of longitudinal studies assessing the bidirectional association between depression and diabetes macrovascular and microvascular complications. A total of 4,592 abstracts were screened for eligibility after searching Embase, Medline, and PsycINFO databases from inception through 27 November, 2017. Multilevel random/mixed-effects models were used for meta-analysis. Newcastle-Ottawa scale was used for quality assessment. 16 of the 22 studies discussed the association between depression and complications related to diabetes. An increased risk of incident macrovascular (HR 1.38; 95% CI 1.30–1.47) and microvascular disease (HR 1.33; 95% CI 1.25–1.41) was observed with depression in diabetes. The association between baseline diabetes complications and subsequent depression was examined by six studies, the results of which showed that diabetes complications increased the risk of incident depressive disorder (HR 1.14; 95% CI 1.07–1.21). Thus, the relationship between depression and diabetes complications seems to be bidirectional. However, depressed diabetics are at higher risk of developing complications related to diabetes than the risk of developing depression in people with diabetic complications. Further research is warranted to understand the underlying mechanisms.

COMMENT

What was Known Prior to this Study?

Bidirectional relationship between diabetes mellitus and depression have been reported in earlier studies and meta-analyses.[49-51] The relative risk (RR) of incident diabetes in patients with depression was found to be 1.6 in a meta-analysis of 13 studies.[52] The data on the development of depression in patients with diabetes is mixed with some studies showing increased incidence and some others showing similar incidence of depression compared to background population.[53-56] A study from Taiwan showed a bidirectional relationship between diabetes and depression, with a stronger association for depression predicting onset of diabetes.[57] A bidirectional longitudinal relationship between diabetes and depression with a modest increased RR (15%) of developing depression in diabetes and a higher RR (60%) for the development of diabetes in depression has been reported.[52]

A complex interplay of biological, psychological and socioeconomic factors can lead to diabetes development in patient with depression. This may include behavioral changes, lack of self-care, lack of access to healthcare, and antidepressants, etc. Often patients suffering from diabetes, suffer diabetes distress. Diabetes distress is a psychological state that is associated with and specific for diabetes and yet do not qualify for the diagnosis of a major psychiatric disorder. The mixed evidence of diabetes leading to depression could be due to lack of clear demarcation between diabetes distress and depression in previous studies.

There is fewer evidence on the relationship between diabetes complications and depression. Earlier, meta-analysis of cross-sectional studies found a significant and consistently positive relationship between diabetes complications and depression.[58] However, the cross-sectional nature of the analyzed study precluded identification of direction of progression.

What Does this Study Add?

About 4,592 longitudinal studies were screened for the meta-analysis to assess the bidirectional association between depression and diabetes, macrovascular and microvascular complications. 22 studies were included in the systematic review. 16 studies examined the relationship between baseline depression and incident diabetes complications, of which nine studies involving over one million participants were suitable for meta-analysis. Six studies examined the association between baseline diabetes complications and subsequent depression, of which two studies involving over 230,000 participants were suitable for meta-analysis. The study used three levels of evidence: Low risk of bias (a score of 7-9), moderate risk of bias (5-6), and a high risk of bias (score < 5).[59]

The relationship between depression and diabetes complications was found to be bidirectional in the present meta-analysis. The presence of depression resulted in a 38% and 33% increase in the risk of development of macrovascular and microvascular complications, respectively. The presence of diabetes complications increased the risk of development of depression by 14%. Thus, the risk of developing diabetes complications in patients with diabetes was higher than the risk of developing depression in patients with diabetes complications.

The important addition in this study is that similar to the bidirectional association of diabetes and depression found in cohort studies and meta-analysis of longitudinal studies; there is also a bidirectional relationship between depression and diabetes in this large meta-analysis of longitudinal studies. This adds to the information regarding the bidirectional association between diabetes complications and depression which was seen in earlier meta-analysis of cross-sectional studies. However, the longitudinal nature of the studies in the meta-analysis adds to information about direction of progression. Also, as in the bidirectional relationship between diabetes and depression; where depression was found to be a stronger predictor of diabetes, compared to diabetes as a predictor of depression; in this meta-analysis too, depression was found to be a stronger determinant of diabetes complications compared to diabetes complications as a determinant of depression.

Major Strengths of the Study

The major strengths are the longitudinal nature of the studies analyzed and the large number of study population.

Limitations of the Study

The studies were heterogenous with some studies having more weight on the meta-analysis than some other. The analyzed studies were not fully free of bias. Of the 22 studies, two showed a high risk of bias, eight showed a moderate risk of bias, and 12 showed a low risk of bias.

Implications of the Findings for the Clinicians

Depression is an important risk factor for the development of diabetes complications. Clinicians should actively look for and treat depression in patients with diabetes to prevent or delay development of diabetes complications. Diabetes complications can also lead to depression. This also needs to be addressed.

Knowledge Gaps Identified and Scope for Future Research

Pathophysiologic mechanism behind the bidirectional link between diabetes complications and depression needs to be studied. Moreover, the reason why depression is a greater determinant of diabetes complications than vice versa needs to be understood.

7. Bone Histomorphometry in Young Patients with Type 2 Diabetes is Affected by Disease Control and Chronic Complications

Ref: Andrade VFC, Chula DC, Sabbag FP, Cavalheiro DDDS, Bavia L, Ambrósio AR, et al. Bone Histomorphometry in Young Patients with Type 2 Diabetes is Affected by Disease Control and Chronic Complications. J Clin Endocrinol Metab. 2020;105(2):dgz070.

ABSTRACT

Introduction: An increased risk of fractures is reported to be associated with type 2 diabetes mellitus (T2DM). Till now, there is no study conducted on premenopausal women with T2DM that assessed the correlation of parameters of bone histomorphometry (BH) with glycemic control and presence of chronic complications (CCs). This study aimed at assessing the BH and correlating them with the degree of glycemic control and presence of CCs.

Methods: This cross-sectional study was carried out at a tertiary medical-center. Total 26 premenopausal women who had T2DM were included, who were divided into two groups. 10 participants with glycated hemoglobin (HbA1c) is <7% were included in good control (GC) group, and 16 participants with HbA1c is >7% in poor control (PC) group, and were further subdivided into groups with CCs ($n = 9$) and without CCs ($n = 17$).

Measurement of BH parameters {i.e., bone volume [bone volume per total volume (BV/TV)]}, trabecular thickness (Tb.Th), trabecular number (Tb.N), trabecular separation (Tb.Sp), osteoid thickness (O.Th), {osteoid surface [osteoid surface per bone surface (OS/BS)]}, mineralizing surface (MS/BS), bone formation rate (BFR), and mineral apposition rate (MAR) was done. Serum pentosidine (PEN) and insulin-like growth factor 1 (IGF-1) were also measured. Comparison of the BH data was done between the groups and with a BH control group (CG) (CG including 15 participants) matched by age, sex, and race.

Results: An increase in the BV/TV was noted in GC ($p < 0.001$) group and PC ($p = 0.05$) group. As compared to the CG group, O.Th was lesser in the PC group ($p = 0.03$). On comparing the groups with and without CCs with the CG, it was demonstrated that in the group with CCs, O.Th was lesser ($p = 0.01$), and BV/TV comparable to the CG ($p = 0.11$). There was a negative correlation between HbA1c and O.Th ($p = 0.02$) and OS/BS ($p = 0.01$). No correlation of BH with PEN and IGF-1 was observed.

Conclusion: Among premenopausal patients who had T2DM, BH was affected by disease control as well as CCs.

COMMENT

What was Known Prior to this Study?

The risk of fracture in type 2 diabetes mellitus (T2DM) is high. This is despite the fact that patients with T2DM have bone mineral density (BMD) that is similar to or higher than the nondiabetes controls. Numerous factors have been associated with the development of fractures in diabetes mellitus (DM). These include poor bone remodeling and poor bone quality; propensity to fall due to neuropathy, retinopathy, and postural hypotension; medications (like glitazones) that impair bone formation and other unknown factors. Poor bone remodeling in diabetes has also been linked to increased sclerostin, an inhibitor of the bone anabolic Wnt/β-catenin pathway.[60] Poorly controlled hyperglycemia can impair bone quality by increasing levels of advanced glycation end-products [e.g., pentosidine (PEN)] thereby increasing the risk of fracture.[61,62]

Bone histomorphometry (BH) analyzes the cortical and trabecular microarchitecture of bone biopsy specimens. This technique is considered the gold standard for the study of bone remodeling and is used in studies on bone metabolism. BH analysis has been sparingly done in T2DM. BH have shown increased bone volume (BV), but reduced bone formation in T2DM.[63-65]

What Does this Study Add?

The study assessed BH in 26 premenopausal women with diabetes. It assessed the association of BH findings with status of glycemic control and with the presence and the absence of complications. The histomorphometric controls were the histomorphometric parameters of 15 bone biopsies obtained postmortem from premenopausal, healthy women.

Bone volume per total volume (BV/TV), a measure of structural volume in increased in patients with diabetes compared to controls. However, the osteoid thickness (O.Th) was lower in the poor glycemic control group compared to the good glycemic control group. The O.Th was smaller in the chronic complication (CC) group compared to the controls but the BV/TV were similar in the two groups. There was a negative correlation between HbA1c and O.Th and osteoid surface per bone surface (OS/BS), a measure of OS. There was no correlation of BH to PEN, a marker of bone advanced glycation end-products and IGF-1. Thus, BH was adversely affected by the presence of diabetes and its complications.

The study re-emphasizes the fact that BH markers are impaired in T2DM even if BV may be increased. The study further adds that the impaired BH markers are a function of poor glycemic control and of presence of CCs of diabetes, namely retinopathy and nephropathy.

Major Strengths of the Study

The major strength is that the study is among the earliest to analyze the BH, a gold standard to study bone remodeling and metabolism, in T2DM. The study by dividing the study population based on glycemic control status and complications, help assess the association of these with BH markers.

Limitations of the Study

Limitations are a small, single-center study. The use of deceased donors as controls, where the anthropometric data and cause of death (at a young age) is not clear, is also a limitation. A cause effect relationship between poor glycemic control and diabetes complications cannot be established form this study, even if an association was established.

Implications of the Findings for the Clinicians

Clinicians need to recognize that there is poor bone quality in patients with diabetes that can increase the risk of fracture. From the study, it appears that poor glycemic control and presence of complications are associated with poorer BH markers. Thus, a good glycemic control and prevention of complications may be associated with improved bone health.

Knowledge Gaps Identified and Scope for Future Research

Greater research is needed to identify the measures and mechanisms of increased bone fragility in diabetes. Larger and longitudinal studies, though extremely challenging, can help establish not only an association but also a cause-effect relationship between poor glycemic control, diabetes complications, and impaired bone health in diabetes.

8. Teriparatide [Recombinant Human Parathyroid Hormone (1-34)] Increases Foot Bone Remodeling in Diabetic Chronic Charcot Neuroarthropathy: A Randomized Double-blind Placebo-controled Study

Ref: Rastogi A, Hajela A, Prakash M, Khandelwal N, Kumar R, Bhattacharya A, et al. Teriparatide [recombinant human parathyroid hormone (1–34)] increases foot bone remodeling in diabetic chronic Charcot neuroarthropathy: a randomized double-blind placebo-controlled study. J Diabetes. 2019;11(9):703-10.

ABSTRACT

Background: There is presently no consensus on the medical treatment of chronic Charcot neuroarthropathy (CN) of foot, with the exception of effective off-loading. Tarsal bones are primarily trabecular; therefore, in chronic CN, teriparatide may result in improvement of the macroarchitecture of foot bones.

Methods: The study included patients with diabetes and chronic CN, who were randomly assigned to receive either 20 μg teriparatide or placebo subcutaneous daily for 12 months. Screening of 38 patients was done, and data of 20 patients were evaluated. Assessment of the maximum standardized uptake (SUV$_{max}$) value of fluorodeoxyglucose-positron emission tomography/computerized tomography) ($_{18}$F-FDG PET/CT) the region of interest, bone turnover markers, and foot bone mineral density (BMD) was done. The primary outcome considered in the study was change in SUV$_{max}$ g/mL.

Results: The most common region involved was midfoot. After 12 months, there was an increase in the SUV$_{max}$ from 30.6 ± 14.7 to 37.7 ± 18.0 ($p = 0.044$) in the teriparatide group, and a decrease with placebo (from 27.6 ± 12.2 to 22.9 ± 10.4, $p = 0.148$).

The estimated treatment difference (ETD) was 11.9 ± 4.3 (95% CI 2.9, 20.8; $p = 0.012$). In the similar manner, there was an increase in procollagen type I N-terminal propeptide (P1NP) with teriparatide (19.8 ± 5.5; $p = 0.006$), but reduction with placebo (−5.1 ± 3.8 ng/mL; $p = 0.219$). ETD was 24.8 ± 6.6 (95% CI 10.8, 38.8; $p < 0.001$). An increase in CTX was noted in teriparatide and placebo groups. With teriparatide, there was an increase in foot BMD by 0.06 ± 0.04 g/cm^2 ($p = 0.192$), but reduced by −0.06 ± 0.08 g/cm^2 with placebo ($p = 0.488$; intergroup comparison, $p = 0.096$).

Conclusion: In patients with CN, teriparatide by an osteoanabolic action results in an increase in foot bone remodeling.

COMMENT

What was Known Prior to this Study?

Charcot's neuroarthropathy (CN) of the foot is a chronic, progressive, and destructive arthropathy of the lower limbs that is potentially limb threatening. Unabated inflammation in the background of peripheral neuropathy resulting in lack of proprioception, sensory-motor neuropathy, and autonomic neuropathy are responsible for its development. An exaggerated local inflammatory response in response to trauma is the initiating event in most. The loss of pain sensation in Charcot's foot results in continued ambulation causing further trauma that heightens the inflammatory response. The proinflammatory milieu promotes the expression receptor activator of nuclear factor-kB ligand (RANKL) which promotes osteoclastogenesis.[66] This increased osteoclastic activity along with the persistent inflammatory response increases bone resorption without increasing formation resulting in disruption of trabecular microarchitecture.[67]

Treatment of CN consists of off-loading in acute phase, followed by gradual weight-bearing and prescription footwear, once the inflammatory changes resolve. Guidelines for management are based on case-series and expert opinion due to lack of randomized studies. Treatment that have been tried for CN include bisphosphonates, calcitonin, teriparatide, and bone growth stimulators with mixed results.[68-73] Therefore, there is no consensus on the choice of medications to improve outcomes in CN.

What Does this Study Add?

The study aimed to investigate the therapeutic efficacy of teriparatide in inactive CN, as the authors postulated that teriparatide being an osteoanabolic agent, may increase the remodeling of foot bones, subsequently improve bone mineral density (BMD), and prevent the progression of deformities. It was a placebo-control double-blind single-center study where 20 patients with inactive CN received 20 μg teriparatide subcutaneously and another 20 with inactive CN received placebo.

The study found that after 12 months the use of teriparatide was associated with a statistically significant increase in the radiotracer [^{18}F-sodium fluoride (^{18}F-NaF)] uptake (a measure of metabolic effect of teriparatide) by the foot bones, whereas there was a decrease uptake in those who were on placebo. Compared to baseline, there was also a statistically significant increase in markers of bone formation (P1NP) in patients who received teriparatide; however, compared to baseline the bone formation markers decreased in patients who received placebo though this was not statistically significant. However, bone resorption markers increased in both teriparatide and placebo. Foot BMD increased in the teriparatide group and decreased in the placebo, though the findings were not statistically significant.

The study demonstrated that the metabolic effect of teriparatide was evident on foot-bones in patients with inactive CN. The increase in the bone formation markers and trend toward improvement in foot BMD in the teriparatide group pointed to an anabolic effect of teriparatide on bones of the foot in CN.

Major Strengths of the Study

In a placebo-controlled study, the study by establishing the anabolic effect of teriparatide in inactive CN widens the scope for possible pharmacotherapeutic options in patients with CN, though larger scale and detailed mechanistic studies are still required.

Limitations of the Study

Single-center study with a small study population.

Implications of the Findings for the Clinicians

Pharmacotherapeutic options for CN are limited but are evolving, based on improved understanding of the pathophysiology of the condition.

Knowledge Gaps Identified and Scope for Future Research

The improved understanding on the pathogenesis of CN needs to be streamlined for better development of pharmacotherapeutics. Research is needed in that field.

REFERENCES (Complications)

1. Malka D, Hammel P, Sauvanet A, Rufat P, O'Toole D, Bardet P, et al. Risk factors for diabetes mellitus in chronic pancreatitis. Gastroenterology. 2000;119(5):1324-32.
2. Wang W, Guo Y, Liao Z, Zou DW, Jin ZD, Zou DJ, et al. Occurrence of and risk factors for diabetes mellitus in Chinese patients with chronic pancreatitis. Pancreas. 2011;40(2):206-12.
3. Howes N, Lerch MM, Greenhalf W, Stocken DD, Ellis I, Simon P, et al. Clinical and genetic characteristics of hereditary pancreatitis in Europe. Clin Gastroenterol Hepatol. 2004;2(3):252-61.
4. Gukovsky I, Li N, Todoric J, Gukovskaya A, Karin M. Inflammation, autophagy, and obesity: Common features in the pathogenesis of pancreatitis and pancreatic cancer. Gastroenterology. 2013;144(6):1199-209.
5. Bensellam M, Jonas JC, Laybutt DR. Mechanisms of -cell dedifferentiation in diabetes: Recent findings and future research directions. J Endocrinol. 2018;236(2):R109-R143.
6. Webb MA, Chen JJ, James RFL, Davies MJ, Dennison AR. Elevated levels of alpha-cells emanating from the pancreatic ducts of a patient with a low BMI and chronic pancreatitis. Cell Transplant. 2018;27(6):902-6.
7. Hennig R, Kekis PB, Friess H, Adrian TE, Büchler MW. Pancreatic polypeptide in pancreatitis. Peptides. 2002;23(2):331-8.
8. Constantino MI, Molyneaux L, Limacher-Gisler F, Al-Saeed A, Luo C, Wu T, et al. Long-term complications and mortality in young-onset diabetes: type 2 diabetes is more hazardous and lethal than type 1 diabetes. Diabetes Care. 2013;36(12):3863-9.
9. Amutha A, Anjana RM, Venkatesan U, Ranjani H, Unnikrishnan R, Narayan KMV, et al. Incidence of complications in young-onset diabetes: Comparing type 2 with type 1 (the young diab study). Diabetes Res Clin Pract. 2017;123:1-8.
10. Ehrmann DA, Temple KA, Rue A, Barengolts E, Mokhlesi B, Cauter EV. Effects of treatment of impaired glucose tolerance or recently diagnosed type 2 diabetes with metformin alone or in combination with insulin glargine on -cell function: Comparison of responses in youth and adults. Diabetes. 2019;68(8):1670-80.
11. Baldi JC, Manning PJ, Hofman PL, Walker RJ. Comment on: TODAY Study Group. Effects of metformin, metformin plus rosiglitazone, and metformin plus lifestyle on insulin sensitivity and -cell function in TODAY. Diabetes Care. 2013;36(12):e223.
12. Zoungas S, Woodward M, Li Q, Cooper ME, Hamet P, Harrap S, et al. Impact of age, age at diagnosis and duration of diabetes on the risk of macrovascular and microvascular complications and death in type 2 diabetes. Diabetologia. 2014;57(12):2465-74.
13. Heng LZ, Comyn O, Peto T, Tadros C, Ng E, Sivaprasad S, et al. Diabetic retinopathy: Pathogenesis, clinical grading, management and future developments. Diabet Med. 2013;30(6):640-50.
14. Bermea KC, Rodríguez-García A, Tsin A, Barrera-Saldaña HA. Somatolactogens and diabetic retinopathy. Growth Horm IGF Res. 2018;41:42-7.
15. Stavropoulos PG, Soura E, Antoniou C. Drug-induced pemphigoid: A review of the literature. J Eur Acad Dermatol Venereol. 2014;28(9):1133-40.
16. Ohnuma K, Dang NH, Morimoto C. Revisiting an old acquaintance: CD26 and its molecular mechanisms in T-cell function. Trends Immunol. 2008;29(6):295-301.
17. van Lingen RG, van De Kerkhof PC, Seyger MM, de Jong EM, van Rens DW, Poll MK, et al. CD26/dipeptidyl-peptidase IV in psoriatic skin: Upregulation and topographical changes. Br J Dermatol. 2008;158(6):1264-72.
18. Yazbeck R, Howarth GS, Abbott CA. Dipeptidyl peptidase inhibitors, an emerging drug class for inflammatory disease? Trends Pharmacol Sci. 2009;30(11):600-7.
19. Remm F, Franz WM, Brenner C. Gliptins and their target dipeptidyl peptidase 4: implications for the treatment of vascular disease. Eur Heart J Cardiovasc Pharmacother. 2016;2(3):185-93.
20. Skandalis K, Spirova M, Gaitanis G, Tsartsarakis A, Bassukas ID. Drug-induced bullous pemphigoid in diabetes mellitus patients receiving dipeptidyl peptidase-IV inhibitors plus metformin. J Eur Acad Dermatol Venereol. 2012;26(2):249-53.
21. García M, Aranburu MA, et al. Dipeptidyl peptidase-IV inhibitors induced bullous pemphigoid: A case report and analysis of cases reported in the European pharmacovigilance database. J Clin Pharm Therapeut. 2016;41(3):368-70.
22. Bene J, Moulis G, Bennani I, Auffret M, Coupe P, Babai S. Bullous pemphigoid and dipeptidyl peptidase IV inhibitors: A case-noncase study in the French pharmacovigilance database. Br J Dermatol. 2016; 175(2):296-301.
23. Varpuluoma O, Försti AK, Jokelainen J, Turpeinen M, Timonen M, Huilaja L. Vildagliptin significantly increases the risk of bullous pemphigoid: A Finnish nationwide registry study. J Invest Dermatol. 2018;138(7):1659-61.
24. Lee SG, Lee HJ, Yoon MS, Kim DH. Association of dipeptidyl peptidase 4 inhibitor use with risk of bullous pemphigoid in patients with diabetes. JAMA Dermatol. 2019;155(2):172-77.
25. Kridin K, Bergman R. Association of bullous pemphigoid with dipeptidylpeptidase 4 inhibitors in patients with diabetes: Estimating the risk of the new agents and characterizing the patients. JAMA Dermatol. 2018;154(10):1152-8.
26. Simo R, Hernandez C, Genescà J, Jardí R, Mesa J. High prevalence of hepatitis C virus infection in diabetic patients. Diabetes Care. 1996;19(9):998-1000.
27. Guo X, Jin M, Yang M, Liu K, Li JW. Type 2 diabetes mellitus and the risk of hepatitis C virus infection: A systematic review. Sci Rep. 2013;3:2981.
28. Petit JM, Bour JB, Galland-Jos C, Minello A, Verges B, Guiguet M, et al. Risk factors for diabetes mellitus and

early insulin resistance in chronic hepatitis C. J Hepatol. 2001;35(2):279-83.
29. Ryu JK, Lee SB, Hong SJ, Lee S. Association of chronic hepatitis C virus infection and diabetes mellitus in Korean patients. Korean J Intern Med. 2001;16(1):18-23.
30. Mason AL, Lau JY, Hoang N, Qian K, Alexander GJ, Xu L, et al Association of diabetes mellitus and chronic hepatitis C virus infection. Hepatology. 1999;29(2):328-33.
31. Mehta SH, Brancati FL, Sulkowski MS, Strathdee SA, Szklo M, Thomas DL. Prevalence of type 2 diabetes mellitus among persons with hepatitis C virus infection in the United States. Ann Intern Med. 2000;133(8):592-9.
32. Hong YS, Chang Y, Ryu S, Cainzos-Achirica M, Kwon MJ, Zhang Y, et al. Hepatitis B and C virus infection and diabetes mellitus: A cohort study. Sci Rep. | 2017;7(1):4606.
33. Sheikh MY, Choi J, Qadri I, Friedman JE, Sanyal AJ. Hepatitis C virus infection: Molecular pathways to metabolic syndrome. Hepatology. 2008;47(6):2127-33.
34. Vanni E, Abate ML, Gentilcore E, Hickman I, Gambino R, Cassader M, et al. Sites and mechanisms of insulin resistance in nonobese, nondiabetic patients with chronic hepatitis C. Hepatology. 2009;50(3):697-706.
35. Schillie SF, Xing J, Murphy TV, Hu DJ. Prevalence of hepatitis B virus infection among people with diagnosed diabetes mellitus in the United States, 1999-2010. J Viral Hepat. 2012;19(9):674-6.
36. Gotz HM, Schutten M, Borsboom GJ, Hendriks B, van Doornum G, de Zwart O. A cluster of hepatitis B infections associated with incorrect use of a capillary blood sampling device in a nursing home in the Netherlands, 2007. Euro Surveill. 2008;13(27):18918.
37. Rajbhandari SM, Jenkins RC, Davies C, Tesfaye S. Charcot neuroarthropathy in diabetes mellitus. Diabetologia. 2002;45(8):1085-96.
38. Uccioli L, Mancini L, Giordano A, Solini A, Magnani P, Manto A. Lower limb arteio-venous shunts, autonomic neuropathy and diabetic foot. Diabetes Res Clin Pract. 1992;16(2):123-30.
39. Lee KH, Jang HJ, Kim YH, Lee EJ, Choe YS, Choi Y. Prognostic value of cardiac autonomic neuropathy independent and incremental to perfusion defects in patients with diabetes and suspected coronary artery disease. Am J Cardiol. 2003;92(12):1458-61.
40. Fabrin J, Larsen K, Holstein PE. Long-term follow up in diabetic Charcot feet with spontaneous onset. Diabetes Care. 2000;23(6):796-800.
41. Pakarinen TK, Laine HJ, Honkonen SE, Peltonen J, Oksala H, Lahtela J. Charcot arthropathy of the diabetic foot. Current concepts and review of 36 cases. Scand J Surg. 2002;91(2):195-201.
42. Petrova NL, Foster AV, Edmonds ME. Difference in presentation of Charcot osteoarthropathy in type 1 compared with type 2 diabetes. Diabetes Care. 2004;27(5):1235-6.
43. Pop-Busui R. Cardiac autonomic neuropathy in diabetes: A clinical perspective. Diabetes Care. 2010;33(2):434-41.
44. Jirkovska A, Boucek P, Wu S, Hosová J, Bém R, Fejfarova V, et al. Power spectral analysis of heart rate variability in patients with Charcot's neuroarthropathy. J Am Podiatr Med Assoc. 2006;96(1):1-8.
45. Stevens MJ, Edmonds ME, Foster AV, Watkins PJ. Selective neuropathy and preserved vascular responses in the diabetic Charcot foot. Diabetologia. 1992;35(2):148-54.
46. Ewing DJ, Martyn CN, Young RJ, Clarke BF. The value of cardiovascular autonomic function tests: 10 years experience in diabetes. Diabetes Care. 1985;8(5):491-8.
47. Ewing DJ, Clarke BF. Diagnosis and management of diabetic autonomic neuropathy. Br Med J (Clin Res Ed). 1982;285(6346):916-8.
48. Stuck RM, Sohn MW, Budiman-Mak E, Lee TA, Weiss KB. Charcot arthropathy risk elevation in the obese diabetic population. Am J Med. 2008;121(11):1008-14.
49. Golden SH, Williams JE, Ford DE, Yeh HC, Paton Sanford C, Nieto FJ, et al. Atherosclerosis Risk in Communities study. Depressive symptoms and the risk of type 2 diabetes: The Atherosclerosis Risk in Communities study. Diabetes Care. 2004;27(2):429-435.
50. Carnethon MR, Kinder LS, Fair JM, Stafford RS, Fortmann SP. Symptoms of depression as a risk factor for incident diabetes: Findings from the National Health and Nutrition Examination Epidemiologic Follow-up Study, 1971-1992. Am J Epidemiol. 2003;158(5):416-23.
51. Palinkas LA, Lee PP, Barrett-Connor E. A prospective study of type 2 diabetes and depressive symptoms in the elderly: The Rancho Bernardo Study. Diabet Med. 2004;21(11):1185-91.
52. Mezuk B, Eaton WW, et al. Depression and type 2 diabetes over the lifespan: A meta-analysis. Diabetes Care. 2008;31(12):2383-2390.
53. Egede LE, Nietert PJ, Zheng D. Depression and all-cause and coronary heart disease mortality among adults with and without diabetes. Diabetes Care. 2005;28(6):1339-45.
54. Brown LC, Majumdar SR, Newman SC, Johnson JA. Type 2 diabetes does not increase risk of depression. CMAJ. 2006;175(1):42-46.
55. Polsky D, Doshi JA, Marcus S, Oslin D, Rothbard A, Thomas N, et al. Long-term risk for depressive symptoms after a medical diagnosis. Arch Intern Med. 2005;165(11):1260-6.
56. Maraldi C, Volpato S, Penninx BW, Yaffe K, Simonsick EM, Strotmeyer ES, et al. Diabetes mellitus, glycemic control, and incident depressive symptoms among 70-to 79-year-old persons: The health, aging, and body composition study. Arch Intern Med. 2007;167(11):1137-44.
57. Chen PC, Chan YT, Chen HF, Ko MC, Li CY. Population-based cohort analyses of the bidirectional relationship between type 2 diabetes and depression. Diabetes Care. 2013;36(2):376-82.
58. de Groot M, Anderson R, Freedland KE, Clouse RE, Lustman PJ. Association of depression and diabetes complications: A meta-analysis. Psychosom Med. 2001;63(4):619-30.
59. McPheeters ML, Kripalani S, Peterson NB, Idowu RT, Jerome RN, Potter SA et al. Closing the quality gap: Revisiting the state of the science (vol. 3: Quality improvement interventions to address health disparities). Evid Rep Technol Assess (Full Rep). 2012;208(3):1-475.

60. García-Martín A, Rozas-Moreno P, Reyes-García R, Morales-Santana S, García-Fontana B, García-Salcedo JA, et al. Circulating levels of sclerostin are increased in patients with type 2 diabetes mellitus. J Clin Endocrinol Metab. 2012;97(1):234-41.
61. Hein GE. Glycation endproducts in osteoporosis—is there a pathophysiologic importance? Clin Chim Acta. 2006;371(1-2):32-6.
62. Saito M, Fujii K, Mori Y, Marumo K. Role of collagen enzymatic and glycation induced cross-links as a determinant of bone quality in spontaneously diabetic WBN/Kob rats. Osteoporos Int. 2006;17(10):1514-23.
63. Krakauer JC, McKenna MJ, Buderer NF, Rao DS, Whitehouse FW, Parfitt AM. Diabetes 1995;44(7):775-82.
64. Armas LA, Akhter MP, Drincic A, Recker RR. Trabecular bone histomorphometry in humans with Type 1 Diabetes Mellitus. Bone. 2012;50(1):91-6.
65. Manavalan JS, Cremers S, Dempster DW, Zhou H, Dworakowski E, Kode A, et al. Circulating osteogenic precursor cells in type 2 diabetes mellitus. J Clin Endocrinol Metab. 2012;97(9):3240-50.
66. Jeffcoate WJ, Game F, Cavanagh PR. The role of proinflammatory cytokines in the cause of neuropathic osteoarthropathy (acute Charcot foot) in diabetes. Lancet. 2005;366(9502):2058-61.
67. La Fontaine J, Shibuya N, Sampson HW, Valderrama P. Trabecular quality and cellular characteristics of normal, diabetic, and Charcot bone. J Foot Ankle Surg. 2011;50(6):648-53.
68. Selby PL, Young MJ, Boulton AJ. Bisphosphonates: A new treatment for diabetic Charcot neuroarthropathy? Diabet Med. 1994;11(1):28-31.
69. Pitocco D, Ruotolo V, Caputo S, Mancini L, Collina CM, Manto A, et al. Six-month treatment with alendronate in acute Charcot neuroarthropathy: A randomized controlled trial. Diabetes Care. 2005;28(5):1214-5.
70. Jude EB, Selby PL, Burgess J, Lilleystone P, Mawer EB, Page SR, et al. Bisphosphonates in the treatment of Charcot neuroarthropathy: A double-blind randomised controlled trial. Diabetologia. 2001;44(11):2032-7.
71. Bem R, Jirkovská A, Fejfarová V, Skibová J, Jude EB. Intranasal calcitonin in the treatment of acute Charcot neuro osteoarthropathy: A randomized controlled trial. Diabetes Care. 2006;29(6):1392-4.
72. Wukich DK, Sung W. Charcot arthropathy of the foot and ankle: Modern concepts and management review. J Diabetes Complications. 2009;23(6):409-26.
73. Hockenbury RT, Gruttadauria M, McKinney I. Use of implantable bone growth stimulation in Charcot ankle arthrodesis. Foot Ankle Int. 2007;28(9):971-6.

Section 5: Type 1 Diabetes Mellitus

Ajitesh Roy, Archana Sarda, Banshi Saboo, Ch Vasanth Kumar

1. Immune Checkpoint Inhibitor-induced Type 1 Diabetes: A Systematic Review and Meta-analysis

Ref: Akturk HK, Kahramangil D, Sarwal A, Hoffecker L, Murad MH, Michels AW. Immune checkpoint inhibitor-induced Type 1 diabetes: a systematic review and meta-analysis. Diabet Med. 2019;36:1075-81.

ABSTRACT

Aim: To conduct systematic review of existing evidence on antiprogrammed cell death protein-1 (PD-1)/antiprogrammed cell death protein-1 ligand (PD-L1) inhibitor-induced type 1 diabetes mellitus (T1DM).

Methods: A total of 71 cases found from 56 publications after searching MEDLINE, EMBASE, SCOPUS, and Cochrane databases (August, 2000–2018) for publications on immune checkpoint inhibitors (CPIs). Fisher's exact and Student's t-tests were used for comparison.

Results: The mean ±SD age at T1DM presentation was 61.7 ± 12.2 years, while the median time to T1DM onset was 49 (5–448) days with ketoacidosis in 76% of cases. 55% of cases were in men, and melanoma (53.5%) was the most frequent cancer. The average ±SD glycated hemoglobin (HbA1c) concentration was 62 ± 0.3 mmol/mol (7.84 ± 1.0%) at presentation. Insulin deficiency was seen in all cases that required permanent exogenous insulin treatment. Type 1 diabetes-associated antibodies was seen at presentation in half of the cases, and they had a more rapid onset ($p = 0.005$) and higher incidence of diabetic ketoacidosis ($p = 0.02$) compared to people without antibodies.

Conclusion: Type 1 diabetes mellitus was observed within 3 months of initial PD-1/PD-L1 inhibitor exposure in many people. Presence of type 1 diabetes-associated antibodies was associated with a more rapid onset and higher incidence of ketoacidosis. Awareness of this potential severe adverse event associated with PD-1/PD-L1 inhibitor exposure is needed.

COMMENT

What was Known Prior to the Study?

The spectrum of cancer therapeutics has been changed with the invention of immune checkpoint inhibitors (CPIs) including agents targeted against cytotoxic T-lymphocyte-associated protein-4 (CTLA-4), programmed cell death-1 (PD-1) and PD-ligand 1 (PD-L1). These immune checks help in maintaining peripheral tolerance at homeostasis. Invasion of these checks by malignant cells enables growth of cancer. Although initially approved of CPIs use was received in treatment of metastatic melanoma, these modalities have been found to be beneficial in a growing number of cancer types and genetic anomalies. Despite their efficacy, frequency of autoimmune complications with the use of CPI has become increasingly apparent. These complications known as immune-related adverse events (irAEs), mainly affects endocrine organs including hypophysitis, thyroiditis and adrenalitis and autoimmune diabetes (CPI-DM). These endocrine events are rarely reversible and do not improve by steroids making them relatively unique to others. Steroids are reported to be failed in reserving β-cell dysfunction and also worsening insulin resistance in CPI-DM similar as in type 1 diabetes mellitus (T1DM). Despite of its rarity, CPI-DM is estimated between 0.2% and 1.4%[1]

of CPI-treated patients. The insight into the factors contributing toward development of conventional T1DM may be gained by studying the incidence of autoimmune diabetes following targeted modulations of immune signaling.

A recent review[2] summarizing 91 case reports institution-specific case-series has been carried out by De Filette and colleagues including an additional independent 53 cases [27 from University of California San Francisco (UCSF) and Yale (five of which were included in De Filette et al.'s case summary),[3] 21 from Mayo Clinic[4] and 10 from Melanoma Institute Australia[5]].

Another study by Marco Zezza et al. showed oncological patients treated with combination therapy of anti-PD1 and anti-CTLA-4 can develop a particular pattern of T1DM, with very rapid onset within a few weeks after starting immune checkpoint inhibitor (ICI) therapy, even in the presence of an existing type 2 diabetes mellitus (T2DM). Compared to patients who received anti-PD-1 or anti-PD-L1 therapy, patients who received anti-CTLA-4 therapy were significantly less likely to experience DM. CPIs-induced T1DM is a medical emergency in presence of severe inaugural diabetic ketoacidosis and requires collaboration between specialists and primary care physicians, as well as patient education, for early diagnosis and supportive care.[6]

What this Study Adds?

- Immune CPI-induced T1DM was reported in majority of the participants within 3 months of treatment initiation demonstrated by this systematic review.
- Rapid onset with higher emergence of diabetic ketoacidosis was reported in people presenting with type 1 diabetes-associated antibodies at presentation.
- No correlation between glycated hemoglobin (HbA1c) and time to new-onset T1DM was reported indicating a short time period of significantly elevated blood glucose prior to diabetes onset.

Major Strengths of the Study

This systematic review included case reports and series exploring duration of onset of T1DM after therapy with immune CPI. This review took into consideration that the duration of first 3 months for emergence of T1DM after therapy initiation reporting development of disease in 71% of the reviewed cases. All of the reviewed cases were reported to be insulin deficient at the time of presentation requiring permanent therapy with exogenous insulin. Presentation within a shorter timeframe with diabetic ketoacidosis was reported in cases with anti-glutamic acid decarboxylase antibody (anti-GAD Ab) presence as compared to those without antibodies. The treatment for melanoma with PD-1 inhibitors was given to the majority of cases developing T1DM. Substantially high blood glucose levels (HbA1c 7.84 ± 1.0%) were reported at presentation and no correlation was found between duration of onset of T1DM after therapy and HbA1c, implying a short timeframe of significant hyperglycemia.

Limitations of the Study

This systematic review and meta-analysis did not indicate whether any variation was present in the development of T1DM in people of different ethnic background. Despite including studies of sufficient number and duration there was no information regarding "honeymoon" phase which is a common phenomenon in T1DM during which time glycemic control is achieved with modest doses of insulin or, rarely, insulin is not needed. Results for other antibodies, such as islet cell antibodies, insulin, islet antigen 2, and zinc transporter 8 were not reported in all the cases.

Implications of the Findings for the Clinicians

The healthcare providers involved in the management of the patients being treated with these therapies should be aware of

T1DM presenting with diabetic ketoacidosis. Additionally, patients should also be counseled and educated regarding about hyperglycemia and diabetic ketoacidosis, their signs and symptoms and the importance of monitoring blood glucose. Initial elevations in blood glucose are required to be identified by routine self-monitoring of blood glucose or the use of continuous glucose monitoring. So effective cooperation between endocrinologists and oncologists can reduce the detrimental effects of antitumor therapies.

Knowledge Gaps Identified

- It is still not clear that whether T1DM antibodies preceded or developed after therapy initiation.
- Why there were no cases reported among the patients treated with ipilimumab as a single agent with new-onset T1DM following therapy?

Scope for Future Research

- All of the traditional antibodies associated with T1DM and those directed against post-translationally modified B-cell proteins are needed to be evaluated thus more research is needed in this area.
- Evaluation of HLA genes and other potential genetic risk factors is also needed to be evaluated in the future studies as HLA typing has been performed only in a limited number of people till date.
- The estimated incidence of immune CPI-induced T1DM is 1%.[3,7-10] It will be difficult to conduct prospective clinical trials to assess PD-1/PD-L1 inhibitor-induced T1DM with this frequency leading to need to have registries and to review cases available in the literature rigorously.
- We have to focus on identification of biomarkers which could help for proper prediction of irAE. Till date B-cell number, baseline neutrophil-to-lymphocyte ratio, and platelet-to-lymphocyte ratio were significantly associated with the development of irAEs.
- Future prospective clinical studies are warranted to screen patients having risk factors of T1DM and being managed with these therapies. This will help to decrease the incidence and risk of life-threatening diabetic ketoacidosis.

2. Serum Urate Lowering with Allopurinol and Kidney Function in Type 1 Diabetes

Ref: Doria A, Galecki AT, Spino C, Pop-Busui R, Cherney DZ, Lingvay I, et al. Serum Urate Lowering with Allopurinol and Kidney Function in Type 1 Diabetes. N Engl J Med. 2020;382:2493-503.

ABSTRACT

Introduction: High levels of serum urate are reported to be associated with an increase in the risk of diabetic kidney disease (DKD). In people who have type 1 diabetes mellitus (T1DM) and early-to-moderate DKD, decreasing the level of serum urate with allopurinol may decelerate the reduction in the glomerular filtration rate (GFR).

Methods: This was a double-blind trial, which included individuals with T1DM, a serum urate level of minimum 4.5 mg/dL, an estimated GFR (eGFR) of 40.0–99.9 mL/min/1.73 m^2 of body-surface area and evidence of DKD. Participants were randomized to receive either allopurinol or placebo. The primary outcome considered in the study was the baseline-adjusted GFR (measured with iohexol), following 3 years in addition to a 2-month washout period. Secondary outcomes were the reduction in the iohexol-based GFR per year as well as the urinary albumin excretion (UAE) rate after washout. Assessment of safety was also done.

Results: Patients were randomized to receive either allopurinol (n = 267) or placebo (n = 263). The mean age of the patients was 51.1 years. The mean duration of diabetes was 34.6 years; the mean glycated hemoglobin level was 8.2%. The mean baseline iohexol-based GFR in the allopurinol group and the placebo group was 68.7 mL/min/1.73 m² and 67.3 mL/min/1.73 m². During the intervention period, there was a decrease in the mean serum urate level from 6.1 to 3.9 mg/dL with allopurinol and stayed at 6.1 mg/dL with placebo. The between-group difference in the mean iohexol-based GFR, after washout, was found to be 0.001 mL/min/1.73 m² [95% confidence interval (CI) −1.9 to 1.9; p = 0.99]. The mean decrease in the iohexol-based GFR with allopurinol and with placebo was −3.0 mL/min/1.73 m² per year and −2.5 mL/min/1.73 m² per year, respectively (between-group difference, −0.6 mL/min/per 1.73 m² per year; 95% CI −1.5 to 0.4). After washout, as compared to placebo, the mean UAE rate was found to be 40% (95% CI 0–80) higher with allopurinol. There was no significant difference in frequency of serious adverse events between the two groups.

Conclusion: In patients with T1DM and early-to-moderate DKD, results of the study showed no evidence of clinically meaningful advantages of reduction of serum urate with allopurinol on kidney outcomes. (Funded by the National Institute of Diabetes and Digestive and Kidney Diseases and others; PERL ClinicalTrials.govnumber, NCT02017171)

COMMENT

What was Known Prior to the Study?

Diabetic nephropathy (DN) is the leading cause of kidney disease in patients starting renal replacement therapy and affects approximately 40% of type 1 diabetic patients. It increases the risk of death, mainly from cardiovascular causes, and is defined by increased urinary albumin excretion (UAE) in the absence of other renal diseases. Current treatment methods, with better control of glycemia, dyslipidemia and blood pressure, use of renin–angiotensin system (RAS) blockade, appear to have slowed the nephropathy progression rate but have not substantially decreased the annual incidence of new end-stage renal disease (ESRD) cases. Thus, new treatment targets are needed.

As an inflammatory factor, uric acid (UA) increases oxidative stress and promotes the activation of the renin–angiotensin–aldosterone system (RAAS).[11,12] Therefore, UA levels are associated with the occurrence and development of DN and are independent risk factors for early kidney disease,[13,14] which also help to predict microalbuminuria progression. In patients with type 1 diabetes mellitus (T1DM) without complications, higher UA levels are associated with lower glomerular filtration rate (GFR), which is due to UA-mediated increased resistance in afferent renal arteriole promoting the renal microcirculation ischemia.[15,16]

In Chinese patients with type 2 diabetes mellitus (T2DM), UA-related alleles may affect susceptibility to diabetic kidney disease (DKD). Xanthine oxidase (XO) is a very important enzyme that is responsible for the conversion of sulfhydryl groups to UA. In diabetes, both XO and uric acid are independently associated with albuminuria.[17]

Historically, few observational studies showed that serum urate could be a potential target involving humans.[18] Two trials involving participants (~25% of whom had diabetes) with moderate chronic kidney disease[19-21] showed reduction in the serum urate level slowed the decline in the GFR, decreases C-reactive protein (CRP) level, and rate of hospitalization.

A post hoc analysis of RENAAL study showed that participants experiencing an UA reduction (a direct effect of losartan) in the first 6 months of the trial had fewer renal events that those in whom UA did not decrease. Also post hoc analysis of EMPA-REG found estimated GFR (eGFR) preservation and reduced renal events which could be due to UA-lowering effect of sodium-glucose cotransporter-2 inhibitors.

What this Study Adds?

With this background, researcher tested in this trial, whether reduction of the serum urate level with allopurinol therapy could slow the decline in GFR in early-to-moderate DKD.[22] It is a double-blind trial, where participants were assigned randomly with T1DM, a serum urate level of at least 4.5 mg/dL, an eGFR of 40.0–99.9 mL/min/1.73 m^2 of body-surface area, and evidence of DKD to receive allopurinol or placebo. The mean decrease in the GFR was –3.0/min/1.73 m^2 per year with allopurinol and –2.5 mL/min/1.73 m^2 per year with placebo. So no evidence of clinically meaningful benefits of serum urate reduction with allopurinol on kidney outcomes among patients with T1DM and early-to-moderate DKD was seen.

The findings of this trial differ from the previously mentioned smaller trials where participants were older, the baseline GFR was lower and the serum urate level higher.[19-21] Although it is possible that a reduction in the serum urate level might have been more effective in slowing the decline in GFR in advanced chronic kidney disease or higher serum urate levels (or both) than the patients in this cohort, but secondary analyses also did not reflect any effect. Another recent trial, CKD-FIX (Controlled Trial of Slowing of Kidney Disease Progression from the Inhibition of Xanthine Oxidase),[23] did not show a beneficial effect of allopurinol therapy on the eGFR decline in persons who had a lower estimated GFR at baseline (mean, 31.7 mL/min/1.73 m^2) and a higher serum urate level at baseline (mean, 8.2 mg/dL).

Major Strengths of the Study

This trial had many strengths including adequate power, high participant adherence, which resulted in sustained reduction (36%) in the serum urate level. Also selection of trial population was perfect as the rate of kidney-function decline was consistent with clinically significant progression of DKD per se.

Iohexol was selected for GFR because studies have indicated that the measured GFR was more sensitive for the detection of GFR change than the GFR estimating equations. Equations could be erroneous due to possible transient renal hemodynamic effects of allopurinol.

Limitations of the Study

However, there are some limitations in this study. A trial of longer duration might be necessary to reveal differences between groups. Treatment without RAS inhibitors could have been a better step to find out actual benefit of allopurinol therapy. Due to lack of proper admixture of population the results may not be fully applicable to other ethnic groups. Similarly, the results should not be generalized to patients with other stages of DKD or in T2DM patients.

Scope for Future Research

A recent understanding is that allopurinol protects glomerular endothelial cells from high glucose-induced ROS generation, p53 overexpression and endothelial dysfunction. These data provide a pathogenetic mechanism that supports the results of experimental and clinical studies about the beneficial effect of XO inhibitors on the development of DN. Also immune cells contribute to the pathogenesis of DN and urate at concentrations above its crystallization threshold boosts cellular and humoral immunity.[24] So large prospective randomized controlled trial (RCT) is much needed to adopt UA reduction as a standard of care for persons with diabetes at increased risk of nephropathy.

3. Profile of Auto-antibodies (Disease Related and Other) in Children with Type 1 Diabetes

Ref: Basu M, Pandit K, Banerjee M, Mondal SA, Mukhopadhyay P, Ghosh S. Profile of Auto-antibodies (Disease Related and Other) in Children with Type 1 Diabetes. Indian J Endocrinol Metab. 2020;24:256-9.

ABSTRACT

Background: Type 1 diabetes mellitus (T1DM) is associated with several disease-related and other organ-specific autoimmune disorders. Data related to various autoantibodies in T1DM in India is limited.

Materials and methods: In this cross-sectional study, 92 subjects with T1DM (33 males, 59 females) were evaluated for T1DM-related antibodies [autoantibodies to anti-glutamic acid decarboxylase (anti-GAD), autoantibodies to protein tyrosine phosphatase islet antigen 2 (anti-IA2), anti-islet cell antibody (ICA), insulin autoantibody (IAA), anti-zinc transporter (ZnT8), and other organ-specific autoantibodies such as anti-thyroid peroxidase (anti-TPO), antithyroglobulin antibody (TgAb), IgA anti-tissue transglutaminase (IgA anti-tTG), anti-21-hydroxylase, and antiovarian antibody (in females)].

Results: Anti-GAD, IA2, ICA, IAAs, and ZnT8 antibody were present in 79.3%, 32.6%, 61.9%, 63%, and 20.65% subjects, respectively. Only 2.2% patients with T1DM were antibody negative. At least one antibody was found in 97.8% and at least two antibodies in 67.3%. The presence of anti-TPO, anti-thyroglobulin, IgA anti-tTG, and anti-21-hydroxylase were found in 51%, 25%, 22.8%, and 2.1%, respectively. Antiovarian antibody was absent in all females of our study population. The duration of diabetes positively correlated with the number of T1DM-specific antibody and also with GAD antibody positivity. Anti-TPO positivity correlated with the age of onset of T1DM, but not with the duration of disease or presence of other T1DM-specific autoantibody.

Conclusion: Type 1 diabetes mellitus is associated with a high prevalence of autoantibodies and antibody-negative T1DM is rare. The association with other organ-specific antibody (especially thyroid and adrenal glands) and celiac disease is also substantial, which reinforces the importance of regular thyroid and celiac disease screening in T1DM subjects. The duration of diabetes positively correlated with number of T1DM-specific antibodies.

COMMENT

Introduction

Type 1 diabetes mellitus (T1DM) is an autoimmune disease with selective destruction of beta cells of pancreas. The most frequently detected antibodies are anti-glutamic acid decarboxylase (GAD) antibody, tyrosine phosphatase associated islet antigen related antibody (IA2), islet cell autoantibody (ICA), zinc transporter (ZnT8) autoantibody.[25,26] The presence of one or more disease-specific autoantibody is required to make immunological diagnosis of T1DM. Apart from these disease-specific autoantibodies, T1DM is also associated with autoimmune thyroid disease (AITD), idiopathic Addison's disease, and celiac disease.[26-28]

What was Known Prior to this Study?

Prevalence of GAD 70–80%, IA2 60–70%, and ZnT8 60–80%, respectively in children with new onset T1DM in western studies.[25] Insulin autoantibody is present in 90% of children who develop T1DM before 5 years while prevalence reduces with increasing age.[25] An Indian study show GAD, IA2, and ZnT8 positivity up to 80%. Another study shows negativity up to 45% when they measured both ZnT8 and IA2. Research showed that the number of antibodies, rather than the individual antibody, is thought to be the most predictive of progression to overt diabetes. Overall risk for development of multiple autoantibodies was independent of antibody type, inversely related to age, and associated with high- and intermediate-risk human leukocyte antigen (HLA) class II genotypes and high GAD titers.

In relatives with IAA, spread of islet autoimmunity mainly occurs in early childhood, whereas immune responses initially directed at GAD can mature over a longer period. These differences are important for monitoring these patients and for designing prevention trials.

Autoimmune markers of other conditions may exist with disease-specific autoantibodies even before clinical onset of disease. Long back, the high incidence of thyroid and gastric autoimmunity in T1DM patients, were described.[29] Autoimmune gastritis is being present in up to 2% of the general population, while in T1DM patients the prevalence is 3- to 5-fold increased. Antibody to thyroid is the most common as noted in earlier studies.[30,31] Anti-thyroid peroxidase (TPO) is much more common compared to antithyroglobulin.

In a German/Austrian multicenter survey, 15% of T1DM patients were found positive for antithyroid antibodies.[32] Celiac disease seems to be less frequent than AITD, but still common among T1DM patients. The prevalence of specific antibodies for celiac disease among T1DM patients in the German/Austrian multicenter survey was 11%.[32]

What this Study Adds?

Autoantibody-negative T1DM is rare in our population. This study shows that if all the antibodies are tested, then the occurrence of antibody-negative T1DM is low. At least one antibody is positive in 96.7% of the cases. Anti-GAD antibody and anti-IA2 antibody is significantly higher than other previous Indian studies.

Duration of diabetes has a positive correlation with number of autoantibodies but there was no correlation with the age of onset of diabetes.

Type 1 diabetes mellitus has high prevalence of other autoantibodies (thyroid, adrenal, and celiac) and thus testing can be done for anti-TPO, antithyroglobulin, anti-tTG antibody IgA, and anti-21-α-hydroxylase antibody. The prevalence of idiopathic Addison's disease and 21-hydroxylase deficiency is at par with other Indian studies. Antiovarian antibody was not found positive in any cases.

Strength and Limitation of this Study

Strength
- All the disease-specific autoantibodies have been used for testing.
- Proper diagnostic methods of T1DM as per American Diabetes Association (ADA) criteria is used.
- The assay methods used are appropriate.

Limitation
- The sample size of the study if larger could have given more appropriate results.
- Since this is a cross-sectional study, age-based changes in autoantibody levels could not be predicted.
- Cost issues can hamper use in routine clinical practice.

Implication of Findings for the Clinicians

- Antibody-negative T1DM is rare and so all the antibodies should ideally be checked for. Anti-GAD and Anti-IA2 antibody are the most common ones.
- We have come to understand a great deal about associated autoimmune diseases that can occur outside the pancreas in patients with T1DM, like idiopathic Addison's disease, AITD, and celiac disease, etc.
- If the associated diseases are in preclinical phase also, early diagnosis and appropriate measures could have profound impact on outcome.

4. Biomarker Panels Associated with Progression of Renal Disease in Type 1 Diabetes

Ref: Colombo M, Valo E, McGurnaghan SJ, Sandholm N, Blackbourn LAK, Dalton RN, et al. Biomarker panels associated with progression of renal disease in type 1 diabetes. Diabetologia. 2019;62:1616-27.

ABSTRACT

Aims/Hypothesis: Identification of a panel of biomarkers associated with progression of renal disease in type 1 diabetes mellitus (T1DM) population.

Methods: Type 2 diabetic patients from the Scottish Diabetes Research Network Type 1 Bioresource (SDRNT1BIO) ($n = 859$) and the Finnish Diabetic Nephropathy (FinnDiane) study ($n = 315$), were included in our study. An entry estimated glomerular filtration rate (eGFR) ranging from 30 to 75 mL/min/1.73 m², was noted in all who were from FinnDiane. A total of 297 circulating biomarkers including 30 proteins, 121 metabolites, and 146 tryptic peptides were measured in serum samples using the Luminex platform and liquid chromatography (LC)-electrospray tandem mass spectrometry (LC-MS/MS). Associations of these biomarkers with final eGFR and with rapid progression of renal disease were analyzed using linear and logistic regression models. Identification of panels of biomarkers was done using a penalized Bayesian approach, and their performance was evaluated through 10-fold cross-validation and comparison was done using clinical record data alone.

Results: There was a significant association between final eGFR, and 16 proteins and 30 metabolites or tryptic peptides in SDRNT1BIO, and nine proteins and five metabolites or tryptic peptides in FinnDiane, beyond age, sex, diabetes duration, study day eGFR and length of follow-up (all at $p < 10^{-4}$). CD27 antigen (CD27), kidney injury molecule 1 (KIM-1), and α1-microglobulin showed the strongest association. The r^2 for prediction of final eGFR increased from 0.47 to 0.58 in SDRNT1BIO and from 0.33 to 0.48 in FinnDiane, on including Luminex biomarkers in addition to baseline covariates. At least 75% of the increment in r^2 was attributable to CD27 and KIM-1. However, using the weighted average of historical eGFR gave similar performance to biomarkers. The LC-MS/MS platform performed less well.

Conclusion/Interpretation: A sparse panel of just CD27 and KIM-1 can be relied upon for the predictive information for eGFR progression. The increment in prediction beyond clinical data can be useful for oversampling individuals with rapid disease progression into clinical trials, especially where there is little information on prior eGFR trajectories.

COMMENT

What was Known Prior to the Study?

Chronic kidney disease (CKD) is emerging as an important public health problem with the estimated prevalence of 8–16% worldwide.[33] In view of global increase in type 2 diabetes mellitus (T2DM), it has emerged as the leading cause of CKD worldwide.[34,35] Diabetic nephropathy is reported to occur in approximately 40% of diabetic patients [type 1 diabetes mellitus (T1DM) or T2DM].[36] There is need to identify patients at risk of diabetic nephropathy and at high risk of progression as there is concomitant increase in cardiovascular morbidity and mortality in addition to significant risk of progression to end-stage renal disease (ESRD) in diabetic patients with diabetic nephropathy.[36] But, there is lack of sensitive and specific biomarker to predict which diabetic patients will progress to diabetic nephropathy or ESRD. Presently, estimated glomerular filtration rate (eGFR) and proteinuria are used commonly as markers for renal disease in clinical practice. Late functional changes are reflected by estimation of GFR. Methodological limitations also compromise estimates of declining GFR.[36,37] Onset and progression of diabetic nephropathy is monitored by albuminuria since long time.[36] Although microalbuminuria has been considered a strong predictor of progression to proteinuria but as there are reports of spontaneous remission of microalbuminuria in majority of diabetic patients, the predictive value of microalbuminuria has been challenged in many recent studies.[36-38] Therefore, there is need of new biomarkers for prediction of renal disease progression. Tubular biomarkers are important predictor of renal dysfunction among other types of biomarkers. Neutrophil gelatinase-associated lipocalin (NGAL), kidney injury molecule 1 (KIM-1), and liver fatty acid-binding protein (L-FABP) are most studied tubular biomarkers. Significant change in biomarker in renal disease was observed by large studies by Bolignano et al.,[39] Yang et al.,[40] Smith et al.,[41] etc.

What this Study Adds?

Tubular biomarkers are now important additional indicator of renal disease progression in T1DM whereas it was previously believed that microalbuminuria was predictor of renal disease progression.

Although a large number of biomarkers were evaluated in this study, highly significant association was reported with eGFR and its decline: (1) Modest marginal increment in prediction was reported using these biomarkers panels; (2) two biomarkers (CD27 and KIM-1) were adequate to provide almost all of the information; and (3) similar prediction performance for using the biomarkers was given by using weighted eGFR and albuminuria.

Strength of the Study

Use of two cohorts with differing characteristics and rates of disease was the major strength of this study. The Finnish Diabetic Nephropathy (FinnDiane) cohort set used was oversampled for albuminuria but the Scottish Diabetes Research Network Type 1 Bioresource (SDRNT1BIO) cohort was not oversampled. Therefore, the rate of progression was higher in FinnDiane for similar starting GFR. Among cases with albuminuria, the associations of biomarkers were stronger with final eGFR. The biomarkers were found to be highly sensitive to storage, an important consideration for their practical use in clinical settings by examination allowed by the storage conditions in the two cohorts (−80°C with no freeze/thaw cycles in SDRNT1BIO and −20°C in FinnDiane). The use of advanced statistical methods including cross-validation and use of penalty parameters accounting for the high number of analyses was another key strength of this study.

Limitation of the Study

Relatively short follow-up and low progression rates in SDRNT1BIO cohort was the main limitation in the study but the similar follow-up time was used in many other trials. This shorter follow-up time resulted in less stable observed slope and rapid progressor status and more misclassification in SDRNT1BIO cohort. So follow-up time needed to be longer.

Implication of the Findings for the Clinicians

Although this study examined a variety of tubular biomarkers extensively but only modest increments in prediction of future eGFR could be demonstrated. The magnitude of resulted increment could be of some use in some trials but not for decision making in routine clinical setting. But it is still possible that other biomarkers or the same biomarkers assayed on other platforms might achieve greater performance.

Knowledge Gap Identified and Scope of Future Research

Further research to be done to find more reliable biomarker that is more consistent with renal disease progression in T1DM.

5. Effect of Continuous Glucose Monitoring on Glycemic Control in Adolescents and Young Adults with Type 1 Diabetes: A Randomized Clinical Trial

Ref: Laffel LM, Kanapka LG, Beck RW, Bergamo K, Clements MA, Criego A, et al. Effect of Continuous Glucose Monitoring on Glycemic Control in Adolescents and Young Adults With Type 1 Diabetes: A Randomized Clinical Trial. JAMA. 2020;323:2388-96.

ABSTRACT

Importance: The worst glycemic control has been reported among type 1 diabetic patients in adolescent and young age group across the lifespan. The benefits of continuous glucose monitoring (CGM) has not been demonstrated in improving the glycemic control among adults although they have shown the improvement in glycemic control.

Objective: To assess the effect of CGM on glycemic control among type 1 diabetic patients in adolescent and young age group.

Design, setting, and participants: This randomized clinical trial conducted enrolled 153 type 1 diabetic patients belonging to age group of 14–24 years with glycated hemoglobin (HbA1c) in the range of 7.5–10.9% from January 2018 to May 2019 at 14 endocrinology practices in the US.

Interventions: Participants were assigned randomly to CGM group ($n = 74$) and BGM (blood glucose monitoring) group using a blood glucose meter ($n = 79$).

Main outcomes and measures: The change in HbA1c was reported to be the primary outcome from baseline to 26 weeks. Twenty secondary outcomes included additional HbA1c outcomes, CGM glucose metrics and patient-reported outcomes with adjustment for multiple comparisons to control for the false discovery rate.

Results: The mean age among the 153 participants was 17 ± 3 years with 76 (50%) female. The mean duration was reported to be 9 ± 5 years. Out of total 153 participants, 142 (93%) completed the trial. 68% of participants in CGM group used CGM at least 5 days per week in month 6. The mean HbA1c was 8.9% in both the groups at baseline. At 26 weeks the mean HbA1c was 8.5% in CGM group whereas it remained 8.9% BGM group [adjusted between-group difference, –0.37% (95% CI –0.66 to –0.08%); $p = .01$]. Out of 20 secondary outcomes, statistically significant differences were reported in 3 of 7 binary HbA1c outcomes, 8 of 9 CGM metrics, and 1 of 4 patient-reported outcomes. The most commonly reported adverse events in both the groups were severe hypoglycemia, hyperglycemia/ketosis, and diabetic ketoacidosis. In CGM group, 3, 1, and 3 participants reported severe hypoglycemia, hyperglycemia/ketosis, and diabetic ketoacidosis, respectively whereas in BGM group, 2, 4, and 1 participants reported severe hypoglycemia, hyperglycemia/ketosis, and diabetic ketoacidosis, respectively.

Conclusion and relevance: A statistically significant although small improvement in glycemic control over 26 weeks was reported with CGM compared with standard BGM among type 1 diabetic adolescents and young adults. Although, further studies are needed to clearly understand the clinical importance of the findings.

COMMENT

What was Known Prior to the Study?

Glycated hemoglobin (HbA1c) is still currently recognized as the key surrogate marker for assessment of glucose control and the development of long-term diabetes complications in people with type 1 diabetes mellitus (T1DM). But HbA1c fails to identify the magnitude and frequency of intra- and interday glucose variation and acute glycemic excursions. Continuous glucose monitoring (CGM) provides a measure of glucose concentrations every 5 minutes, yielding a more complete picture of glycemic excursion.

Improvements in sensor accuracy, greater convenience, and ease of use led to growing adoption of CGM. However, successful utilization of CGM technology in routine clinical practice remains relatively low due to lack of evidences particularly in younger age group.

In 2012, the Helmsley Charitable Trust sponsored the first expert panel to recommend the standardization of CGM metrics and CGM report visualization.[42]

In February 2019, the Advanced Technologies and Treatments for Diabetes (ATTD) Congress convened an international panel of physicians, researchers, and individuals with diabetes who are expert in CGM technologies to address issues related to CGM.

There are few studies done previously to find out the evidences in younger age group.[43-45] The largest and most referenced randomized trial that examined CGM use in this age group was the JDRF (Juvenile Diabetes Research Foundation) CGM randomized clinical trial.[46] In this study all the participants were stratified into three groups according to age. The changes in HbA1c were significantly seen among patients 25 years of age or older that favored CGM (mean difference in change, -0.53%; 95% CI -0.71 to -0.35; $p < 0.001$). However, only 30% used CGM regularly (6-7 day/week), which is substantially less than observed in the current trial.

What this Study Adds?

This randomized controlled trial (RCT) was done to determine the effect of CGM on glycemic control in adolescents and young adults aged 14-24 years with T1DM and HbA1c of 7.5-10.9%. The primary outcome was change in HbA1c from baseline to 26 weeks. Mean HbA1c was 8.9% at baseline and 8.5% at 26 weeks in the blood glucose monitoring (CGM) group and 8.9% at both baseline and 26 weeks in the blood glucose monitoring (BGM) group. The percentages of time in target glucose range during daytime and nighttime hours are significant. Mean time in hypoglycemia was significantly lower in the CGM group than the BGM group. Regarding patient-reported outcomes CGM group reported significantly higher glucose monitoring satisfaction, measured via the glucose monitoring satisfaction survey score.

Strength of this Study

The strengths of this study include enrollment of a diverse population including minorities. Also CGM use was significantly high though with time decreasing trend noticed to some extent.

Limitation of this Study

There are several limitations of the study.

First, in view of the eligibility criteria, the results may not be applicable to individuals below 14 years. In our country, we treat significant percentage of patients below this age category. Second, results will not be applicable if HbA1c outside the eligibility range of HbA1c of 7.5-10.9%. Third, the study included a relatively short intervention period of 6 months. Fourth, when the patients on CGM were regularly counseled on the benefits the other cohort could have been counseled rigorously on the same way to monitor sugar levels at least for this 26 weeks.

Implication of Findings for the Clinicians

Use of CGM provides the ability to obtain immediate result on current glucose levels as well as gives information regarding time in ranges (within target range, below range, above range). This information allows patients to optimize dietary intake and exercise, make informed therapy decisions regarding mealtime and correction of insulin dosing, and, react immediately to acute glycemic events.

Scope for Future Research

In clinical practice, widespread use of CGM is much needed in management of T1DM for day-to-day treatment decision making. In economically compromised countries like

India, it is quite difficult to advise CGM for every patient but we can hope for the best. In future, we are expecting intelligent CGM device that promises to be smaller, less-invasive, long-lasting, and lower cost than anything on the market now.

6. Continuous Glucose Monitoring in People with Type 1 Diabetes on Multiple-dose Injection Therapy: The Relationship between Glycemic Control and Hypoglycemia

Ref: Oliver N, Gimenez M, Calhoun P, Cohen N, Moscardo V, Hermanns N, et al. Continuous Glucose Monitoring in People With Type 1 Diabetes on Multiple-Dose Injection Therapy: The Relationship Between Glycemic Control and Hypoglycemia. Diabetes Care. 2020;43:53-58.

ABSTRACT

Objective: To determine the relationship between glycemic control and hypoglycemia in people with type 1 diabetes mellitus (T1DM) taking multiple-dose injection (MDI) regimens.

Research design and methods: Analysis of continuous glucose monitoring (CGM) data from the intervention [real-time continuous glucose monitoring (rtCGM)] and control [self-monitored blood glucose (SMBG)] phases of the Multiple Daily Injections and Continuous Glucose Monitoring in Diabetes (DIAMOND) and HypoDE studies was done. The relationship between glycemic control [glycated hemoglobin (HbA1c) and mean rtCGM glucose levels] and percentage time spent in hypoglycemia was determined for thresholds of 3.9 mmol/L (70 mg/dL) and 3.0 mmol/L (54 mg/dL). Analysis of variance (ANOVA) across the range of HbA1c and mean glucose was performed.

Results: We identified a nonlinear relationship between mean glucose and hypoglycemia at baseline. The relationship curve between overall glucose and hypoglycemia flattened with the use of rtCGM, and the most evident impact was seen at lower values of mean glucose and HbA1c.

Conclusion: The relationship between overall glucose control and hypoglycemia flattens using rtCGM with greater effects at lower values of HbA1c and mean glucose in type 1 diabetics patients using MDI regimens.

COMMENT

What was Known Prior to the Study?

The Diabetes Control and Complications Trial (DCCT) study[47] demonstrated a substantial reduction in microvascular complication risk in an intensely treated group of adults with type 1 diabetes mellitus (T1DM). However, the intensively treated group had significantly increase risk of severe hypoglycemia and there was inverse relationship found between glycated hemoglobin (HbA1c) and severe hypoglycemia. It is well appreciated that hypoglycemia is associated with significant morbidity.

Reduction in hypoglycemia risk independently of the glycemic control has been achieved in due to therapeutic and technological advances in the management of diabetes in the modern era. The outcomes of type 1 diabetes have improved due to invention of insulin analogs, insulin pump therapy improvement, and use of continuous glucose monitoring (CGM). More precise definition of hypoglycemia which requires a minimum duration of 15 minutes below threshold with events separated by at least 30 minutes has been formulated due to CGM.[48] A reduction in the frequency of severe hypoglycemia has been demonstrated with the follow-up data from the DCCT/EDIC (Epidemiology of Diabetes Interventions and Complications) cohort over time.

A previous 26-week randomized controlled trial (RCT), Juvenile Diabetes Research Foundation (JDRF) CGM study, published in 2008 and carried out in children and adults with T1DM to evaluate the efficacy and safety of CGM[46,49-50] demonstrated the improvement in glycemic control with the continuous use of real-time continuous glucose monitoring (rtCGM) devices clearly. The time in hypoglycemia was assessed from the baseline blinded CGM data in all individuals. The risk of hypoglycemia was lowest in participants with HbA1c values between 8.1% and 8.6% and J-shaped relationships were reported for all biochemical hypoglycemia thresholds. CGM was concluded to decrease the percentage duration of hypoglycemia, changing HbA1c, and hypoglycemia relationship.

What this Study Adds?

This study assessed the relationship between glucose control and hypoglycemia in type 1 diabetic patients using multiple-dose injection (MDI) regimens. Data from the DIAMOND[51] and HypoDE[52] studies were analyzed. The relationship of percentage duration of hypoglycemia with glucose control (HbA1c and mean rtCGM glucose levels) was explored for thresholds of 3.9 mmol/L (70 mg/dL) and 3.0 mmol/L (54 mg/dL). Analysis of variance (ANOVA) was applied across the range of HbA1c and mean glucose. At baseline, there was a nonlinear relationship between mean glucose and hypoglycemia and the steepest relationship was observed at lower values of mean glucose. The ability of rtCGM to convert this relationship from nonlinear at the lower end of glucose to an approximately linear relationship was observed which demonstrated usefulness of use of rtCGM on the risk of hypoglycemia at lower HbA1c values.

The relationship between hypoglycemia and mean glucose was found to unchange from baseline for participants randomized to self-monitored blood glucose (SMBG) and similarly a nonlinear relationship also emerged between hypoglycemia and HbA1c.

This study suggested the usefulness of rtCGM usage in achieving target glycemia without remarkable increase in hypoglycemia. Furthermore, it also showed the effective reduction in hypoglycemia in patients with above target HbA1c as hypoglycemia was reported to decrease continuously at higher HbA1c levels in the rtCGM group with highest risk of hypoglycemia at the lower extreme of HbA1c such as JDRF data set.

Strength and Limitation of this Study

The strengths of this study include the data taken from two large-scale rtCGM studies with participants using MDI. Also including patients with impaired awareness of hypoglycemia or a history of severe hypoglycemia addresses a gap in the evidence base.

One limitation of this study may be that it was difficult to assess the relationship between glycemia and hypoglycemia in the CGM group because of very less time spent in hypoglycemia among most patients. Also in contrast to the other landmark studies, the J-shaped association was not confirmed in this analysis, with no demonstrable increase in hypoglycemia risk at higher overall glucose values which could be due to exclusive use of MDI rather than insulin pump.

Implication of Findings for the Clinicians

As per Guidelines, to minimize the risk of severe hypoglycemia we adopt a HbA1c target of <8% but after this study we could think of lowering the cut off of HbA1c because of much lower risk of hypoglycemia at lower end of HbA1c with the use of CGM. Extensive use of CGM with newer modifications is much needed for better control of glycemia in T1DM patients.

7. The Efficacy of Technology in Type 1 DM: A Systemic Review, Network Meta-analysis, and Narrative Synthesis

Ref: Pease A, Lo C, Earnest A, Kiriakova V, Liew D, Zoungas S. The Efficacy of Technology in Type 1 Diabetes: A Systematic Review, Network Meta-analysis, and Narrative Synthesis. Diabetes Technol Ther. 2020;22:411-21.

ABSTRACT

Background: There is scarcity of previous studies that compared the available technologies for type 1 diabetes mellitus (T1DM) with the full range of alternative devices. For evaluating technologies, multiple metrics of glycemia as well as outcomes reported by patients also need to be considered. This systematic review, network meta-analysis, and narrative synthesis aimed at comparing the relative efficacy of existing technologies for T1DM management.

Methods: In this review, PubMed, MEDLINE, EMBASE, MEDLINE In-Process, and other nonindexed citations, all evidence-based medicine reviews, PsycINFO, Web of Science, PROSPERO, and CINAHL (inception—April 24, 2019) were searched. Review included randomized controlled trials (RCTs), conducted for duration of >6 weeks, which compared technologies for management of T1DM in nonpregnant adults of >18 years of age. Extraction of data was done by using a predefined tool. Primary outcomes considered in the study included glycated hemoglobin (HbA1c) (%), rates of hypoglycemia, and quality of life (QoL). The mean difference for HbA1c and nonsevere hypoglycemia, rate ratio for severe hypoglycemia, and standardized mean difference for QoL in network meta-analysis with random effects were evaluated.

Results: Total 16,772 publications were identified. Out of these, 52 eligible studies compared 12 diabetes management technologies; total 3,975 participants in network meta-analysis were included. This was observed that the integrated insulin pump and continuous glucose monitoring (CGM) systems with low-glucose suspend or hybrid closed-loop algorithms lead to HbA1c levels 0.96% [predictive interval (95% PrI) 0.04–1.89] and 0.87% (95% PrI 0.12–1.63) lower compared to the multiple daily injections with either flash glucose monitoring or capillary glucose testing, respectively. Also, integrated systems demonstrated the best ranking for reduction of HbA1c using the surface under the cumulative ranking curve (SUCRA-96.4). There were nonsignificant treatment effects for several technology comparisons in terms of severe hypoglycemia and QoL. However, simultaneous assessment of outcomes in cluster analyses and narrative synthesis seemed to prefer integrated insulin pump as well as continuous glucose monitors. The overall risk of bias was found to be moderate-high, and the certainty of evidence was observed to be very low.

Conclusion: The best technologies for HbA1c reduction, composite ranking for HbA1c and severe hypoglycemia, and QoL seemed to be integrated insulin pump and CGM systems along with low-glucose suspend or hybrid closed-loop capability. (Registration: PROSPERO, number CRD42017077221)

COMMENT

What was Known Prior to the Study?

Technologies pertaining to and aiming for better glycemic management and prevention of complications have been in existence for over four decades and evolving continuously. The knowledge of and comparisons between various closed loop devices and segregated insulin delivery or monitoring systems has existed[53-57] before but the parameters compared have been limited. In 2014, safety and effectiveness of a bionic pancreas under unrestricted outpatient conditions were published by Russel et al.[53] There have also been researches regarding inhaled insulin and various insulin pump devices but most of those chiefly compared (HbA1c) as the primary outcome over a period of time.

What this Study Adds?

This study that utilized a systematic review, network meta-analysis, and narrative synthesis compared the relative efficacies of available technologies for the management of type 1 diabetes mellitus (T1DM). Study population selected was nonpregnant adult >18 years of age and the primary outcomes compared were not only the HbA1c, but also the rates of severe as well as nonsevere hypoglycemia, and the aspects of improvement of the quality of life (QoL). Also this has been the first network meta-analysis of its kind to integrate the comparison of technologies for insulin delivery, glucose monitoring, and insulin dose calculations in the management of T1DM. The uniformity of reporting outcomes including hypoglycemia would also assist in making direct and indirect treatment comparisons. The study enforced upon the fact that integrated continuous subcutaneous insulin infusion (CSII) and continuous glucose monitoring (CGM) with low glucose suspend or hybrid closed loop algorithms was the best overall option for majority of outcomes, with an evidence strongest for HbA1c reduction.

Major Strengths of the Study

The study compared the relative efficacies of various available technologies in the management of T1DM. The key strength of the study was to rank the efficacies of the techniques against their key outcomes. Another strength of the study was about the parameters included for comparison of the key outcomes, viz., HbA1c, rates of both severe as well as nonsevere hypoglycemia and overall QoL.

Limitations of the Study

The study excluded adolescents and children as subjects and study was limited only to nonpregnant adults >18 years of age. Therefore, the study lacked generalizability. Also none of the techniques was sufficient to compare the QoL with precision. The time in range could not be meta-analyzed properly because of inconsistent reporting. Although nonserious hypoglycemia was taken as a parameter for primary outcome but could not be defined properly.

Implications of the Findings for the Clinicians

The study brings out important conclusions and implications for the clinicians regarding management in cases of T1DM. The study has brought home a point quite clear and loud that integrated systems comprising low glucose suspends or hybrid closed loop algorithms such as CSIIs or continuous glucose monitors were best for HbA1c reduction, preventing episodes of hyperglycemia, diabetic ketoacidosis, and other diabetes-related complications. Hence, making the management of T1DM more practical and fruitful both for the patient and clinicians.

Scope for Future Research

Though the role of integrated or hybrid closed loop systems was well demonstrated with respect to issues of better glycemic control, youth may not wear CGM/pump in view of many reasons: Requirement of significant patient input in CGM use (sensor insertion, calibration, response to sensor alarms, etc.) and insulin dosing in ongoing self-monitoring of blood glucose (SMBG). There are reports of pain during sensor insertion, skin reactions, and frustration with sensor alarms by the Juvenile Diabetes Research Foundation CGM trial.[58] Additionally, CGM use was found to be associated with higher educational level, higher income, private insurance, and longer diabetes duration as per the T1DM Exchange registry. Also, most of the patients do not download it regularly so may not get its full benefit and the retrospective review of the data from the device as shown in the recent data.[59] Patients compliance is also affected by the lack of a proper education, low motivation, deliberate insulin omission, and altered attitude. Therefore, the adherence and the treatment satisfaction can be enhanced by ensuring behavioral therapy in training which will result in better glycemic control outcomes. If the new technologies are not used as expected, they can underperformance even if they may have positive outcomes. At last, we can hope for a fully automated artificial pancreas for every T1DM patients in the near future but it is crucial to implement the use of technological advances that are currently available in correct fashion.

8. Use of Sensor-integrated Pump Therapy to Reduce Hypoglycemia in People with Type 1 Diabetes: A Real-world Study in the UK

Ref: Choudhary P, de Portu S, Arrieta A, Castañeda J, Campbell FM. Use of sensor-integrated pump therapy to reduce hypoglycaemia in people with Type 1 diabetes: a real-world study in the UK. Diabet Med. 2019;36:1100-8.

ABSTRACT

Aim: Assessment of effectiveness of sensor-integrated insulin pump system in real-world setting.

Methods: Anonymized data uploaded to CareLink™ by 920 type 1 diabetic patients between February, 2016 and June, 2018, who were using the MiniMed Paradigm Veo system and the MiniMed 640G system (Medtronic International Trading S`arl, Tolochanez, Switzerland) with SmartGuard technology, were analyzed. Users who had ≥70% sensor-wear time and data of ≥15 days were categorized into three groups: Group I had sensor-augmented pump (SAP) alone, group II had sensor-integrated pump with low glucose suspend enabled, while the group III had sensor-integrated pump with predictive low glucose management enabled.

Results: The median number of days for which the system was used was 161 (58–348). 0.8 (0.3–1.7)%, 0.3 (0.1–0.7)%, and 0.3 (0.1–0.5)% were the median time spent with sensor glucose values ≤3 mmol/L was in the groups I, II, and III, respectively. The monthly rate of hypoglycemic events <3 mmol/L [rate ratio 0.63, 95% confidence interval (CI) 0.45–0.89; $p = 0.009$] and the percentage of time with glucose values ≤3 mmol/L reduced significantly, on switching from group I to group II ($n = 31$) [group I: 0.63% (95% CI 0.34–1.29), group II: 0.33% (95% CI 0.16–0.64); $p = 0.001$]. Also, there was further decrease in the monthly rate of hypoglycemic events in individuals ($n = 139$) when switched from group II to group III [rate ratio 0.82 (95% CI 0.69–0.98); $p < 0.0274$]. For sensor glucose values <3.9 mmol/L, we observed same pattern of results.

Conclusion: Automation of insulin suspension can reduce the occurrence to hypoglycemia in patients with type 1 diabetes mellitus (T1DM).

COMMENT

Introduction

Type 1 diabetes mellitus (T1DM) is the result of interactions of genetic, environmental, and immunologic factors that ultimately lead to immune-mediated destruction of the pancreatic β cells. Insulin is the mainstay of therapy of T1DM management. Although there is well-established role of tight glycemic control in reducing the vascular complications of T1DM but such control achievement can be complicated by hypoglycemia. Now days, continuous glucose monitoring (CGM) has transformed the management of T1DM. CGM can be used with or without insulin pump therapy. Although glycemic control can be improved potentially by CGM alone and hypoglycemia can be reduced, but the risk of harm resulting from hypoglycemia can be prevented or minimized by combining it with continuous subcutaneous insulin infusion (CSII) with real-time CGM, i.e., sensor-integrated pump therapy offering the opportunity for automated insulin suspension. Recent studies demonstrated the superiority of sensor-augmented pump (SAP) therapy versus multiple daily injections[60,61] with a mean decrease of 0.8–1.2% in glycated hemoglobin (HbA1c) levels, without increasing the risk of hypoglycemia. The INTERPRET Study, largest and longest multicenter prospective observational study providing real-life data on SAP showed the effectiveness of CGM in pump users.[62]

What this Study Adds?

The effectiveness of automated insulin suspension systems was assessed in this one of the first real-world studies. In the group of predictive low glucose management, the median time with sensor glucose values <3 mmol/L in the SAP group was reported to be 0.8%, in the sensor-integrated pump with low glucose suspend group was 0.3% and in the sensor-integrated pump with group was 0.3%. Significant reductions were found in the monthly hypoglycemic events <3 mmol/L in patients who switched to sensor-integrated pump with low glucose suspend from SAP. It was demonstrated in this study that the burden of hypoglycemia in the real clinical setting by using automated insulin suspension in response to hypoglycemia. There was no loss of mean glucose control with the reductions in hypoglycemia. An incremental value is added to the threshold suspend system by predictive suspension of insulin.

Major Strength of the Study

Strengths of the present study include the large dataset and the real-world setting.

Limitations of the Study

The demographic data was lacking in the database. Additionally, it was a nonrandomized study. Additionally, the data of the patients who consented the use of their anonymized data for research could only be used. The treatment groups of different sizes and durations of treatment were analyzed initially and there was no data of the factors which affected their choice for device. Similarly, no data were available for the reasons for using SAP therapy without any suspension mode activated and switching to low glucose suspend.

Implications of the Findings for the Clinicians

The generalizability of the usefulness of pump therapy with insulin suspension technologies to the real-world clinical setting is clearly of great clinical relevance. The data generated from the study may influence the clinicians to motivate the patients to use sensor-integrated pump which will reduce the hypoglycemic events and cause less clinical manifestations due to hypoglycemia. Substantial savings could be possible by reducing rates of severe hypoglycemia by decreasing the number of visits to emergency department and paramedic call-outs and the quality of life may also be improved resulting from decreased anxiety about nocturnal hypoglycemia.

Knowledge Gaps and Scope for Future Research

We have to prepare more advanced devices which have the facility to monitor glucose continuously, use an algorithm to change the basal insulin rate, and give automated corrective boluses and suspend insulin release predicting hypoglycemia even before actual hypoglycemia occurs.

Though various new inventions have arrived in the market, insulin along with delivery pumps is costly in countries such as India. We have to try to make cheaper devices for insulin delivery so that a larger population can use it and help from government sectors is of high demand for these situations.

REFERENCES (Type 1 Diabetes Mellitus)

1. June CH, Warshauer JT, Bluestone JA. Is autoimmunity the Achilles' heel of cancer immunotherapy? Nat Med. 2017;23(5):540-7.
2. De Filette J, Jansen Y, Schreuer M, Everaert H, Velkeniers B, Neyns B, et al. Incidence of thyroid-related adverse events in melanoma patients treated with pembrolizumab. J Clin Endocrinol Metab. 2016;101:4431-9.
3. Stamatouli AM, Quandt Z, Perdigoto AL, Clark PL, Kluger H, Weiss SA, et al. Collateral damage: insulin-dependent diabetes induced with checkpoint inhibitors. Diabetes. 2018;67(8):1471-80.
4. Kotwal A, Haddox C, Block M, Kudva YC. Immune checkpoint inhibitors: an emerging cause of insulin-dependent diabetes. BMJ Open Diabetes Res Care. 2019;7(1):e000591.
5. Tsang VH, McGrath RT, Clifton-Bligh RJ, Scolyer RA, Jakrot V, Guminski AD, et al. Checkpoint Inhibitor–Associated Autoimmune Diabetes Is Distinct From Type 1 Diabetes. J Clin Endocrinol Metab. 2019;104(11):5499-506.
6. Zezza M, Kosinski C, Mekoguem C, Marino L, Chtioui H, Pitteloud N, et al. Combined immune checkpoint inhibitor therapy with nivolumab and ipilimumab causing acute-onset type 1 diabetes mellitus following a single administration: two case reports. BMC Endocr Disord. 2019;19(1):144.
7. Accessdata.fda.gov. (2019). Avelumab label information. [online] Available from https://www.accessdata.fda.gov/drugsatfda_docs/label/2017/761049s000lbl.pdf [Last accessed February, 2021].
8. Accessdata.fda.gov. (2019). Durvalumab label information. [online] Available from https://www.accessdata.fda.gov/drugsatfda_docs/label/2017/761069s000lbl.pdf [Last accessed February, 2021].
9. Merck.com. (2019). Pembrolizumab label information. [online] Available from https://www.merck.com/product/usa/pi_circulars/k/keytruda/keytruda_pi.pdf [Last accessed February, 2021].
10. Packageinserts. (2019). Nivolumab label information. [online] Available from https://packageinserts.bms.com/pi/pi_opdivo.pdf [Last accessed February, 2021].
11. Chaudhary K, Malhotra K, Sowers J, Aroor A. Uric acid—key ingredient in the recipe for cardiorenal metabolic syndrome. Cardiorenal Med. 2013;3:208-20.
12. Filiopoulos V, Hadjiyannakos D, Vlassopoulos D. New insights into uric acid effects on the progression and prognosis of chronic kidney disease. Ren Fail. 2012;34:510-20.
13. De Cosmo S, Viazzi F, Pacilli A, Giorda C, Ceriello A, Gentile S, et al. Serum uric acid and risk of CKD in type 2 diabetes. Clin J Am Soc Nephrol. 2015;10:1921-9.
14. Cheng XB, Zhang T, Zhu HJ, Ma N, Sun XD, Wang SH, et al. Correlations between blood uric acid and the incidence and progression of type 2 diabetes nephropathy. Eur Rev Med Pharmacol Sci. 2018;22:506-11.
15. Lytvyn Y, Škrti M, Yang GK, Yip PM, Perkins BA, Cherney DZ. Glycosuria-mediated urinary uric acid excretion in patients with uncomplicated type 1 diabetes mellitus. Am J Physiol Renal Physiol. 2015;308:F77-83.
16. Lytvyn Y, Škrti M, Yang GK, Lai V, Scholey JW, Yip PM, et al. Plasma uric acid effects on glomerular haemodynamic profile of patients with uncomplicated Type 1 diabetes mellitus. Diabet Med. 2016;33:1102-11.
17. Klisic A, Kocic G, Kavaric N, Jovanovic M, Stanisic V, Ninic A. Xanthine oxidase and uric acid as independent predictors of albuminuria in patients with diabetes mellitus type 2. Clin Exp Med. 2018;18:283-90.
18. Mauer M, Doria A. Uric acid and diabetic nephropathy risk. Contrib Nephrol. 2018;192:103-9.
19. Goicoechea M, de Vinuesa SG, Verdalles U, Ruiz-Caro C, Ampuero J, Rincón A, et al. Effect of allopurinol in chronic kidney disease progression and cardiovascular risk. Clin J Am Soc Nephrol. 2010;5:1388-93.
20. Goicoechea M, Garcia de Vinuesa S, Verdalles U, Verde E, Macias N, Santos A, et al. Allopurinol and progression of CKD and cardiovascular events: long-term follow-up of a randomized clinical trial. Am J Kidney Dis. 2015;65:543-9.
21. Siu YP, Leung KT, Tong MK, Kwan TH. Use of allopurinol in slowing the progression of renal disease through its ability to lower serum uric acid level. Am J Kidney Dis. 2006;47:51-9.
22. Afkarian M, Polsky S, Parsa A, Aronson R, Caramori ML, Cherney DZ, et al. Preventing Early Renal Loss in Diabetes (PERL) study: a randomized double-blinded trial of allopurinol—rationale, design, and baseline data. Diabetes Care. 2019;42:1454-63.
23. Badve SV, Pascoe EM, Tiku A, Boudville N, Brown FG, Cass A, et al. Effects of allopurinol on the progression of chronic kidney disease. N Engl J Med. 2020;382:2504-13.
24. Eleftheriadis T, Pissas G, Sounidaki M, Antoniadi G, Antoniadis N, Liakopoulos V, et al. Uric acid increases cellular and humoral alloimmunity in primary human peripheral blood mononuclear cells. Nephrology (Carlton). 2017;23:610-5.
25. Alshiekh S, Larsson HE, Ivarsson SA, Lernmark Š. Autoimmune type 1 diabetes. In: Holt RIG, Cockram CS, Flyvbjerg A, Goldstein BJ (Eds). Textbook of Diabetes, 5th edition. West Sussex, UK: Wiley Blackwell; 2017.
26. American Diabetes Association. Standards of medical care in diabetes—2019. Diabetes Care. 2019;42(Suppl 1):S16-S152.
27. Bottazzo GF, Florin-Christensen A, Doniach D. Islet-cell antibodies in diabetes mellitus with autoimmune polyendocrine deficiencies. Lancet. 1974;2:1279-83.
28. Leslie RDG, Atkinson MA, Notkins AL. Autoantigens IA-2 and GAD in type I (insulin-dependent) diabetes. Diabetologia. 1999;42:3-14.
29. Irivine WJ, Clarke BF, Scarth L, Duncan LJ. The incidence of thyroid and gastric autoimmunity in patients with diabetes mellitus. Clin Sci. 1969;37:570.
30. Menon PS, Vaidyanathan B, Kaur M. Autoimmune thyroid disease in Indian children with type 1 diabetes mellitus. J Pediatr Endocrinol Metab. 2001;14:279-86.
31. Sharma B, Nehara HR, Saran S, Bhavi VK, Singh AK, Mathur SK. Coexistence of autoimmune disorders and type

1 diabetes mellitus in children: An observation from western part of India. Indian J Endocrinol Metab. 2019;23:22-6.
32. Frohlich-Reiterer EE, Hofer S, Kaspers S, Herbst A, Kordonouri O, Schwarz HP, et al. Screening frequency for celiac disease and autoimmune thyroiditis in children and adolescents with type 1 diabetes mellitus—data from a German/Austrian multicentre survey. Pediatr Diabetes. 2008;9:546-53.
33. Jha V, Garcia-Garcia G, Iseki K, Li Z, Naicker S, Plattner B, et al. Chronic kidney disease: global dimension and perspectives. Lancet. 2013;382:260-72.
34. Anand S, Bitton A, Gaziano T. The gap between estimated incidence of end-stage renal disease and use of therapy. PLoS One. 2013;8:e72860.
35. KDOQI. KDOQI Clinical Practice Guidelines and Clinical Practice Recommendations for Diabetes and Chronic Kidney Disease. Am J Kidney Dis. 2007;49:S12-154.
36. MacIsaac RJ, Ekinci EI, Jerums G. Markers of and risk factors for the development and progression of diabetic kidney disease. Am J Kidney Dis. 2014;63:S39-62.
37. Levey AS, Coresh J. Chronic kidney disease. Lancet. 2012;379:165-80.
38. Perkins BA, Ficociello LH, Silva KH, Finkelstein DM, Warram JH, Krolewski AS. Regression of microalbuminuria in type 1 diabetes. N Engl J Med. 2003;348:2285-93.
39. Bolignano D, Lacquaniti A, Coppolino G, Donato V, Campo S, Fazio MR, et al. Neutrophil gelatinase-associated lipocalin (NGAL) and progression of chronic kidney disease. Clin J Am Soc Nephrol. 2009;4:337-44.
40. Yang YH, He XJ, Chen SR, Wang L, Li EM, Xu LY. Changes of serum and urine neutrophil gelatinase-associated lipocalin in type-2 diabetic patients with nephropathy: one year observational follow-up study. Endocrine. 2009;36:45-51.
41. Smith ER, Lee D, Cai MM, Tomlinson LA, Ford ML, McMahon LP, et al. Urinary neutrophil gelatinase-associated lipocalin may aid prediction of renal decline in patients with non-proteinuric Stages 3 and 4 chronic kidney disease (CKD). Nephrol Dial Transplant. 2013;28:1569-79.
42. Bergenstal RM, Ahmann AJ, Bailey T, Beck RW, Bissen J, Buckingham B, et al. Recommendations for standardizing glucose reporting and analysis to optimize clinical decision making in diabetes: the Ambulatory Glucose Profile (AGP). Diabetes Technol Ther. 2013;15:198-211.
43. Diabetes Research in Children Network (DirecNet) Study Group; Buckingham B, Beck RW, Tamborlane WV, Xing D, Kollman C, et al. Continuous glucose monitoring in children with type 1 diabetes. J Pediatr. 2007; 151:388-93, 393.e1-2.
44. Weinzimer S, Xing D, Tansey M, Fiallo-Scharer R, Mauras N, Wysocki T, et al. FreeStyle navigator continuous glucose monitoring system use in children with type 1 diabetes using glargine-based multiple daily dose regimens: results of a pilot trial Diabetes Research in Children Network (DirecNet) Study Group. Diabetes Care. 2008;31:525-7.
45. Wilson DM, Beck RW, Tamborlane WV, Dontchev MJ, Kollman C, Chase P, et al. The accuracy of the FreeStyle Navigator continuous glucose monitoring system in children with type 1 diabetes. Diabetes Care. 2007;30(1):59-64.
46. Juvenile Diabetes Research Foundation Continuous Glucose Monitoring Study Group; Tamborlane WV, Beck RW, Bode BW, Buckingham B, Chase HP, et al. Continuous glucose monitoring and intensive treatment of type 1 diabetes. N Engl J Med. 2008;359:1464-76.
47. Diabetes Control and Complications Trial Research Group, Nathan DM, Genuth S, Lachin J, Cleary P, Crofford O, et al. The effect of intensive treatment of diabetes on the development and progression of long-term complications in insulin-dependent diabetes mellitus. N Engl J Med. 1993;329:977-86
48. Schnell O, Barnard K, Bergenstal R, Bosi E, Garg S, Guerci B, et al. Role of continuous glucose monitoring in clinical trials: recommendations on reporting. Diabetes Technol Ther. 2017;19:391-9.
49. JDRF CGM Study Group. JDRF randomized clinical trial to assess the efficacy of real-time continuous glucose monitoring in the management of type 1 diabetes: research design and methods. Diabetes Technol Ther. 2008;10: 310-21.
50. Juvenile Diabetes Research Foundation Continuous Glucose Monitoring Study Group, Beck RW, Hirsch IB, Laffel L, Tamborlane WV, Bode BW, et al. The effect of continuous glucose monitoring in well-controlled type 1 diabetes. Diabetes Care. 2009;32:1378-83.
51. Beck RW, Riddlesworth T, Ruedy K, Ahmann A, Bergenstal R, Haller S, et al. Effect of continuous glucose monitoring on glycemic control in adults with type 1 diabetes using insulin injections: the DIAMOND randomized clinical trial. JAMA. 2017;317:371-8.
52. Heinemann L, Freckmann G, Ehrmann D, Faber-Heinemann G, Guerra S, Waldenmaier D, et al. Real-time continuous glucose monitoring in adults with type 1 diabetes and impaired hypoglycaemia awareness or severe hypoglycaemia treated with multiple daily insulin injections (HypoDE): a multicentre, randomised controlled trial. Lancet. 2018;391:1367-77.
53. Russell SJ, El-Khatib FH, Sinha M, Magyar KL, McKeon K, Goergen LG, et al. Outpatient glycemic control with a bionic pancreas in type 1 diabetes. N Engl J Med. 2014;371:313-25.
54. Kovatchev BP, Renard E, Cobelli C, Zisser HC, Keith-Hynes P, Anderson SM, et al. Safety of outpatient closed-loop control: first randomized crossover trials of a wearable artificial pancreas. Diabetes Care. 2014;37:1789-96.
55. Ly TT, Breton MD, Keith-Hynes P, De Salvo D, Clinton P, Benassi K, et al. Overnight glucose control with an automated, unified safety system in children and adolescents with type 1 diabetes at diabetes camp. Diabetes Care. 2014;37:2310-6.
56. Thabit H, Lubina-Solomon A, Stadler M, Leelarathna L, Walkinshaw E, Pernet A, et al. Home use of closed-loop insulin delivery for overnight glucose control in adults with type 1 diabetes: a 4-week, multicentre, randomised crossover study. Lancet Diabetes Endocrinol. 2014;2:701-9.

57. Nimri R, Muller I, Atlas E, Miller S, Fogel A, Bratina N, et al. MD-Logic overnight control for 6 weeks of home use in patients with type 1 diabetes: randomized crossover trial. Diabetes Care. 2014;37:3025-32.
58. Juvenile Diabetes Research Foundation Continuous Glucose Monitoring Study Group. Validation of measures of satisfaction with and impact of continuous and conventional glucose monitoring. Diabetes Technol Ther. 2010;12: 679-84.
59. Liberman A, Buckingham B, Phillip M. Diabetes technology and the human factor. Int J Clin Pract Suppl. 2012;175: 79-84.
60. Bergenstal RM, Tamborlane WV, Ahmann A, Buse JB, Dai-ley G, Davis SN, et al. Effectiveness of sensor-augmented insulin-pump therapy in type 1 diabetes. N Engl J Med. 2010;363:311-320.
61. Hermanides J, Nørgaard K, Bruttomesso D, Mathieu C, Frid A, Dayan CM, et al. Sensor-augmented pump therapy lowers HbA1c in suboptimally controlled type 1 diabetes; a randomized controlled trial. Diabet Med. 2011;28:1158-67.
62. Nørgaard K, Scaramuzza A, Bratina N, Lalić NM, Jarosz-Chobot P, Kocsis G, et al. Routine sensor-augmented pump therapy in type 1 diabetes: the INTERPRET study. Diabetes Technol Ther. 2013;15:273-80.

Section 6: Gestational Diabetes Mellitus

Rana Bhattacharjee, Purvi Chawla, Sunil Surajprasad Gupta, Rajeev Chawla

1. Prevention of Gestational Diabetes Mellitus in Overweight or Obese Pregnant Women: A Network Meta-analysis

Ref: Chatzakis C, Goulis DG, Mareti E, Eleftheriades M, Zavlanos A, Dinas K, et al. Prevention of gestational diabetes mellitus in overweight or obese pregnant women: A network meta-analysis. Diabetes Res Clin Pract. 2019;158:107924.

ABSTRACT

Aim: Overweight or obese pregnant women are prone to develop gestational diabetes mellitus (GDM). This network meta-analysis aimed to compare the effect of different interventions in prevention of GDM that include promoting physical activities, use of metformin, vitamin D supplements, and probiotics.

Materials: Four electronic databases and grey literature sources were searched for randomized trials and a network meta-analysis was performed, with the primary outcome being the development of GDM. Any other complications of pregnancy were taken as secondary outcomes.

Results: Out of the 23 studies (4,237 participants) included, none of the interventions were found superior to placebo/no intervention. For gestational weight gain, metformin, and increased physical activities were effective compared to placebo/no intervention [mean difference (MD) −1.21, 95% confidence interval (CI) −2.14 to −0.28 and MD −0.96, 95% CI −1.69 to −0.22, respectively]. Metformin was better in reducing caesarean sections and admission to neonatal intensive care unit (NICU) compared to placebo/no intervention.

Conclusion: The interventions could not prevent the development of GDM in overweight/obese pregnant women.

COMMENT

What was Known Prior to this Study?

The prevalence of obesity is increasing globally affecting primarily younger people, especially women in the reproductive age group. In parallel, the incidence of gestational diabetes mellitus (GDM) has also increased. It has been estimated that currently one in six births is affected by gestational diabetes.[1] To prevent GDM, interventions like physical exercise and drugs (metformin, vitamin D, and probiotics) have been tested against no intervention in overweight and obese pregnant women.[2-5]

What this Study Adds?

There was no head-to-head comparison between these interventions. The authors of the study used network meta-analysis to compare these interventions with each other or no interventions and find out the most effective way to prevent GDM in overweight and obese pregnant women. A total of 23 studies with 4,237 participants were included.

None of the interventions studied here, i.e., physical activity, metformin, vitamin D, and probiotics were found to be effective in the prevention of GDM, which was the primary outcome. Among secondary outcomes in terms of other pregnancy complications, none of the interventions were found to be effective in prevention of pre-eclampsia, large for gestational age fetus, intrauterine death, or macrosomia although metformin was found to be superior for the prevention of caesarean section and admission to neonatal intensive care unit (NICU). Both metformin and physical exercise were effective in the reduction of gestational weight gain, and physical exercise was more effective than metformin in reducing gestational weight gain.

Major Strengths of the Study

This is the first study comparing the effectiveness of multiple important interventions for prevention of GDM in overweight and obese pregnant women. The authors ranked different interventions in terms of efficacy by applying the GRADE (Grading of Recommendations Assessment, Development and Evaluation) criteria for the quality of the current evidence. The inclusion criteria were more rigorous than any meta-analyses undertaken earlier. The magnitude of the reduction in the gestational weight gain with the type and duration of the physical activity intervention has also not been reported to enable understanding the impact of weight management in preventing GDM in the overweight and obese pregnant women.

Limitations of the Study

The authors did not include dietary intervention as these are difficult to quantify for the purpose of meta-analysis. Thus far, the only intervention that prevents GDM in overweight/obese pregnant women is the Mediterranean diet as reported in the St Carlos Study.[6] The overall evidence from the available studies was moderate-to-low giving rise to trends in results and requiring high quality evidence to make definitive conclusions.

Implications of the Findings for the Clinicians

Adequate physical activity should be advised to the overweight and obese pregnant women to prevent excessive gestational weight gain. Continuation of metformin after conception in cases where it was given pregestationally has a limited role in this population and should be discontinued. Vitamin D and probiotics are also not effective in prevention of obesity-related complications in pregnancy.

Knowledge Gaps Identified and Scope for Future Research

The quality of evidence for prevention of GDM in the non-diabetic, overweight, and obese pregnant women is moderate-to-low for the interventions studied in this network meta-analyses, i.e., physical activity, metformin, vitamin D, and probiotics. Future research should focus on this area.

---

2. Maternal Age and the Risk of Gestational Diabetes Mellitus: A Systematic Review and Meta-analysis of Over 120 Million Participants

Ref: Li Y, Ren X, He L, Li J, Zhang S, Chen W. Maternal age and the risk of gestational diabetes mellitus: A systematic review and meta-analysis of over 120 million participants. Diabetes Res Clin Pract. 2020;162:108044.

ABSTRACT

Aim: Evaluation and quantification of risk of gestational diabetes mellitus (GDM) in pregnant females with increasing age.

Methods: Publications were searched from inception to July, 2018 in three electronic databases. Odds ratio (OR) and 95% confidence interval (95% CI) were calculated. Generalized least squares regression was used for dose-response analysis. To explore the source of identified heterogeneity among studies, we conducted subgroup and meta-regression analyses.

Results: We included 24 studies in the meta-analysis. The ORs and 95% CIs were compared across different age-groups: Women <20 years versus 25–29 years, 30–34 years, 35–39 years, and ≥40 years. The values were 0.60 (95% CI 0.50–0.72), 1.69 (95% CI 1.49–1.93), 2.73 (95% CI 2.28–3.27), 3.54 (95% CI 2.88–4.34), and 4.86 (95% CI = 3.78–6.24), respectively. A linear relationship of risk of GDM with maternal age (Ptrend < 0.001) was observed in the dose-response analysis. The risk in overall population increased by 7.90%, while for Asian and European population, it was 12.74% and 6.52%, respectively, for each one-year increase in maternal age at the time of conception from 18 years onward. Subgroup analyses showed that in women >25 years, risk of developing GDM was more in Asian women as compared to the European women (all $P_{interactions}$ < 0.001).

Conclusion: This meta-analysis concluded that risk of developing GDM increases with increasing maternal age at the time of conception in a linear fashion and is also more pronounced in Asian women as compared to their European counterparts.

COMMENT

What was Known Prior to this Study?

The average age of childbearing has been increasing over the years due to a myriad of socioeconomic determinants.[7] Advanced maternal age is considered as an independent risk factor for gestational diabetes mellitus (GDM) although the evidence is conflicting.[8-11]

What this Study Adds?

The authors did a meta-analysis of 24 cohort studies involving 127,275,067 participants, where the participants were grouped according to the maternal age categories (≥3 groups) and screened for GDM. A linear increase in the incidence of GDM with successive age-groups was observed indicating a strong positive association between rising maternal age at the time of conception and the GDM risk. Moreover, Asian women had a significantly higher risk of developing GDM than European women, above the age of 25 years.

Major Strengths of the Study

Exclusive inclusion of cohort studies and large sample size are the major strengths of this study. Sensitivity analysis was done which found that the combined OR remained significant for all comparisons.

Limitations of the Study

Definition of GDM and the cut-off glycemic criteria were different across the studies. Classification of the participants in different age categories was also heterogeneous.

Implications of the Findings for the Clinicians

This study emphasized the need for GDM screening in pregnant women, particularly for those above 25 years of age at the time of conception, with highlighting the higher risk in pregnant women of Asian origin in comparison with those of European origin. This study underscores the importance of preconceptional counseling as early as possible by physicians.

3. Gestational Diabetes Mellitus in HIV-infected Pregnant Women: A Systematic Review and Meta-analysis

Ref: Biadgo B, Ambachew S, Abebe M, Melku M. Gestational diabetes mellitus in HIV-infected pregnant women: A systematic review and meta-analysis. Diabetes Res Clin Pract. 2019;155:107800.

ABSTRACT

Background: Impaired glucose metabolism during pregnancy is associated with significant adverse outcomes. Antiretroviral therapy (ART) in human immunodeficiency virus (HIV)-infected pregnant women can lead to impaired glucose tolerance and gestational diabetes mellitus (GDM), as reported by previous studies.

Methods: This systematic review and meta-analysis followed the PRISMA (Preferred Reporting Items for Systematic Reviews and Meta-Analyses) guidelines. For calculating the pooled prevalence of GDM using the random effect model and 95% confidence interval (CI), the STATA version 11 was used. Subgroup analysis was conducted by geographical regions. For demonstrating the publication bias, visual inspection of the funnel plot and Egger's regression test statistic were used.

Results: Twenty one publications met the inclusion criteria, out of a total of 13,517 articles. Among the HIV-infected pregnant women, the pooled prevalence of GDM was 4.42% (95% CI 3.48, 5.35). The subgroup analysis revealed that the pooled prevalence of GDM among HIV-infected pregnant women was 7.1% (95% CI 3.38, 10.76) in Asia, 5.83% (95% CI 2.61, 9.04) in Europe, 3.58% (95% CI 2.67, 4.50) in America, and 3.19% (95% CI −2.89, 9.27) in Africa.

Conclusion: Early screening of HIV-infected pregnant women for GDM is crucial to reduce its complications as the pooled prevalence is expectedly high among them.

COMMENT

What was Known Prior to this Study?

The introduction of highly active antiretroviral therapy (HAART) has revolutionized the management of HIV-infected pregnant women. Protease inhibitors (PI), one of the important components of HAART increase the likelihood of development of diabetes,[12] although the propensity varies between various PIs.[13] The evidence of increased incidence of gestational diabetes mellitus (GDM) among HIV-infected pregnant women is conflicting and many studies did not find such association.[14-17] Moreover, there was a dearth of data regarding the global prevalence of GDM in women with HIV infection.

What this Study Adds?

The pooled prevalence of GDM among HIV-infected pregnant women was found to be 4.42% (95% CI 3.48, 5.35). This estimated prevalence was lower than the estimation of GDM among the general population by the World Health Organization (8.5%)[18] and the International Diabetes Federation (IDF) (14%).[19] Upon further subgroup analysis of this study, the prevalence of GDM among HIV-infected pregnant women was 7.07% (95% CI 3.38, 10.76) in Asia, 5.83% (95% CI 2.61, 9.04) in Europe, 3.58% (95% CI 2.67, 4.50) in America, and 3.19% (95% CI 2.89, 9.27) in Africa; the trend consistent with that reported in the IDF Atlas. A higher incidence of GDM among those exposed to PI was observed as compared to other Antiretroviral therapy (ART) users.

Major Strengths of the Study

This is the first study that synthesized data on the prevalence of GDM among HIV-infected women in a global perspective.

Limitations of the Study

This study has several limitations. Approximately, one-third of the included studies did not report the GDM diagnostic criteria; even when reported, they were varied in the different studies, rendering them difficult to compare. Moreover, there was substantial heterogeneity between the studies regarding the prevalence of GDM. Although the authors reported that the prevalence of GDM was high in HIV-infected women, the prevalence is lower than the general population by most of the estimates. Other factors like pre-gestational weight and BMI and status of pre-diabetes that are important drivers of GDM, were not reported here.

Implications of the Findings for the Clinicians

Clinicians should screen the HIV-infected pregnant women for GDM, particularly those on PI best therapy.

Knowledge Gaps Identified and Scope for Future Research

Despite the higher prevalence of diabetes among HIV-infected nonpregnant population, increased incidence of GDM was not found in HIV-infected pregnant women in comparison to noninfected ones. There is a scope of research to find out the cause of this discrepancy.

4. Continuous Glucose Monitoring in Pregnancy: Importance of Analyzing Temporal Profiles to Understand Clinical Outcomes

Ref: Scott EM, Feig DS, Murphy HR, Law GR. Continuous glucose monitoring in pregnancy: Importance of analysing temporal profiles to understand clinical outcomes. Diabetes Care. 2020;43(6):1178-84.

ABSTRACT

Aim: To determine the difference of temporal glucose profiles in different clinical interventions and monitoring settings in pregnancy.

Research design and methods: Pregnant women with type 1 diabetes mellitu (T1DM) from the continuous glucose monitoring in women with T1DM in pregnancy trial [CONCEPTT (Continuous Glucose Monitoring in Women With Type 1 Diabetes in Pregnancy Trial)] were categorized as: (1) those who were randomized to real-time continuous glucose monitoring (RT-CGM) or self-monitored blood glucose (SMBG), (2) those who used insulin pumps or multiple daily insulin injections (MDIs), and (3) women whose infants were born large for gestational age (LGA). CGM data were taken at baseline and at 24- and 34-weeks' gestation. Multivariable regression analysis was done if temporal differences in 24 hour glucose profiles occurred between comparators in each of the three groups.

Results: A significantly lower glucose [0.4–0.8 mmol/L (7–14 mg/dL)] for 7 h/day (08:00 h to 12:00 h and 16:00 h to 19:00 h) was observed in RT-CGM group as compared with those with SMBG. Women using pumps had significantly higher glucose [0.4–0.9 mmol/L (7–16 mg/dL)] for 12 h/day at 24 weeks compared with MDI. A significantly higher glucose for 4.5 h/day at baseline, for 16 h/day at 24 weeks, and for 14 h/day at 34 weeks, was observed in women who had an LGA infant. The increase was by 0.4–0.7 mmol/L (7–13 mg/dL), 0.4–0.9 mmol/L (7–16 mg/dL) and 0.4–0.7 mmol/L (7–13 mg/dL), respectively.

Conclusion: Better daytime glycemic control can be achieved using RT-CGM, reducing exposure of fetus to higher levels of maternal plasma glucose.

COMMENT

What was Known Prior to this Study?

Maternal glucose levels are dynamic. In addition to the diurnal variation in insulin resistance,[20] factors like diet, physical activity, energy expenditure, stress, sleep, and shift work add to this glycemic variability with even more impact during gestation.[21] The fetus is exposed to this fluctuating glycemic levels. Continuous glucose monitoring (CGM) is one of the most effective ways/tools to measure this blood glucose variability.[22] Standard summary metrics (SSM) are recommended for the reporting of CGM which includes mean CGM glucose levels, the percentage of time spent within the target range (63–140 mg/dL) recommended during pregnancy, and time spent above and below that target range. It also provides the measures of glycemic variability [interquartile range (IQR); mean amplitude of glucose excursions (MAGE); and mean of daily differences (MODD)].[22] A recent trial on type 1 diabetes mellitus (T1DM) showed that RT-CGM was associated with improved neonatal outcomes like a lower incidence of LGA newborns, neonatal hypoglycemia, and neonatal intensive care unit (NICU) admissions as compared to those who used only SMBG. Although, these improvements were likely due to better glucose control, SSM showed no difference in mean glucose levels between these two groups studied. RT-CGM users spent more time in the target glucose range recommended during pregnancy and less time above the range.[23] Another study showed that in patients with T1DM, pump use was associated with an increased incidence of neonatal hypoglycemia and NICU admissions than those who used multiple subcutaneous injections (MSI). The SSM showed that the pump group spent only 5% more time as compared to MSI users.[24] The small differences in SSM reported with significant differences in neonatal outcomes in these studies indicated that there may be differences in temporal glucose profiles, undetected by SSM.

What this Study Adds?

The authors have applied functional data analysis on CGM data to extract information regarding temporal glucose dysregulation that cannot be measured with SSM. They have analyzed data of 200 participants from the CONCEPTT trial[23] in whom >96 hours of CGM and birth weight data were available. For each individual, the mean of the four or more days of temporal CGM data obtained at each glucose time point across the 24 h/day was taken for the analysis. Each of the glucose values at baseline and at 24- and 34-weeks' gestation was recorded. Sequential glucose measurements from each measurement episode were modeled as trajectories by calculating continuous mathematical functions of CGM-derived glucose measurements collected every 5 minutes throughout that measurement episode. By applying the functional data analyses to the CGM data, the authors were able to identify differences in maternal glucose patterns and determine when and for how long during the 24 hours interval were these occurring, even when standard CGM metrics failed to detect a variation. They were able to demonstrate that pregnant women randomized to RT-CGM in the CONCEPTT trial had improved glycemic control during the daytime than women using SMBG alone. This finding suggested that RT-CGM data assisted pregnant women in understanding the impact of behavioral changes on the glycemic profiles, i.e., effect of carbohydrate intake, much better than SMBG does, and better equipped to make informed choices for improved glycemic control. This analysis also demonstrated that the women on insulin pump therapy started pregnancy with better glucose control. However, the 24 weeks' gestation data showed worse daytime glucose control, which possibly contributed to worse neonatal outcomes in the pump users.

Major Strengths of the Study

This trial used data from a large multinational randomized control trial, i.e., thirty trial centers located across six countries—Canada, UK, Spain, Italy, US, and Ireland. Thus, the results are applicable to pregnant women with T1DM from different geographies and ethnic backgrounds. It was one of the largest randomized trials of T1DM patients evaluating the efficacy and safety of RT-CGM in pregnant patients with diabetes for the first time.

Limitations of the Study

As CGM uses interstitial glucose values, the correlation with blood glucose levels during the rapid change of blood glucose levels may not be accurate. In this study, CGM data were obtained only at baseline, and at 24- and 34-weeks' gestation, which do not represent the glycemic status throughout the pregnancy. Moreover, current guideline[22] recommends that 2 weeks of CGM data should be preferred for analysis. The study did not have data of carbohydrate intake which was possibly responsible for the difference in daytime glucose values.

Implications of the Findings for the Clinicians

As this study has demonstrated that daytime hyperglycemia is associated with adverse neonatal outcome in women with T1DM, addressing this may lead to an improved neonatal outcome. Daytime hyperglycemia may be impacted by including more complex carbohydrates in the food intake replacing refined carbohydrates, incorporating post-prandial physical activity, or earlier/timely administration of prandial insulin in relation to meals.[25]

Knowledge Gaps Identified and Scope for Future Research

There is more research required linking the various novel CGM parameters with maternal/neonatal outcomes in patients of T1DM. A larger sample size, detailed record of meal and exercise patterns along with the CGM data will help in identifying measures to improve the glycemic parameters in pregnant women with T1DM.

5. Urinary and Serum Angiogenic Markers in Women with Pre-existing Diabetes During Pregnancy and their Role in Pre-eclampsia Prediction

Ref: Zen M, Padmanabhan S, Zhang K, Kirby A, Cheung NW, Lee VW, et al. Urinary and Serum Angiogenic Markers in Women With Preexisting Diabetes During Pregnancy and Their Role in Pre-eclampsia Prediction. Diabetes Care. 2020;43(1):67-73.

ABSTRACT

Objective: To determine the correlation between urinary and serum placental growth factor (PlGF) and investigate the predictive value as pregnancy progresses of urinary PlGF compared with serum PlGF, soluble fms-like tyrosine kinase-1 (sFLT-1), and the sFLT-1–to–PlGF ratio for the outcome of pre-eclampsia in women with preexisting diabetes.

Research design and methods: A multicenter prospective cohort study was conducted in 158 women with preexisting diabetes (41 with type 1 diabetes mellitus (T1DM) and 117 with type 2 diabetes mellitus (T2DM)) on insulin therapy. Urinary PlGF and serum PlGF, sFLT-1, and the sFLT-1–to–PlGF ratio were assessed four times (14, 24, 30, and 36 weeks' gestation) throughout pregnancy, and the development of pre-eclampsia was recorded and analyzed.

Results: A correlation between urinary and serum PlGF was demonstrated from 24 weeks' gestation onward ($p < 0.001$). At all time-points, those who developed pre-eclampsia had lower serum PlGF levels ($p < 0.05$), and receiver operating characteristic curves demonstrated that serum PlGF in this cohort performed better than the serum sFLT-1–to–PlGF ratio as a predictive test for pre-eclampsia. Preconception glycated hemoglobin (HbA1c) ≥6.5% (48 mmol/mol) was an important factor in predicting pre-eclampsia ($p = 0.01$).

Conclusions: This study prospectively describes the longitudinal changes in urinary PlGF alongside serum angiogenic markers throughout pregnancy in women with preexisting diabetes. We demonstrate correlation between urinary and serum PlGF and that in women with preexisting diabetes in pregnancy, serum PlGF is a better predictor of pre-eclampsia than the sFLT-1–to–PlGF ratio.

COMMENT

What was Known Prior to this Study?

Pre-eclampsia is about four times more common in pregnant women with pregestational diabetes than those who do not have that condition.[26] Identification of biomarkers to help predict the subset of pregnant women at a higher risk of developing pre-eclampsia will help adequate precautionary measures and management. The underlying pathophysiological process of pre-eclampsia appears to be an imbalance between angiogenic and antiangiogenic factors, leading to the development of aberrant placental vasculature and subsequent placental ischemia.[27] Vascular endothelial growth factor (VEGF) and placental growth factor (PlGF) plays a key role in placental angiogenesis during pregnancy. Pre-eclampsia is associated with elevated serum levels of the soluble receptor for VEGF or sFLT-1, which binds to and decreases free levels of VEGF and PlGF.[28,29] Women with diabetes and pre-eclampsia have increased sFLT-1, decreased PlGF, and an increased sFLT-1–to–PlGF ratio;[30,31] however, no study of urinary biomarkers for the prediction of pre-eclampsia in women with type 1 diabetes mellitus (T1DM) has been undertaken before.

What this Study Adds?

This was a hospital-based, multi-center cohort study done across three hospitals in Western Sydney, Australia. The study included women over the age of 16 with singleton pregnancies and a diagnosis of preexisting T1DM or type 2 diabetes mellitus (T2DM) or a new diagnosis of overt diabetes post a 75 g oral glucose tolerance test before 20 weeks' gestation, urinary, and serum PlGF both increased between 14- and 24-weeks' gestation, then remained relatively unchanged by 30 weeks' gestation and slightly decreased at 36 weeks' gestation. In contrast, the sFLT-1–to–PlGF ratio showed an inverse trend. There was a correlation between urinary and serum PlGF. Despite this correlation, urine PlGF was found to be inferior to serum PlGF in predicting pre-eclampsia. Moreover, serum PlGF performed better as a predictive marker than sFLT-1–to–PlGF ratio. Furthermore, serum PlGF was the only biomarker with significantly lower levels throughout pregnancy for women who went on to develop other features of placental insufficiency in addition to pre-eclampsia, i.e., small for gestational age, stillbirth, and premature delivery. Thus, serum PlGF was found to be useful in any trimester in predicting pre-eclampsia with the potential for early implementation of preventative strategies. This study also confirmed that preconception HbA1c ≥6.5% (48 mmol/mol) is an important predictor for pre-eclampsia.

Major Strengths of the Study

As it was a longitudinal study, the predictive potential of various biomarkers could be tested.

Limitations of the Study

They have combined women with mellitus (T1DM), T2DM, and newly diagnosed diabetes before 20 weeks' of pregnancy in the cohort. The sample size for biomarker standardization and predictive value potential should be large and they should be separately studied in different populations of diabetes. However, they performed a subgroup analysis and found the study findings and trends were robust across the subtypes.

Implications of the Findings for the Clinicians

Clinicians are aware of the traditional risk factors for pre-eclampsia in pregestational diabetes, e.g., preconception HbA1c ≥6.5%; nevertheless, biomarkers may help further consolidate the risk of pre-eclampsia in these patients. These will help stratifying the patients based on the level of their risk and preventive measures may be undertaken. Standardization of the biomarkers is a really important aspect to understand the practical implications of the same.

Knowledge Gaps Identified and Scope for Future Research

Larger studies, which include one or the other type of diabetes exclusively to test the biomarkers for prediction of placental hypoperfusion and its clinical consequences. Development of more sensitive kits for serum and urinary PlGF would also be very helpful. Research can also be directed at the development of predictive models of pre-eclampsia by including both traditional and novel biomarkers.

REFERENCES (Gestational Diabetes Mellitus)

1. International Diabetes Federation. (2020). Gestational diabetes. [online] Available from https://www.idf.org/our-activities/care-prevention/gdm [Last accessed February, 2021].
2. Du MC, Ouyang YQ, Nie XF, Huang Y, Redding SR. Effects of physical exercise during pregnancy on maternal and infant outcomes in overweight and obese pregnant women: A meta-analysis. Birth. 2019;46(2):211-21.
3. Dodd JM, Grivell RM, Deussen AR, Hague WM. Metformin for women who are overweight or obese during pregnancy for improving maternal and infant outcomes. Cochrane Database Syst Rev. 2018;7(7):CD010564.
4. Pellonperä O, Mokkala K, Houttu N, Vahlberg T, Koivuniemi E, Tertti K, et al. Efficacy of Fish Oil and/or Probiotic Intervention on the Incidence of Gestational Diabetes Mellitus in an At-Risk Group of Overweight and Obese Women: A Randomized, Placebo-Controlled, Double-Blind Clinical Trial. Diabetes Care. 2019;42(6):1009-17.
5. Corcoy R, Mendoza LC, Simmons D, Desoye G, Adelantado JM, Chico A, et al. The DALI vitamin D randomized controlled trial for gestational diabetes mellitus prevention: No major benefit shown besides vitamin D sufficiency. Clin Nutr. 2020;39(3):976-84.
6. Assaf-Balut C, García de la Torre N, Durán A, Fuentes M, Bordiú E, del Valle L, et al. A Mediterranean diet with additional extra virgin olive oil and pistachios reduces the incidence of gestational diabetes mellitus (GDM): A randomized controlled trial: The St. Carlos GDM prevention study. PLoS One. 2017;12(10):e0185873.
7. Matthews TJ, Hamilton BE. First births to older women continue to rise. NCHS Data Brief. 2014;152:1-8.
8. Liu X, Zou L, Chen Y, Ruan Y, Liu Y, Zhang W. Effects of maternal age on pregnancy: A retrospective cohort study. Zhonghua Yi Xue Za Zhi. 2014;94(25):1984-8.
9. Schummers L, Hutcheon JA, Hacker MR, VanderWeele TJ, Williams PL, McElrath TF, et al. Absolute risks of obstetric outcomes by maternal age at first birth: A population-based cohort. Epidemiology. 2018;29(3):379-87.
10. Wang Y, Chen L, Xiao K, Horswell R, Besse J, Johnson J, et al. Increasing incidence of gestational diabetes mellitus in Louisiana, 1997-2009. J Womens Health. 2012;21(3):319-25.
11. Zhang F, Dong L, Zhang CP, Li B, Wen J, Gao W, et al. Increasing prevalence of gestational diabetes mellitus in Chinese women from 1999 to 2008. Diabet Med. 2011;28(6):652-7.
12. Monroe A. HIV/AIDS and diabetes: Minimizing risk, optimizing care. BETA. 2009;21(2):38-44.
13. Noor MA. The role of protease inhibitors in the pathogenesis of HIV-associated insulin resistance: Cellular mechanisms and clinical implications. Curr HIV/AIDS Rep. 2007;4(3):126-34.
14. Moore R, Adler H, Jackson V, Lawless M, Byrne M, Eogan M, Lambert JS. Impaired glucose metabolism in HIV-infected pregnant women: a retrospective analysis. Int J STD AIDS. 2016;27(7):581-5.
15. Jao J, Wong M, Van Dyke RB, Geffner M, Nshom E, Palmer D, et al. Gestational diabetes mellitus in HIV-infected and -uninfected pregnant women in Cameroon. Diabetes Care. 2013;36(9):e141-2.
16. Soepnel LM, Norris SA, Schrier VJ, Browne JL, Rijken MJ, Gray G, et al. The association between HIV, antiretroviral therapy, and gestational diabetes mellitus. AIDS. 2017;31(1):113-25.
17. González-Tomé MI, Ramos Amador JT, Guillen S, Solís I, Fernández-Ibieta M, Muñoz E, et al. Gestational diabetes mellitus in a cohort of HIV-1 infected women. HIV Med. 2008;9(10):868-74.

18. World Health Organization. Global report on diabetes. 2016.
19. Cho NH, Shaw JE, Karuranga S, Huang Y, da Rocha Fernandes JD, Ohlrogge AW, et al. IDF Diabetes Atlas: Global estimates of diabetes prevalence for 2017 and projections for 2045. Diabetes Res Clin Pract. 2018;138:271-81.
20. Tan E, Scott EM. Circadian rhythms, insulin action, and glucose homeostasis. Curr Opin Clin Nutr Metab Care. 2014;17(4):343-8.
21. Catalano PM, Huston L, Amini SB, Kalhan SC. Longitudinal changes in glucose metabolism during pregnancy in obese women with normal glucose tolerance and gestational diabetes mellitus. Am J Obstet Gynecol. 1999;180(4):903-16.
22. Danne T, Nimri R, Battelino T, Bergenstal RM, Close KL, DeVries JH, et al. International consensus on use of continuous glucose monitoring. Diabetes Care. 2017;40(12):1631-40.
23. Feig DS, Donovan LE, Corcoy R, Murphy KE, Amiel SA, Hunt KF, et al. CONCEPTT Collaborative Group. Continuous glucose monitoring in pregnant women with type 1 diabetes (CONCEPTT): a multicenter international randomised controlled trial. Lancet. 2017;390(10110):2347-59.
24. Feig DS, Corcoy R, Donovan LE, Murphy KE, Barrett JFR, Sanchez JJ, et al. Pumps or multiple daily injections in pregnancy involving type 1 diabetes: A prespecified analysis of the CONCEPTT randomized trial. Diabetes Care. 2018;41(12):2471-9.
25. Luijf YM, van Bon AC, Hoekstra JB, Devries JH. Premeal injection of rapid-acting insulin reduces postprandial glycemic excursions in type 1 diabetes. Diabetes Care. 2010;33(10):2152-5.
26. Bartsch E, Medcalf KE, Park AL, Ray JG, High risk of preeclampsia identification group. Clinical risk factors for preeclampsia determined in early pregnancy: Systematic review and meta-analysis of large cohort studies. BMJ. 2016;353:i1753.
27. Bdolah Y, Sukhatme VP, Karumanchi SA. Angiogenic imbalance in the pathophysiology of preeclampsia: Newer insights. Semin Nephrol. 2004;24(6):548-56.
28. Rana S, Powe CE, Salahuddin S, Verlohren S, Perschel FH, Levine RJ, et al. Angiogenic factors and the risk of adverse outcomes in women with suspected preeclampsia. Circulation. 2012;125(7):911-9.
29. Maynard SE, Venkatesha S, Thadhani R, Karumanchi SA. Soluble Fms-like tyrosine kinase 1 and endothelial dysfunction in the pathogenesis of preeclampsia. Pediatr Res. 2005;57(5):1R-7R.
30. Yu Y, Jenkins AJ, Nankervis AJ, Hanssen KF, Scholz H, Henriksen T, et al. Anti-angiogenic factors and pre-eclampsia in type 1 diabetic women. Diabetologia. 2009;52(1):160-8.
31. Cohen AL, Wenger JB, James-Todd T, Lamparello BM, Halprin E, Serdy S, et al. The association of circulating angiogenic factors and HbA1c with the risk of preeclampsia in women with preexisting diabetes. Hypertens Pregnancy. 2014;33(1):81-92.

Section 7: Drugs and Therapeutics

Sayantan Ray, Pratap Jethwani, Anuj Maheshwari, Sudhir Bhandari

1. Effect of Dapagliflozin on Worsening Heart Failure and Cardiovascular Death in Patients with Heart Failure with and without Diabetes

Ref: Petrie MC, Verma S, Docherty KF, Inzucchi SE, Anand I, Belohlávek J, et al. Effect of Dapagliflozin on Worsening Heart Failure and Cardiovascular Death in Patients With Heart Failure With and Without Diabetes. JAMA. 2020;323(14):1353-68.

ABSTRACT

Importance: There is paucity of literature regarding the additional treatments required in patients of heart failure with reduced ejection fraction (HFrEF). Sodium-glucose cotransporter-2 (SGLT-2) inhibitors may be useful for the treatment in such scenario irrespective of the diabetic status of the patients.

Objective: To explore the effectiveness of dapagliflozin in heart failure (HF) with HFrEF in both diabetic and nondiabetic patients.

Design setting and participants: This exploratory trial was conducted in 20 countries with 410 sites. This phase 3 randomized trial planned for 1 year recruited patients with New York Heart Association (NYHA) classification II to IV with an ejection fraction of ≤40% and elevated plasma N-terminal pro B-type natriuretic peptide from February 15, 2017 to August 17, 2018. The final follow-up was conducted on June 6, 2019.

Interventions: Supplementation of 10 mg dapagliflozin once a day or placebo to the recommended therapy.

Main outcomes and measures: The primary outcome, i.e., an episode of worsening of HF or cardiovascular death, was analyzed and compared based on the diabetic status, i.e., diabetic and nondiabetic as well as on the level of glycated hemoglobin (HbA1c), i.e., HbA1c ≥ 5.7% and HbA1c level < 5.7%.

Results: Total 4,744 patients were enrolled in the trial with mean age of 66 years and 1,109 (23%) women. 2,605 participants (55%) were nondiabetic patients. Among all the participants, 4,742 completed the trial. Among the nondiabetic participants, the primary outcome occurred in 171 of 1,298 (13.2%) in dapagliflozin receiving group and 231 of 1,307 (17.7%) in placebo receiving group [hazard ratio (HR) 0.73 (95% CI 0.60–0.88)]. Whereas among the diabetic participants, the primary outcome occurred in 215 of 1,075 (20.0%) in dapagliflozin receiving group and 271 of 1,064 (25.5%) in placebo receiving group [HR 0.75 (95% CI 0.63–0.90)] (P value for interaction = 0.80). Among patients with HbA1c < 5.7%, the primary outcome occurred in 53 of 438 patients (12.1%) in dapagliflozin receiving group and 71 of 419 (16.9%) in placebo receiving group [HR 0.67 (95% CI 0.47–0.96)]. Whereas in patients with a HbA1c of ≥5.7%, the primary outcome occurred in 118 of 860 patients (13.7%) in dapagliflozin receiving group and 160 of 888 (18.0%) in placebo receiving group [HR 0.74 (95% CI 0.59–0.94)) (P value for interaction = 0.72). Among nondiabetic patients, volume depletion was seen in 7.3% patients in dapagliflozin receiving group and 6.1% in placebo receiving group. Whereas among diabetic patients, it was seen in 7.8% patients in dapagliflozin receiving group and 7.8% in placebo receiving group. Another adverse event related to kidney was reported in 4.8% patients in dapagliflozin receiving group and 6.0% in placebo receiving group among patients and among nondiabetic patients. Whereas in 8.5% of patients in dapagliflozin receiving group and 8.7% in placebo receiving group among diabetic patients.

Conclusion and relevance: This randomized trial concluded that addition of dapagliflozin to recommended therapy significantly reduced the risk of worsening HF or cardiovascular death in patients with HFrEF as compared to placebo irrespective of their diabetes status.

COMMENT

What was Known Prior to this Study?

The profound effects of sodium-glucose cotransporter-2 (SGLT-2) inhibition on the risks of cardiovascular (CV) complications in patients with diabetes have provided for rapid and substantive changes to diabetes guidelines. Dapagliflozin and Prevention of Adverse Outcomes in Heart Failure (DAPA-HF) trial[1] was the first large-scale trial of an SGLT-2 inhibitor designed particularly to assess the effects of the drug on CV endpoints in patients with heart failure (HF). The high-quality trial showed definitive evidence of protection against a broad range of CV and kidney complications for patients with HF and reduced ejection fraction (HFrEF). The design feature of the DAPA-HF trial that distinguished it from its predecessors was the inclusion of patients without diabetes.

What this Study Adds?

Petrie and colleagues[2] report findings from a highly informative exploratory analysis of this recent large-scale clinical trial of dapagliflozin. They defined the effects of SGLT-2 inhibition on various outcomes among patients with diabetes versus those without diabetes. The investigators enrolled 4,744 patients with HFrEF from 410 sites in 20 countries. The majority of participants [2,605 (55%)] had no history of diabetes at baseline. The primary outcome was a composite of worsening HF or CV death. Among patients with diabetes, the primary outcome occurred in 215 of 1,075 patients (20.0%) in the dapagliflozin group and 271 of 1,064 patients (25.5%) in the placebo group. Among participants without diabetes, the primary outcome occurred in 171 of 1,298 (13.2%) patients in the dapagliflozin group and 231 of 1,307 patients (17.7%) in the placebo group. Results were similarly consistent across those with and without diabetes for each individual component of the primary composite endpoint, for secondary measures assessing effects on kidney function, and for death from any cause (P value for heterogeneity for all ≥0.22).

Strengths and Limitations of the Study

Although these findings are based on post hoc and exploratory analyses, they are compelling. The study was large; the effects of the drug were clinically meaningful; and, unlike many subgroup analyses of randomized trials, there was reasonable statistical power to address the questions posed. Consequently, the likelihood that the benefits observed for the subgroup of patients without diabetes arose by chance is small. The conclusion of benefits irrespective of the presence of diabetes in the DAPA-HF trial is further strengthened by this exploratory analysis by Petrie et al.

Implications of the Findings for the Clinicians

The observation of benefit for the patients without diabetes in DAPA-HF trial may have the most far-reaching implications. These results may suggest the next chapter for this class of drugs—the transition from a glucose-lowering agent that provides cardioprotection agent to a cardioprotective agent that happens to lower blood glucose.[3] It may also mark the beginning of a new treatment option for patients with HFrEF without T2DM.

Knowledge Gaps Identified and Scope for Future Research

A key outstanding question regarding the role of SGLT-2 inhibition in HF is whether the benefits observed for patients with HFrEF will also be observed in patients with HF and preserved ejection fraction. The DELIVER (Dapagliflozin Evaluation to Improve the LIVEs of Patients with Preserved Ejection Fraction Heart Failure; NCT03619213) study will specifically address this question.

2. Glycemic Efficacy and Safety of Glucagon-like Peptide-1 Receptor Agonist on Top of Sodium-glucose Cotransporter-2 Inhibitor Treatment Compared to Sodium-glucose Cotransporter-2 Inhibitor Alone: A Systematic Review and Meta-analysis of Randomized Controlled Trials

Ref: Patoulias D, Stavropoulos K, Imprialos K, Katsimardou A, Kalogirou MS, Koutsampasopoulos K, et al. Glycemic efficacy and safety of glucagon-like peptide-1 receptor agonist on top of sodium-glucose cotransporter-2 inhibitor treatment compared to sodium-glucose cotransporter-2 inhibitor alone: A systematic review and meta-analysis of randomized controlled trials. Diabetes Res Clin Pract. 2019;158:107927.

ABSTRACT

Objective: This meta-analysis evaluates the glycemic efficacy and safety of addition of glucagon-like peptide-1 receptor agonists (GLP-1RA) in patients with type 2 diabetes mellitus (T2DM) who are already receiving sodium-glucose cotransporter-2 (SGLT-2) inhibitors for glycemic control.

Research design and methods: Randomized controlled trials (RCTs) of ≥12 weeks duration on patients of T2DM that evaluated the safety and efficacy of supplementing a GLP-1RA with a SGLT-2 inhibitors compared to SGLT-2 inhibitors alone were searched in PubMed and CENTRAL, along with gray literature till May, 2019. The credibility of the summary estimates were evaluated using Grading of Recommendations Assessment, Development and Evaluation (GRADE) approach.

Results: Pooled data of 1,042 patients from three selected RCTs were retrieved. GLP-1RA (maximum dose) and SGLT-2 inhibitors treatment compared to SGLT-2 inhibitors only, resulted in statistically significant reduction in glycated hemoglobin (HbA1c) by 0.91% (95% CI −1.41 to −0.42) (GRADE: moderate). Body weight reduced by 1.95 kg (95% CI −3.83 to −0.07) (GRADE: moderate), and fasting plasma glucose reduced by 1.53 mmol/L (95% CI −2.17 to −0.88) (GRADE: moderate). The systolic blood pressure levels fall by 3.64 mm Hg (95% CI −6.24 to −1.03). No such effect was seen on lipid profile and diastolic blood pressure. The risk for any hypoglycemia [relative risk (RR) 2.62, 95% CI 1.15–5.96, $I^2 = 33\%$] (GRADE: moderate) and nausea (RR 3.21, 95% CI 1.36–7.54, $I^2 = 63\%$) (GRADE: moderate) increased significantly. An increase in the risk for diarrhea (RR 1.64, 95% CI 0.98–2.75, $I^2 = 0\%$) (GRADE: low) was not significant.

Conclusions: GLP-1RA/SGLT-2 inhibitors combination showed improved glycemic control and body weight loss, if tolerated well. However, it can increase risk for any hypoglycemia and gastrointestinal adverse events.

COMMENT

What was Known Prior to this Study?

Glucagon-like peptide-1 receptor agonists (GLP-1RA) and sodium-dependent glucose cotransporter-2 inhibitors (SGLT-2i) have shown clinically significant benefits on hemoglobin A1c (HbA1c), weight, blood pressure, and cardiorenal outcomes. Both GLP-1RAs and SGLT-2i are associated with minimal risk of hypoglycemia.[4] The distinct and complementary advantages of these two drug classes provide a compelling argument for combining GLP-1RA with SGLT-2i therapy. This concept has already been examined in various randomized controlled trials (RCTs) to determine the efficacy and safety profiles of this combination of antidiabetic agents.[5-7]

What this Study Adds?

This systematic review was done for the identification and critical appraisal of the RCTs relevant to the study and to summarize and provide the effect estimates of the safety and efficacy of the addition of a GLP-1RA (injectable or oral) to the antidiabetic regimen of type 2 diabetic patients including a SGLT-2i.[8] Three trials were included by Patoulias et al. in this meta-analysis, i.e., the DURATION-8,[6] AWARD-10[7] and SUSTAIN 9[9] clinical trials. The data comparing addition of GLP-1RA or placebo to SGLT-2i were extracted. The glycemic efficacy of GLP-1RA and SGLT-2i combination were compared to SGLT-2i alone as the primary efficacy outcome by the absolute change in HbA1c levels (%). This meta-analysis demonstrated a significant decrease in glycemic parameters, i.e., HbA1c and fasting plasma glucose by adding a GLP-1RA at the maximum dose to the antidiabetic regimen including a SGLT-2i in type 2 diabetic patients. This combination also resulted in a significant decrease by 1.95 kg in weight and decrease in systolic blood pressure (SBP) levels by 3.64 mm Hg as compared to SGLT-2i alone. On the other hands, the odds for any hypoglycemia and the incidence of minor gastrointestinal adverse events, i.e., nausea and diarrhea were reported to increase by the GLP-1RA/SGLT-2i combination.

Strengths and Limitations of the Study

The precise effect estimates on key safety and efficacy outcomes of a GLP-1RA and SGLT-2i combination were provided by this systematic review and meta-analysis first which included all the available, relevant RCTs in type 2 diabetic patients receiving an antidiabetic regimen including a SGLT-2i. By in list of limitations, high heterogeneity was observed in this study and subgroup analyses could not be performed in the participants according to the different SGLT-2i. Additionally, the data regarding the safety and efficacy of GLP-1RA/SGLT-2i combination of the participants according to age, gender, ethnicity, and baseline HbA1c were not provided by the author.

Implications of the Findings for the Clinicians

A recent updated meta-analysis[10] confirmed these observations[8] regarding the therapeutic potential of the SGLT-2i/GLP-1RA combination and its effect on cardiometabolic risk factors, although data on mortality and cardiovascular (CV) outcomes were scarce.

Knowledge Gaps Identified and Scope for Future Research

It remains under question whether the improvements in established CV risk factors, such as body weight and SBP, are translated into a benefit for those patients. No such data regarding the CV efficacy of that combination, questioning whether those two drug classes exhibit additive cardioprotective effects or not. Adequately powered trials assessing other indices, besides the established, "classic" ones, will shed light on the potential CV synergy of these two drug classes, which has to be proven.

3. Once-weekly Insulin for Type 2 Diabetes without Previous Insulin Treatment

Ref: Rosenstock J, Bajaj HS, Janež A, Silver R, Begtrup K, Hansen MV, et al. Once-weekly insulin for type 2 diabetes without previous insulin treatment. N Engl J Med. 2020;383(22):2107-16.

ABSTRACT

Introduction: In patients who have type 2 diabetes mellitus (T2DM), decreasing the frequency of basal insulin injections is believed to increase treatment acceptance as well as adherence. Insulin icodec, a basal insulin analog, is designed for administration once a week; it is still in developmental stage for the treatment of diabetes.

Methods: This was a randomized, double-blind, double-dummy, and phase 2 trial conducted for evaluating the efficacy as well as safety of once-weekly insulin icodec in comparison to once-daily insulin glargine U100; this study was conducted for a duration of 26 weeks. The study population included patients who had not received insulin treatment for a long-term previously and whose T2DM was not effectively controlled [level of glycated hemoglobin (HbA1c), 7.0–9.5%] at the time of receiving metformin along with or without a dipeptidyl peptidase-4 (DPP-4) inhibitor. The change in HbA1c level from baseline to 26th week was considered as the primary endpoint. Evaluation of safety endpoints, consisting of episodes of hypoglycemia as well as insulin-related adverse events, was done.

Results: Study population included 247 participants, who were randomized (1:1) to receive either icodec or glargine. There was no significant difference in baseline characteristics between the two groups. The mean baseline HbA1c level in the icodec group and the glargine group was 8.09% and 7.96%, respectively. The estimated mean change from baseline in the HbA1c level in the icodec group was −1.33% points and in the glargine group was −1.15% points, to estimated means of 6.69% and 6.87%, respectively. At week 26; the estimated between-group difference in the change from baseline was −0.18% points [95% confidence interval (CI) −0.38–0.02, $p = 0.08$]. This was found that the rates of hypoglycemia with severity of level 2 (i.e., level of blood glucose, <54 mg/dL) or level 3 (i.e., severe cognitive impairment) were low (in the icodec group 0.53 events per patient-year and in the glargine group 0.46 events per patient-year; estimated rate ratio, 1.09; 95% CI 0.45–2.65). No between-group difference in insulin-related key adverse events was noted. There were low rates of hypersensitivity as well as injection site reactions. Majority of the adverse events were mild; no serious events were appeared to be associated with the medications of the trial.

Conclusion: In patients who have T2DM, treatment with once-weekly insulin icodec demonstrated to be glucose-lowering efficacy as well as a safety profile comparable to once-daily insulin glargine U100. (Funded by Novo Nordisk; NN1436-4383 ClinicalTrials.gov number, NCT03751657. opens in new tab).

COMMENT

What was Known Prior to this Study?

The increasing incidence of type 2 diabetes mellitus (T2DM) and of health consequences related to complications from poor glycemic control is of major concern. Even with the introduction of new adjunctive medicines, recombinant insulins, and the ability to monitor blood glucose in real time, treatment for diabetes remains less than ideal.[11] Patients for whom oral agents such as metformin, sulfonylureas, and dipeptidyl peptidase-4 (DPP-4) inhibitors have become ineffective may now be offered a choice of one of the newer therapies or once daily basal insulin treatment.

Nevertheless, insulin therapy is cumbersome and requires at least daily injections, which may result in poor compliance and clinical inertia. Therefore, longer-acting basal insulins that provide glycemic control with fewer injections are needed.

What this Study Adds?

In this context, Rosenstock et al. present an attempt to simplify the delivery of basal insulin therapy for T2DM patients with a once-weekly formulation of insulin icodec. Insulin icodec is a novel insulin with a half-life of 196 hours that allows for once-weekly dosing.[12] The investigators compared weekly insulin icodec with daily insulin glargine U100 in a rigorous double-blind, double-dummy trial in which the effects of these insulins were examined for 26 weeks. The trial population included patients whose diabetes was inadequately controlled with metformin with or without a DPP-4 inhibitors and who had not previously received long-term insulin treatment. The authors used treat-to-target algorithms that aggressively increased the dose of each type of insulin to reach fasting blood glucose (FBG) targets. The glycated hemoglobin (HbA1c) level in the icodec group decreased from 8.1% to 6.7%, and that in the glargine group decreased from 8.0% to 6.9%; icodec achieved these glycemic targets with a lower overall dose of insulin. Icodec was associated with no major adverse events.

Strengths and Limitations of the Study

A strength of this study was the double-blind, double-dummy design. The high number of patients who completed therapy during the 26 week treatment period was another strength. Regarding limitations, this phase 2 trial was not powered to detect significant differences between treatments for any endpoint. The incidence of mild hypoglycemia was slightly higher in the icodec group, but the trial was not powered to detect significance. Further investigation will be needed in a larger and more diverse patient population to evaluate the hypoglycemic profile of icodec.

Implications of the Findings for the Clinicians

Once-weekly insulin therapy would be easier than daily therapy for patients with T2DM who are planning to incorporate insulin into their treatment regimens. However, since there is an expanding number of a therapeutic option for T2DM patients, the particular population included in the trial may not represent the typical patient with diabetes. Further studies are therefore warranted to determine how once-weekly insulin can be incorporated into treatment algorithms.

Knowledge Gaps Identified and Scope for Future Research

Although the simplicity of a once-weekly therapy is an advantage, the inability to vary the dose might make it harder for patients who are trying to incorporate exercise into their care regimens. This is equally relevant for patients with type 1 diabetes mellitus (T1DM), especially those who are very physically active.[13] The pharmacokinetics of icodec are being investigated in patients with T1DM (ClinicalTrials.gov number, NCT03723772). Overall, this trial represents an advance that may eventually add another agent to our armamentarium for the treatment of diabetes. Real world pragmatic studies assessing quality of life and feasibility of weekly insulin are still needed in people with T1DM and in people with a history of poor compliance with insulin therapy before icodec can be widely used.

4. Efficacy and Safety of the Glucagon Receptor Antagonist RVT-1502 in Type 2 Diabetes Uncontrolled on Metformin Monotherapy: A 12-Week Dose-ranging Study

Ref: Pettus JH, D'Alessio D, Frias JP, Vajda EG, Pipkin JD, Rosenstock J, et al. Efficacy and safety of the glucagon receptor antagonist RVT-1502 in type 2 diabetes uncontrolled on metformin monotherapy: A 12-week dose-ranging study. Diabetes Care. 2020;43(1):161-8.

ABSTRACT

Background: For type 2 diabetic patients where metformin is insufficient to maintain the optimum sugar levels, RVT-1502, a glucagon receptor antagonist (GRA), can be useful for improving glycemic control.

Research design and methods: We conducted a phase 2, double-blind, randomized, placebo-controlled study with 166 patients of type 2 diabetes mellitus (T2DM) on a fixed dose of metformin. They were randomly divided into four groups (1:1:1:1) to receive placebo, 5 mg, 10 mg, and 15 mg of RVT-1502 once daily for 12 weeks. Any change from baseline values of hemoglobin A1c (HbA1c) for each dose of RVT-1502 received, compared with placebo was taken as the primary endpoint. Change from baseline values of fasting glucose and safety assessments were the secondary endpoints.

Results: There was a reduction HbA1c and fasting plasma glucose (FPG) by 0.74% and 2.1 mmol/L relative to placebo in 5 mg group of RVT-1502 over 12 weeks ($p < 0.001$), respectively. For 10 mg group, reduction was 0.76% and 2.2 mmol/L, while for 15 mg group, it was 1.05% and 2.6 mmol/L ($p < 0.001$), respectively. An HbA1c < 7.0% was achieved in 19.5%, 39.5%, 39.5%, and 45.0% in the four groups, respectively ($p \leq 0.02$ vs. placebo). None of the episodes of hypoglycemia were severe. Mild reversible elevation of mean aminotransferase levels, unrelated to dose, was observed with RVT-1502. No significant difference in weight and lipid levels were observed across the groups. Mild elevation of blood pressure was inconsistent and unrelated to dose.

Conclusion: RVT-1502 has a great potential to lower HbA1c and FPG. Further longer duration studies are warranted to establish its safety profile and support further clinical development. (NCT02851849).

COMMENT

What was Known Prior to this Study?

Pancreatic α-cells are the major source of glucagon, a hormone that counteracts the hypoglycemic action of insulin and strongly contributes to the correction of acute hypoglycemia. Patients with diabetes mellitus (DM) display two main alterations of glucagon secretion: A relative hyperglucagonemia that aggravates hyperglycemia, and an impaired glucagon response to hypoglycemia.[14] Actions of dipeptidyl peptidase-4 (DPP-4) inhibitors and glucagon-like peptide-1 receptor agonists (GLP-1RAs) on hepatic glucose output suggest that targeting glucagon metabolism can improve glycemic control. Glucagon and GLP-1 act on their own receptors, glucagon receptor (GR), and GLP-1R, respectively, which are both coupled to Gs and, to a lesser extent, to Gq.[15] GR inhibition could be an attractive way to normalize blood glucose. The antiglucagon treatment with glucagon receptor antagonists (GRAs) is very efficient to decrease glycemia and several animal studies have even been performed.[16-18] Early clinical trials evaluating GRAs show these agents reduce fasting plasma glucose (FPG) and hemoglobin A1c (HbA1c) in type 2 diabetes mellitus (T2DM).[19,20] However, GRA treatment has been associated with dose-dependent adverse effects on lipids, BP, weight, and liver enzymes and increases in hypoglycemia which have so far hampered clinical development of GRAs.[21]

RVT-1502 is a novel, orally bioavailable small molecule GRA being developed to improve glycemic control in adults with diabetes. It is structurally distinct from other small molecule GRAs, containing a sulfonic acid tail rather than a carboxylic acid tail. Pharmacological activity of RVT-1502 appears to be mediated primarily by GR signaling, with minimal evidence of off-target pharmacological effects. In vitro, RVT-1502 binds to the GR with high affinity and selectivity and suppresses glucagon-stimulated cyclic adenosine monophosphate (cAMP) and glucose production.[22] In phase 1 studies, RVT-1502 demonstrated favorable safety, tolerability, and pharmacokinetics in healthy volunteers and subjects with T2DM.[23]

What this Study Adds?

Pettus et al. describe the results of a 12-week, phase 2 dose-ranging study of RVT-1502 5 mg, 10 mg, or 15 mg once daily versus placebo in subjects with T2DM on a stable dose of metformin.[24] In this phase 2 study of RVT-1502, all doses of the drug were well tolerated and significantly reduced HbA1c and FPG over 12 weeks relative to placebo. The incidence of hypoglycemia was low, and no severe events occurred during the study. Weight increased modestly but significantly in the PF-06291874 study.[25] However, in this trial, weight remained stable in all treatment groups.

Strengths and Limitations of the Study

Glucagon receptor antagonism to treat hyperglycemia in T2DM has been pursued for several decades, but no drugs with this mechanism of action are currently available for clinical use. RVT-1502 shows similar HbA1c reductions at lower doses than other GRAs tested to date, which could potentially reduce the risk of off-target adverse effects during chronic therapy. Thus, the results of the current study support continued clinical development of RVT-1502 in subjects with T2DM.

Implications of the Findings for the Clinicians

Inhibition of the glucagon response by RVT-1502 in the fasted state may abrogate the increased overnight gluconeogenesis found in early T2DM, as reflected by the decrease in FPG, while the potential concomitant improvements in fasting insulin sensitivity and insulin secretion in response to an oral glucose load may address the impaired insulin action in the fed state in clinically manifest T2DM.[24] These results support this GRA as a potential novel treatment for T2DM.

Knowledge Gaps Identified and Scope for Future Research

Preclinical models have demonstrated that GLP-1 contributes to the improved glucose tolerance in the setting of reduced GR signaling.[26] In this study, there were increases in total and active GLP-1 relative to baseline with some doses of RVT-1502, and a significant increase in total GLP-1 with RVT-1502 10 mg compared with placebo. Taken together, these findings suggest a mechanism that merits further investigation. GR antagonism may be associated with worsening underlying disease [cardiovascular outcomes, nonalcoholic steatohepatitis (NASH)] in individuals with T2DM, long-term GRA treatment should only be implemented for T2DM if these safety concerns can be mitigated. In this context, possible endpoints to be considered for future clinical trials would include measurement of liver fat, 24-hour blood pressure (BP) monitoring and continuous glucose monitoring.

5. Optimization of Metformin in the GRADE Cohort: Effect on Glycemia and Body Weight

Ref: Sivitz WI, Phillips LS, Wexler DJ, Fortmann SP, Camp AW, Tiktin M, et al. Optimization of Metformin in the GRADE Cohort: Effect on Glycemia and Body Weight. Diabetes Care. 2020;43(5):940-7.

ABSTRACT

Objective: Optimization of metformin dosing by evaluating the effect on glycemia and body weight in type 2 diabetes mellitus (T2DM).

Research design and methods: A total of 6,823 participants were included in the Glycemia Reduction Approaches in Diabetes: A Comparative Effectiveness Study (GRADE). The participants took only metformin as antidiabetic drug and completed a 4- to 14-week (mean ± SD 7.9 ± 2.4) run-in dose adjustment to 2,000 mg/day or a maximally tolerated lower dose. They had T2DM for <10 years and a hemoglobin A1c (HbA1c) ≥ 6.8% (51 mmol/mol) while taking ≥500 mg of metformin/day. Counseling on diet and exercises was provided. Change in HbA1c during run-in was the primary outcome.

Results: On increasing the dose by 1,000 mg/day, change in HbA1c was −0.65 ± 0.02%. HbA1c varied by −0.48 ± 0.02% and by −0.23 ± 0.07% when the dose was unchanged or decreased, respectively. Higher HbA1c at entry predicted greater reduction in HbA1c ($p < 0.001$) in univariate and multivariate analyses. Weight loss adjusted for duration of run-in averaged 0.91 ± 0.05 kg in participants who increased metformin by ≥1,000 mg/day (n = 1,894).

Conclusion: Glycemia and HbA1c values in T2DM can be improved by optimizing dose of metformin to either 2,000 mg/day or a maximally tolerated lower dose. This should be in combination with compliance to medication and lifestyle modifications.

COMMENT

What was Known Prior to this Study?

The incremental effect of metformin when the dose is increased in persons taking less than a maximum dose is not clear. This is a relevant clinical issue, particularly for patients taking <2,000 mg/day who may have hemoglobin A1c (HbA1c) values within a designated target range but still above normal and hence, have suboptimal glycemic control. To better define the extent to which average glycemia can be improved by optimizing metformin dosing can improve our understanding of this issue. The ongoing Glycemia Reduction Approaches in Diabetes: A Comparative Effectiveness Study (GRADE) offers insight in this respect.

What this Study Adds?

GRADE (Glycemia Reduction Approaches in Diabetes: A Comparative Effectiveness Study) is designed to determine the relative effectiveness of four commonly used glucose-lowering medications when added to metformin.[27] Authors report the impact of optimizing metformin dose during the run-in phase of the GRADE study on glycemic control and body weight and evaluate predictors of glycemic response. To enter run-in, participants had to be taking metformin as the sole glucose-lowering medication and to have HbA1c levels ≥6.8%. For participants taking a dose <2,000 mg/day or >2,000 mg/day, the dose was adjusted to 2,000 mg/day as tolerated. The primary outcome was the change in HbA1c between the screening and final run-in visits. Secondary outcome was change in weight, measured twice in light clothing. Adjusting dosage to 2,000 mg/day or to a maximally tolerated lower dose was associated with a mean decrease in HbA1c of 0.52 ± 0.94%. Greater increases in dosing were associated with greater reductions in HbA1c. Authors observed that in participants whose metformin dose was reduced, either because they were taking >2,000 mg at the time of initial run-in or because of intolerance, HbA1c improved less than in participants whose dose was unchanged. There were no reports of severe hypoglycemia during the GRADE run-in.

Strengths and Limitations of the Study

In this study, authors adjusted metformin dosing in persons already taking the drug, typical of what would be done in clinical practice. The unique feature of this study that distinguished it from others was that it compared the effects of differential adjustments in metformin dosage in participants already taking the drug and not using another glucose lowering drug. Nonadherence was lower in this study than in other reports.[28] A total of 90.7% of participants were at 2,000 mg/day, supporting tolerance to metformin. Participants with no change in metformin dosing also exhibited decreases in HbA1c levels, suggesting that improvement in adherence to the medication and/or lifestyle behavior also contributed. The run-in period was variable and as low as 4 weeks for participants entering the study already taking 2,000 mg/day. Therefore, changes in HbA1c in those with short duration of follow-up may have underestimated the effect.

Implications of the Findings for the Clinicians

There may be benefit from metformin dose adjustment in many patients with type 2 diabetes mellitus (T2DM). The improvement is likely to be greater in those with a higher initial HbA1c. In persons on submaximal metformin therapy, these study findings serve as a guide that could help to improve management.

---

6. Combined GLP-1, Oxyntomodulin, and Peptide YY Improves Body Weight and Glycemia in Obesity and Prediabetes/Type 2 Diabetes: A Randomized, Single-blinded, Placebo-controlled Study

Ref: Behary P, Tharakan G, Alexiadou K, Johnson N, Wewer Albrechtsen NJ, Kenkre J, et al. Combined GLP-1, Oxyntomodulin, and Peptide YY Improves Body Weight and Glycemia in Obesity and Prediabetes/Type 2 Diabetes: A Randomized, Single-Blinded, Placebo-Controlled Study. Diabetes Care. 2019;42(8):1446-53.

ABSTRACT

Objective: To study the effects of glucagon-like peptide-1 (GLP-1), oxyntomodulin (OXM), and peptide YY (PYY) ("GOP") infusion on glycemia and body weight in patients with diabetes and obesity.

Research design and methods: A total of 15 obese patients with prediabetes/diabetes were randomly infused GOP or 11 were infused saline infusion for 4 weeks, in this single-blinded mechanistic study. 21 patients who had undergone Roux-en-Y gastric bypass (RYGB) and 22 patients who followed a very low-calorie diet (VLCD) as unblinded comparators, were also included in the study. Outcomes measured were—(1) body weight, (2) fructosamine levels, (3) glucose and insulin during a mixed meal test (MMT), (4) energy expenditure (EE), (5) energy intake (EI), and (6) mean glucose and measures of glucose variability (GV) during continuous glucose monitoring (CGM).

Results: Weight loss with GOP infusion was more than saline infusion {[mean change −4.4 (95% CI −5.3, −3.5) kg] vs. [−2.5 (−4.1, −0.9) kg]} ($p = 0.025$). Also, fructosamine levels improved more with GOP ($p = 0.0026$) [−44.1 (−62.7, −25.5) µmol/L]. There was a reduction in glycemic variability and better glucose tolerance compared to RYGB and VLCD.

Conclusion: There was an improvement in glycemia control and reduction in body weight over 4 weeks of GOP infusion. Superior glucose tolerance and reduced GV compared with RYGB and VLCD was achieved. GOP is a viable alternative for the treatment of diabetes with favorable effects on body weight.

COMMENT

What was Known Prior to this Study?

Glycemic improvement after bariatric surgery is superior to intensive medical management and is sustained.[29] Roux-en-Y gastric bypass (RYGB) in particular, exerts many of its beneficial effects by activating the exaggerated release of glucagon-like peptide-1 (GLP-1), peptide YY (PYY), and oxyntomodulin (OXM) after eating, leading to improvements in glucose metabolism, suppression of appetite, and reductions in body weight.[30,31] These observations suggest alterations in gut hormone secretion contribute to sustained weight loss and glucose control.[30,32] An alternate approach has been to attempt to mimic the results of bariatric surgery with infusions of native gut peptides at concentrations similar to the ones observed after bariatric surgery. Acute studies that coinfused GLP-1, PYY, and OXM into obese volunteers showed promising results on food intake.[33]

What this Study Adds?

Behary et al.[34] present a mechanistic study using an infusion of combination of GLP-1, OXM, and PYY (GOP). It was a single-blinded randomized controlled study comparing two infusion groups (GOP or saline) in patients with obesity and prediabetes or T2DM. Two further similar nonblinded groups of patients undergoing RYGB and patients following a very low-calorie diet (VLCD) diet were recruited. The primary outcome of the study was the change in body weight at 4 weeks. Secondary outcomes were change in glycemia (as assessed by fructosamine measurement), change in ad libitum and 24-hour total energy expenditure (EE) [energy intake (EI)], fasting and postprandial glucose and insulin levels in response to a mixed meal test (MMT), glucose variability (GV) as assessed by continuous glucose monitoring (CGM); and EE. GOP infusion at home was feasible and well tolerated over a 4-week period. It led to a substantial mean weight loss of 4.4 kg. GOP achieves superior glucose tolerance to VLCD, reduces GV, and lowers the risk of provoking hypoglycemia compared with RYGB.

Strengths and Limitations of the Study

The study is limited by a relatively small sample size and short duration. It was not powered to show differences in the secondary endpoints or in safety and tolerability characteristics. Lastly, the study was not designed to examine the contribution of the individual hormones to the overall effect.

Implications of the Findings for the Clinicians

Glucagon-like peptide-1, OXM, and PYY achieved these improvements with a smaller weight loss compared with RYGB and VLCD. This proof-of-concept study suggests that triple agonism of the GLP-1, glucagon, and Y2 receptors using the GOP combination may possess advantages even over RYGB.

Knowledge Gaps Identified and Scope for Future Research

Dual and triple hormone combinations are emerging as a promising strategy for such development.[35] However, further studies are required to explore the doses and combinations to obtain optimal efficacies. Moreover, GOP replicates only postsurgical postprandial gut hormone levels but not the surgical anatomical changes. It also seems fair to say that academic researchers and pharmaceutical industry have not yet struck on the optimal combination for treatment at this present moment.

7. Hypoglycemia is Reduced with Use of Inhaled Technosphere® Insulin Relative to Insulin Aspart in Type 1 Diabetes Mellitus

Ref: Seaquist ER, Blonde L, McGill JB, Heller SR, Kendall DM, Bumpass JB, et al. Hypoglycaemia is reduced with use of inhaled Technosphere® Insulin relative to insulin aspart in type 1 diabetes mellitus. Diabet Med. 2020;37(5):752-9.

ABSTRACT

Aim: To evaluate the effect of inhaled Technosphere® insulin (TI) relative to subcutaneous insulin aspart, on the incidence of hypoglycemia in type 1 diabetic patients in accordance with the recommendations of the International Hypoglycemia Study Group.

Methods: A randomized, phase 3, multicenter AFFINITY-1 study was conducted that included 375 adults with type 1 diabetics of ≥12 months duration and a hemoglobin A1c (HbA1c) level of 7.5–10.0%. They received basal insulin plus either inhaled TI or subcutaneous insulin aspart, in a randomized order. Three levels of hypoglycemia were defined as blood glucose levels of ≤3.9 mmol/L, <3.0 mmol/L, or requiring external assistance for recovery. Primary outcome measures were incidence rates of the three levels and number of hypoglycemic events.

Results: Technosphere insulin had fewer level 1 and 2 hypoglycemic events and a lower incidence of level 3 hypoglycemia, observed across the range of end-of-treatment HbA1c levels. Also, higher rates of hypoglycemia were observed after 30–60 minutes of meals, that reduced significantly after 2–6 hours of meal.

Conclusion: Technosphere insulin is associated with a clinically noninferior glycemic control and lower hypoglycemia rates across a range of HbA1c levels than insulin aspart.

COMMENT

What was Known Prior to this Study?

Technosphere insulin (TI), a dry powder formulation of recombinant human insulin adsorbed onto Technosphere microparticles for oral inhalation, is an ultra-rapid-acting prandial inhaled insulin that has a faster onset (~12 min) and shorter duration (<3 h) of action than currently available subcutaneously injected insulins.[36,37] The 24-week, phase 3 AFFINITY-1 study in type 1 diabetic patients demonstrated noninferior glycemic control of prandial TI to prandial insulin aspart.[38] The categorization of hypoglycemia in clinical trials as level 1 (blood glucose level ≤ 3.9 mmol/L), level 2 (blood glucose < 3.0 mmol/L), or level 3 hypoglycemia (severe cognitive impairment requiring outside assistance for recovery) has been suggested by the International Hypoglycemia Study Group since publication of the AFFINITY-1 trial.[39] The data collected during AFFINITY-1 were needed to be interpreted from the perspective of these new recommendations.

What this Study Adds

The incidence and event rates of level 1, 2, and 3 hypoglycemia were compared as the primary objective of this post-hoc regression analysis by Seaquist et al.[40] on the basis of final hemoglobin A1c (HbA1c) levels which were measured at 24 weeks in type 1 diabetic patients treated with inhaled TI or subcutaneous insulin aspart. Additionally, seven-point self-monitored blood glucose (SMBG) curves were obtained in addition to regular testing of blood glucose at least three times during the week preceding visits at weeks 0, 12, and 24. Significantly, fewer rates of hypoglycemia with noninferior glycemic control were reported in participants receiving the ultra-rapid-acting inhaled insulin TI as compared to subcutaneous insulin aspart during the course of the study. These findings were particularly for statistically significantly fewer level 1 and 2 hypoglycemic events among participants receiving ultra-rapid-acting inhaled insulin TI than participants receiving insulin aspart. After the initial 1.5 hours, substantially fewer hypoglycemic events were seen in TI group than aspart group (2–6 h after meals), translating to a lower overall rate of postprandial hypoglycemia.

Strengths and Limitations of the Study

The direct comparison was limited by the different glycemic targets of the participants in the TI and insulin aspart groups in the AFFINITY-1 study.[38] There may be a possibility of providing more comprehensive information about postprandial hypoglycemia than SMBG values alone with the use of continuous glucose monitors. Additionally, the mean baseline and end-of-treatment HbA1c levels were reported to be higher in TI group as compared to aspart group, in-spite of no clinically statistical treatment difference was found.

Implications of the Findings for the Clinicians

Inhaled insulin offers numerous potential advantages over subcutaneously injected insulin, including faster insulin absorption rates, more rapid onset, and offset of action, improved postprandial glucose control, and a lower risk of latent hypoglycemia. The results of this regression analysis have shown comparable glycemic control and lower rates of hypoglycemia across a range of HbA1c levels at mealtime in inhaled TI group as compared to subcutaneous aspart group. There may be benefit among patients who have already reached their HbA1c goals of switching from subcutaneous rapid-acting insulin analogues to TI by reducing the frequency of hypoglycemic events. The convenience of between meal dosing is provided by the ultra-rapid time-action profile of TI by offering the flexibility to dose at the beginning of or 20 minutes after starting a meal with a lower risk of hypoglycemic events.

Knowledge Gaps Identified and Scope for Future Research

There is need to conduct more studies having comparable glucose targets in both the treatment groups suggested by the promising results of the present study. Given the pulmonary administration route, it is also clinically important to assess and understand effects of TI on pulmonary safety/function.

8. Systematic Review and Meta-analysis of Clinical Trials Examining the Effect of Hyperbaric Oxygen Therapy in People with Diabetes-related Lower Limb Ulcers

Ref: Golledge J, Singh TP. Systematic review and meta-analysis of clinical trials examining the effect of hyperbaric oxygen therapy in people with diabetes-related lower limb ulcers. Diabet Med. 2019;36(7):813-26.

ABSTRACT

Aim: Assessment of effectiveness of hyperbaric oxygen therapy (HBOT) in healing diabetes-related lower limb ulcers.

Methods: Appropriate clinical trials were identified by conducting literature search. Randomized studies that reported the proportion of healed diabetes-related lower limb ulcers were included and a meta-analysis was performed to assess the effectiveness of HBOT in healing diabetes-related ulcers. Minor and major amputations were taken as secondary outcomes.

Results: A total of nine randomized trials were included in the meta-analysis. Complete ulcer healing was more likely to be observed in those who were allocated to HBOT [relative risk (RR) 1.95; 95% confidence interval (CI) 1.51–2.52; $p < 0.001$]. They were also less likely to require major (RR 0.54; 95% CI 0.36–0.81; $p = 0.003$) or minor (RR 0.68; 95% CI 0.48–0.98; $p = 0.040$) amputations than the control groups. Adverse events included an ear barotrauma and a seizure. Absence of blinding of outcome assessors, lack of a justifiable sample size calculation, and limited follow-up were methodological limitations of many trials.

Conclusion: This meta-analysis suggests healing of diabetes-related lower limb ulcers can be improved by HBOT. This therapy can also reduce the need for amputation. A more rigorous assessment of the efficacy of HBOT is needed, as many of these trials had methodological limitations.

COMMENT

What was Known Prior to this Study?

In general, chronic wounds are characterized by hypoxia, impaired angiogenesis, and prolonged inflammation, all of which may theoretically be ameliorated by hyperbaric oxygen therapy (HBOT). The current evidence in the field of chronic wounds suggests that HBOT may have favorable effects on ischemic, infected diabetes-associated foot ulcers (DFUs).[41] However, the results of several trials and systematic reviews have had conflicting results with regard to the value of HBOT for DFU.[42,43] Furthermore, up to one-third of subjects considered for treatment are unsuitable or intolerant of HBOT because of comorbidities.[44]

What this Study Adds?

Most recently, in 2019, Golledge and Singh[45] carried out a systematic review and meta-analysis of nine clinical trials in the field of DFUs. The main finding of the present meta-analysis was that HBOT improved the healing of diabetes-related lower limb ulcers, evidenced by an approximate doubling in the likelihood of an ulcer healing during follow-up and an approximate halving in the requirement for major amputations. The findings for the primary outcome of complete ulcer healing still significantly favored HBOT after removal of any individual study. However, removal of the trial reported by Duzgun et al.[46] substantially reduced the relative risk (RR).

Authors concluded that HBOT improves the healing of DFUs and reduces the amputation rate.

Strengths and Limitations of the Study

The present meta-analysis suggests benefit of HBOT, but findings were dependent on the inclusion of one highly positive study. A number of methodological weaknesses of prior trials, in addition to the heterogeneity of the findings reported, suggest only moderate confidence in these findings. Author could not perform subanalyses to better define whether HBOT may be most effective for ischemic ulcers. It was not possible for the authors to conclude on the cost-effectiveness of HBOT.

Knowledge Gaps Identified and Scope for Future Research

Overall, the paucity of high-quality randomized controlled trials makes it difficult to properly assess the efficacy of HBOT. To accurately validate the potential benefits of HBOT, more vigorous investigations with adequately powered sample sizes are warranted. Having said that, there are inherent impediments to an ideal study design investigating HBOT. To make the matter even worse, there have been contradictory reports on economics and cost-effectiveness of HBOT in the field of chronic wounds. This should be an important focus for future trials.

9. Oral Semaglutide and Cardiovascular Outcomes in Patients with Type 2 Diabetes

Ref: Husain M, Birkenfeld AL, Donsmark M, Dungan K, Eliaschewitz FG, Franco DR, et al. Oral semaglutide and cardiovascular outcomes in patients with type 2 diabetes. N Engl J Med. 2019;381(9):841-51.

ABSTRACT

Introduction: It is significant to establish cardiovascular (CV) safety of the novel therapies for type 2 diabetes mellitus (T2DM). Data related to the subcutaneous form of the glucagon-like peptide-1 (GLP-1) receptor agonist semaglutide are available, but are required for oral semaglutide.

Methods: This was an event-driven, randomized, double-blind, placebo-controlled trial. The CV outcomes of once-daily oral semaglutide were evaluated in patients who were at high CV risk. Patients were at the age of 50 or more years along with established CV or chronic kidney disease (CKD), or age of 60 years or above along with CV risk factors only. The primary outcome in a time-to-event analysis was the first occurrence of a major adverse CV event (which included death due to then on fatal stroke, nonfatal myocardial infarction, or CV causes). The trial was designed to rule out 80% excess CV risk in comparison to the placebo [noninferiority margin of 1.8 for the upper boundary of the 95% confidence interval (CI) for the hazard ratio (HR) for the primary outcome].

Results: Total 3,183 patients were included in the study. Patients were randomized to receive either oral semaglutide or placebo; the mean age was 66 years. Majority of the patients (84.7%, n = 2,695) were ≥50 years of age with CV or CKD. In the trial, the median time was 15.9 months. There were major adverse CV events in 3.8% (61/1,591) patients in the oral semaglutide group and in 4.8% (76/1,592) in the placebo group (HR 0.79; 95% CI 0.57–1.11; $p < 0.001$ for noninferiority). Findings related to the components of the primary outcome were as follows: death due to the CV causes, 0.9% (15/1,591) patients in the oral semaglutide group and 1.9% (30/1,592) in the placebo group (HR 0.49; 95% CI 0.27–0.92); nonfatal myocardial infarction, 2.3% (37/1,591) patients and 1.9% (31/1,592), respectively (HR 1.18; 95% CI 0.73–1.90); and nonfatal stroke, 0.8% (12/1,591) patients and 1.0% (16/1,592), respectively (HR 0.74; 95% CI 0.35–1.57). In the oral semaglutide group and the placebo group, death due to any cause occurred in 1.4% (23/1,591) patients and 2.8% (45/1,592) patients, respectively (HR 0.51; 95% CI 0.31–0.84). With oral semaglutide, there were more gastrointestinal adverse events resulting in discontinuation of oral semaglutide or placebo.

Conclusion: In patients who have T2DM, results indicated no inferiority of oral semaglutide over placebo in terms of the CV risk profile [Funded by Novo Nordisk; PIONEER 6 (Peptide Innovation for Early Diabetes Treatment) ClinicalTrials.gov number, NCT02692716].

COMMENT

What was Known Prior to this Study?

Preventive strategies for cardiovascular (CV) complications in type 2 diabetes mellitus (T2DM) are essential. Glucagon-like peptide-1 (GLP-1) receptor agonists have significantly decreased CV risk in 4 of 6 published outcome trials.[47] All currently approved GLP-1 receptor agonists are administered subcutaneously. Oral semaglutide has been developed as a once-daily tablet, which may alleviate concerns about injections among some patients and clinicians.[48]

What this Study Adds?

In the Peptide Innovation for Early Diabetes Treatment (PIONEER) 6 trial,[49] the first oral GLP-1 receptor agonist (semaglutide) yielded a reduction in CV risk. A total of 3,183 patients were randomly assigned to receive oral semaglutide or placebo. The mean age of the patients was 66 years. This CV outcomes trial met its primary objective of ruling out an 80% excess CV risk with oral semaglutide, confirming noninferiority to placebo for the primary outcome [hazard ratio (HR) 0.79; 95% CI 0.57–1.11]. No unexpected adverse events were identified with oral semaglutide. Authors observed no apparent imbalance between the trial groups in adverse event reporting of diabetic retinopathy.

Strengths and Limitations of the Study

A high completion rate (99.7%), a high percentage of patients who continued to receive oral semaglutide (>80%), and full vital status known at trial end for all randomly assigned patients indicate high validity for the conduct of the trial and the results.

Implications of the Findings for the Clinicians

The question that how does oral semaglutide perform compared with the subcutaneous GLP-1 receptor agonists has been addressed by the authors. Exposure–response relationships for both glycated hemoglobin (HbA1c) level and body weight are similar with oral and subcutaneous semaglutide, which indicates that the efficacy of the molecule is independent of the route of administration. Although fewer events were observed in this trial (in 137 of 3,183 patients) than in SUSTAIN-6 (in 254 of 3,297),[50] the HRs were similar in the present trial and SUSTAIN-6 which may suggest that the CV effect of semaglutide is independent of the route of administration. Indeed, recent European Society of Cardiology guidelines do not distinguish between the oral and subcutaneous formulations of semaglutide when recommending the agent.[51]

10. Effects of Probiotic Supplementation during Pregnancy on Metabolic Outcomes: A Systematic Review and Meta-analysis of Randomized Controlled Trials

Ref: Masulli M, Vitacolonna E, Fraticelli F, Della Pepa G, Mannucci E, Monami M. Effects of probiotic supplementation during pregnancy on metabolic outcomes: A systematic review and meta-analysis of randomized controlled trials. Diabetes Res Clin Pract. 2020;162:108111.

ABSTRACT

Aim: Evaluation of the effect of probiotics on the metabolic outcomes in pregnancy in reference to incidence of gestational diabetes mellitus (GDM) and fasting glucose levels.

Methods: Randomized control trials (RCTs) comparing probiotics with placebo/active comparators in pregnant women were identified from MEDLINE, EMBASE, Scopus, and Cochrane search (up to May 30th, 2019). Incidence of GDM and the change of fasting plasma glucose (FPG) were the primary endpoints, while other maternal and fetal outcomes were secondary endpoints. For dichotomous outcomes, Mantel-Haenszel odds ratio (MH-OR) with 95% CI was calculated, and for continuous variables standardized differences in means was calculated. (PROSPERO registration CRD42019139889).

Findings: We identified 17 RCTs that compared probiotics with placebo for prevention of GDM in pregnancy. Although a small and significant reduction of fasting glucose levels [mean difference −1.01 (−1.96, −0.06) mg/dL; $p = 0.02$; $I^2 = 46\%$] was observed, incidence of GDM [MH-OR 0.77 (0.51, 1.16); $p = 0.21$; $I^2 = 62\%$] was not affected. Maternal insulin decreased significantly in the probiotics group.

Interpretation: Probiotics during pregnancy do not have a role in reducing the incidence of GDM, and do not lead to a clinically significant decrease in fasting glucose levels.

COMMENT

What was Known Prior to this Study?

The effect of microbiota on glucose metabolism in pregnant women may be different than in nonpregnant women. The beneficial effects of probiotic supplementation in pregnant women with gestational diabetes mellitus (GDM) may arise from the fact that, according to Crusell et al.,[52] the gut microbiota composition of those women differs from that of pregnant women without GDM. Probiotic supplementation during pregnancy seems to have some benefits on metabolic health: Results of some randomized controlled trials (RCTs) suggest that probiotics reduce the incidence of GDM[53,54] and reduce fasting plasma glucose (FPG); on the contrary, other RCTs showed that probiotics had no influence.[55] Although the last 2 years has seen the publication of five meta-analyses and systematic reviews aimed at determining the effect of modifications of the gut microbiota composition on glucose metabolism in pregnant women, three of them were restricted only to pregnant women with GDM.[56-58] Moreover, larger RCTs have emerged since the publication of these meta-analyses.

What this Study Adds?

Masulli and colleagues[59] performed a systematic review and meta-analysis of RCTs aimed to evaluate the health effects of probiotic supplementation in pregnant women with or without diabetes. In women without diabetes, the principal outcome was the incidence of GDM; in women with GDM, the principal outcome was the effect on FPG. This meta-analysis showed that probiotic supplementation during pregnancy did not reduce the incidence of GDM, whereas a very little (statistically but not clinically significant) reduction of FPG is observed in women taking probiotics. The concurrent reduction of fasting insulinemia, and the consequent improvement of the homeostasis model assessment (HOMA) index, suggest that this effect is attributable to an increase in insulin sensitivity, rather than to an enhancement of insulin secretion. The reduction of fasting glucose is not significant in separate analyses performed on women either with or without GDM; however, sample sizes could be too small to detect differences in subgroup analyses.

Strengths and Limitations of the Study

Certain limitations of the present meta-analysis should be considered. The reliability of the assessment of publication bias is questionable, because of the small number of available trials. For the same reason, it is not possible to explore factors that determine heterogeneity, which is relevant for both the principal outcomes. Besides, probiotics used differ across trials, adding uncertainty to the interpretation of results.

Implications of the Findings for the Clinicians

Probiotic supplementation during pregnancy is associated with no benefits on the incidence of GDM but it produces a minimal improvement of fasting glucose, which appears to be determined by an increase in insulin sensitivity. Although safe, this treatment does not show, on the basis of currently available trials, sufficient clinical benefits for recommending its widespread use.

Knowledge Gaps Identified and Scope for Future Research

There is a need for RCTs of women with and without GDM, with larger sample sizes, in order to better determine the effect of probiotic supplementation on glucose metabolism. Moreover, it is necessary to determine the best timing, duration, composition, and dose of such supplementation. Dietary intake and baseline gut microbiota composition should also be examined in such studies, as the effectiveness of probiotic supplementation may depend on these factors.

11. Dapagliflozin in Patients with Heart Failure and Reduced Ejection Fraction

Ref: McMurray JJV, Solomon SD, Inzucchi SE, Køber L, Kosiborod MN, Martinez FA, et al. Dapagliflozin in Patients with Heart Failure and Reduced Ejection Fraction. N Engl J Med. 2019;381(21):1995-2008.

ABSTRACT

Introduction: Among the patients who have type 2 diabetes mellitus (T2DM), the risk of a first hospitalization for heart failure (HF) is decreased by the inhibitors of sodium-glucose cotransporter-2 (SGLT-2), probably by glucose-independent mechanisms. There is a requirement of further information related to the effects of SGLT-2 inhibitors among patients who have established HF and a reduced ejection fraction, irrespective of the presence or absence of T2DM.

Methods: This phase 3, placebo-controlled trial included 4,744 patients with New York Heart Association (NYHA) class II, III, or IV HF and an ejection fraction of ≤40%, who were randomized to receive either dapagliflozin (at a dose of 10 mg once daily) or placebo, along with recommended therapy. The primary outcome considered in the study was a composite of worsening HF (i.e., hospitalization or an urgent visit leading to intravenous therapy for HF) or cardiovascular (CV) death.

Results: After the median of 18.2 months, the primary outcome was noted in 16.3% (386/2,373) patients in the dapagliflozin group and in 21.2% (502/2,371) patients in the placebo group [hazard ratio (HR) 0.74; 95% confidence interval (CI) 0.65–0.85; $p < 0.001$]. A first worsening HF event was noted in 10% ($n = 237$) patients in the dapagliflozin group and in 13.7% ($n = 326$) patients in the placebo group (HR 0.70; 95% CI 0.59–0.83). Death due to CV causes in the dapagliflozin group and the placebo group occurred in 9.6% ($n = 227$) patients and in 11.5% ($n = 273$) patients, respectively (HR 0.82; 95% CI 0.69–0.98); in the dapagliflozin group, 11.6% ($n = 276$) patients and in placebo group, 13.9% ($n = 329$) patients, died due to any cause (HR 0.83; 95% CI 0.71–0.97). There was no significant difference in the findings in patients who had diabetes and in patients without diabetes. The frequency of adverse events regarding volume depletion, hypoglycemia, and renal dysfunction were comparable among the treatment groups.

Conclusion: In patients who have HF and a reduced ejection fraction, when compared to individuals who received placebo, those who received dapagliflozin had lower risk of worsening HF or death from CV causes, irrespective of the presence or absence of diabetes.

COMMENT

What was Known Prior to this Study?

In patients with type 2 diabetes mellitus (T2DM), inhibitors of sodium-glucose cotransporter-2 (SGLT-2) have been linked with lower rates of hospitalization for heart failure (HF). However, whether these antidiabetic drugs are effective for treating HF in patients without diabetes was unclear. Dapagliflozin and Prevention of Adverse Outcomes in HF (DAPA-HF) investigators hypothesized that the SGLT-2 inhibitor dapagliflozin might be effective for the treatment of HF and reduced ejection fraction (HFrEF), even in patients without T2DM.

What this Study Adds?

Dapagliflozin and Prevention of Adverse Outcomes in Heart Failure was a phase III, placebo-controlled trial that included patients with an ejection fraction ≤40% and New York Heart Association (NYHA) class II, III, or IV symptoms.[60] Participants were randomly assigned to receive dapagliflozin or placebo, in addition to standard therapy. The primary outcome was a composite of worsening HF or death from cardiovascular (CV) causes. Over the median follow-up duration of 18.2 months, the primary composite outcome occurred in 386 patients (16.3%) in the dapagliflozin group and in 502 patients (21.2%) in the placebo group (HR 0.74; 95% CI 0.65–0.85; $p < 0.001$). Importantly, this reduction in the primary outcome was similar in patients with or without T2DM. Among patients with HFrEF, dapagliflozin is associated with a lower risk of worsening HF or CV death than placebo, regardless of the presence or absence of diabetes.

Strengths and Limitations of the Study

This trial has some limitations. Authors used specific inclusion and exclusion criteria, which may have limited the generalizability of the findings. Most patients had NYHA class II to III symptoms, which limits conclusions about the effects in patients hospitalized with decompensated HF or acute myocardial infarction complicated by symptomatic HF.[61] Less than 5% of the patients were black, and relatively few were very elderly with multiple coexisting illnesses. Although, only 11% of patients were receiving sacubitril/valsartan, post hoc subgroup analysis suggested added benefit.

Implications of the Findings for the Clinicians

These data from the DAPA-HF trial present a new perspective for the care of patients with HF. Although, the primary mediator of the benefits observed in the DAPA-HF trial remains uncertain, the trial provides the clearest evidence yet that glucose lowering per se is of little relevance.[62] However, a precise knowledge of certain details is important in understanding the major practice changing results of the trial.[63]

12. Associations between Metformin Use and Vitamin B12 Levels, Anemia, and Neuropathy in Patients with Diabetes: A Meta-analysis

Ref: Yang W, Cai X, Wu H, Ji L. Associations between metformin use and vitamin B12 levels, anemia, and neuropathy in patients with diabetes: A meta-analysis. J Diabetes. 2019;11:729-43.

ABSTRACT

Background: In diabetic patients, metformin is considered to be the first-line therapy. It may, however, reduce the levels of vitamin B12, which can have hematological or neurological effects. This meta-analysis included existing studies that evaluated the associations between use of metformin and vitamin B12 levels, anemia, and neuropathy in diabetic patients.

Methods: A search was conducted for recognizing all appropriate studies published in English before March, 2018 in Cochrane Library, Embase, PubMed, and web of Knowledge. For dichotomous outcomes, calculation of pooled risk ratios (RRs) and 95% confidence intervals (CIs) was done. For continuous outcomes, calculation of pooled mean differences (MDs) and 95% CIs was done.

Results: Total 31 were included in the meta-analyses. In comparison to patients with diabetes not on metformin, those receiving metformin had a significantly greater risk of vitamin B12 deficiency (RR 2.09; 95% CI 1.49, 2.93; $p < 0.0001$; $I^2 = 64\%$) and significantly lower serum vitamin B12 levels (MD −63.70; 95% CI −74.35, −53.05 pM; $p < 0.00001$; $I^2 = 87\%$), which was dependent on dose as well as duration of treatment. An association between use of metformin with significantly higher percentage reduction in serum vitamin B12 levels from baseline in patients with diabetes was observed (MD −14.68%; 95% CI −17.98%, −11.39%; $p < 0.00001$; $I^2 = 33\%$). On analyses, use of metformin was not significantly associated with the prevalence of anemia or neuropathy.

Conclusion: In patients with diabetes, use of metformin resulted in significantly lower vitamin B12 levels and significantly increased risk of vitamin B12 deficiency. Further good quality studies should be conducted for evaluating the associations between use of metformin and anemia and neuropathy in diabetic patients. In diabetic patients taking metformin, annual assessment of vitamin B12 is recommended.

COMMENT

What was Known Prior to this Study?

Metformin is the first-line therapy for treatment of type 2 diabetes mellitus (T2DM) in most individuals and the most widely prescribed oral antidiabetic medication. Numerous studies have reported associations between metformin use and lower vitamin B12 levels and/or a higher prevalence of vitamin B12 deficiency, although a few studies have not found any such association. A meta-analysis[64] of six randomized controlled trials (RCTs) concluded that metformin use led to dose-dependent reductions in vitamin B12 levels in patients with T2DM. Whether metformin-related vitamin B12 deficiency has clinical implications has also been debated.[65] The main clinical manifestations of vitamin B12 deficiency include anemia and neuropathy.[65] There has been no meta-analysis of the relationship between metformin use and neuropathy or anemia.

What this Study Adds?

A recent meta-analysis by Yang et al. reviewed all available studies on associations between metformin use and vitamin B12 levels, anemia, and neuropathy in individuals with T2DM.[66] Compared with diabetic patients not taking metformin, patients taking metformin had a significantly higher risk of vitamin B12 deficiency. Subgroup analyses revealed that only patients who have a mean duration of >3 years metformin therapy or patients on mean daily dose >2,000 mg metformin had significantly increased risk of vitamin B12 deficiency compared with patients not taking metformin, whereas patients with a mean duration of therapy ≤3 years or receiving a mean daily dose of ≤2,000 mg metformin did not. Although this meta-analysis reported no significant associations between metformin use and the risk of anemia in patients with diabetes, it is important to note that there were only four eligible studies regarding anemia risk, and most of these were cross-sectional or case-control, which did not have anemia as their primary endpoint.[67-70]

Strengths and Limitations of the Study

Since, this meta-analysis included studies on patients who visited primary, secondary, or tertiary care, such a diverse context and the large number of studies included indicate that the results are generalizable. This study has the additional strength derived from subgroup analyses based on mean metformin treatment duration and mean daily metformin dose. Additionally, findings of this meta-analysis could be useful for patients taking metformin for other indications. This study was limited by a lack of high-quality studies. Furthermore, studies included in the analyses used different methods to measure serum vitamin B12 concentrations and such lack of standardization could potentially affect the results. Finally, different studies used somewhat different cut-off values for vitamin B12 deficiency and this could potentially result in over- or underestimation of the incidence of vitamin B12 deficiency.

Implications of the Findings for the Clinicians

The meta-analysis confirmed individuals taking metformin had a significantly higher risk of vitamin B12 deficiency than those not taking metformin and significantly lower serum B12 concentrations, which depended on dose and duration of treatment. Annual assessment of vitamin B12 levels in diabetic patients taking metformin is recommended and appropriate preventive and therapeutic measures should be taken when necessary.

Knowledge Gaps Identified and Scope for Future Research

The meta-analysis did not find significant associations between metformin use and the risk of anemia or neuropathy in patients with diabetes. There is, therefore uncertainty about whether metformin causes anemia and whether or not this is mediated by B12 deficiency in metformin-treated individuals with T2DM. Prospective RCTs with a sufficiently large sample size and a long duration of metformin treatment are needed to further explore the association between metformin use and anemia and neuropathy.

13. Risk of Severe Hypoglycemia and its Impact in Type 2 Diabetes in DEVOTE

Ref: Heller S, Lingvay I, Marso SP, Philis-Tsimikas A, Pieber TR, Poulter NR, et al. Risk of severe hypoglycaemia and its impact in type 2 diabetes in DEVOTE. Diabetes Obes Metab. 2020;22(12):2241-7.

ABSTRACT

Aim: To determine the risk of severe hypoglycemia by conducting a post-hoc analysis DEVOTE trial data.

Materials and methods: For every subject included in the trial, hypoglycemia risk scores were calculated, based on which the trial population was divided into quartiles. The incidence of severe hypoglycemia observed in each quartile, along with major adverse cardiovascular event (MACE) and all-cause mortality were determined. Further, differences within each quartile [insulin degludec (degludec) vs. insulin glargine 100 units/mL (glargine U100)] with respect to severe hypoglycemia, MACE and all-cause mortality were assessed.

Results: The incidence of severe hypoglycemia, MACE and all-cause mortality was higher in those with higher risk scores. Treatment ratios between degludec and glargine U100 in the highest risk quartile were 95% confidence interval (CI) 0.56 (0.39; 0.80) (severe hypoglycemia), 95% CI 0.76 (0.58; 0.99) (MACE), and 95% CI 0.77 (0.55; 1.07) (all-cause mortality).

Conclusion: Those at high risk of severe hypoglycemia as demonstrated by high risk scores are also at risk of increased incidence of MACE and all-cause mortality. However, MACE was less frequent in those treated with degludec.

COMMENT

What was Known Prior to this Study?

DEVOTE demonstrated that degludec was noninferior to glargine U100 in terms of a three-point major adverse cardiovascular event (MACE), including cardiovascular death, nonfatal myocardial infarction or nonfatal stroke, and was superior with regard to hypoglycemia risk, with lower rates of both severe and nocturnal severe hypoglycemia at equivalent glycemic control.[71]

What this Study Adds?

Whether, a high risk of severe hypoglycemia was associated with an increased risk of cardiovascular events. The study concluded that the risk score demonstrated that a high risk of severe hypoglycemia was associated with a high incidence of MACE and all-cause mortality and that, in this high-risk group, those treated with degludec had a lower incidence of MACE.

Major Strengths of the Study

Strengths of this analysis include use of a large, double-blind trial with a high retention rate, independent adjudication of cardiovascular and severe hypoglycemic events, and use of a standard, robust definition of severe hypoglycemia according to international guidelines. To allow the translation of the hypoglycemia risk score to the clinical setting, it was digitized into an online tool (http://www.hyporiskscore.com/). This tool provides patients and healthcare providers with both the level of risk of a patient experiencing a severe hypoglycemic event within 2 years and the observed risk of MACE within the risk quartile.

Limitations of the Study

DEVOTE only collected severe hypoglycemic events, and therefore the contribution of nonsevere events, which have also been shown to be associated with a higher risk of cardiovascular events, hospitalization and all-cause mortality, could not be assessed.

Implications of the Findings for the Clinicians

The observations of the study support the hypothesis that hypoglycemia is a risk factor for cardiovascular events and those patients with the highest hypoglycemia risk had a lower incidence of MACE with degludec compared with glargine U100.

Knowledge Gaps Identified and Scope for Future Research

DEVOTE included a large number of patients at high risk of cardiovascular events, these patients were selected for inclusion in a randomized trial setting and may therefore not be representative of a real-world patient cohort. These findings must be substantiated with long-term real-world evidence (RWE) studies.

14. Switching to Degludec is Associated with Reduced Hypoglycemia, Irrespective of Definition Used or Patient Characteristics: Secondary Analysis of the ReFLeCT Prospective, Observational Study

Ref: de Valk HW, Feher M, Hansen TK, Jendle J, Koefoed MM, Rizi EP, et al. Switching to Degludec is Associated with Reduced Hypoglycaemia, Irrespective of Definition Used or Patient Characteristics: Secondary Analysis of the ReFLeCT Prospective, Observational Study. Diabetes Ther. 2020;11(9):2159-67.

ABSTRACT

Aim: To assess the impact of long-acting insulin, degludec on the incidence of hypoglycemia.

Methods: We conducted a secondary analysis of the REFLECT study, which was a prospective observational study done on patients with type 1 diabetes mellitus (T1DM) and type 2 diabetes mellitus (T2DM). Data of hypoglycemic events were collected from the patients' diary who changed to insulin degludec after physicians' recommendation. To determine the change in number of hypoglycemic events, we conducted two secondary analyses. A post-hoc analysis was undertaken using the level 1, 2, and 3 hypoglycemia definitions recommended by American Diabetes Association (ADA). A pre-specified analysis was done using patient characteristics including baseline HbA1c, duration of disease, and physician's grounds for starting degludec.

Results: Incidence of hypoglycemic events reduced significantly with degludec for all definitions in T1DM, and level 1 and 2 in T2DM. This was not influenced by the patient characteristics.

Conclusion: Change to degludec was associated with reduced incidence of hypoglycemia, and this reduction was independent of baseline characteristics of the patient and definitions used.

COMMENT

What was Known Prior to this Study?
Hypoglycemia is a common and potentially serious treatment side effect of insulin therapy in both type 1 diabetes mellitus (T1DM) and type 2 diabetes mellitus (T2DM). Randomized controlled trials (RCTs) have demonstrated a hypoglycemia risk reduction with insulin degludec, a new-generation long-acting basal insulin analog, compared with insulin glargine 100 units/mL (U100) in both T1DM and T2DM. In the REFLECT study, switching to degludec from other basal insulins was associated with significantly reduced rates of hypoglycemia in insulin-treated adults with diabetes.

What this Study Adds?
The results of the study demonstrated that switching to degludec from other basal insulins was associated with reduced rates of hypoglycemia, irrespective of the definition [level 1, 2, and 3 hypoglycemia American Diabetes Association (ADA) definitions] used or baseline patient characteristics (baseline HbA1c, diabetes duration, and physician's rationale for initiating degludec).

Major Strengths of the Study
The use of prospective data collection was a strength of this study, reducing potential memory recall bias. Additionally, definitions for level 1, 2, and 3 hypoglycemias were well represented in the rate of events and for the change between the baseline and follow-up periods (except for level 3 hypoglycemia for T2DM), strengthening the generalizability of these results.

Limitations of the Study
Study limitations include the observational design precluding randomization, and that a comparator arm was not included; this makes it difficult to determine if reductions in hypoglycemia were a treatment or study effect. As in the primary analysis, change in hypoglycemia was not assessed by baseline insulin group. The proportion of patients receiving glargine U100 versus U300 was not recorded, and it is unclear if differences in their profiles of action may have affected results for each group when switching to degludec.

Implications of the Findings for the Clinicians
These secondary analyses corroborated the findings of the primary REFLECT study, and demonstrated that, irrespective of the hypoglycemia definition used or prespecified patient characteristics, switching to degludec from other basal insulins was associated with reduced rates of hypoglycemia in patients with T1DM or T2DM.[72]

Knowledge Gaps Identified and Scope for Future Research
These patients were selected for inclusion in a randomized trial setting and may therefore not be representative of a real-world patient cohort. Real-world evidence (RWE) studies along with RCT data will provide robust evidence.

15. A Survey of Physician Experience and Treatment Satisfaction using Fast-acting Insulin aspart in People with Type 1 or Type 2 Diabetes

Ref: Baru A, Amir S, Ekelund M, Montagnoli R, Da Rocha Fernandes JD. A survey of physician experience and treatment satisfaction using fast-acting insulin aspart in people with type 1 or type 2 diabetes. Postgrad Med. 2020;132(4):320-7.

ABSTRACT

Aim: To analyze the experience and treatment satisfaction of physician while prescribing insulin aspart in clinical practice.

Materials and methods: Physicians treating diabetic patients who were prescribing insulin aspart were surveyed and interviewed.

Results: A total of 191 physicians took part in the survey. About 68% of type 1 diabetic patients and 63% of type 2 diabetic patients had received insulin before faster aspart. The driving factors for this switch were faster onset of action, better postprandial glycemic control, and dosing flexibility of faster aspart. A good response to current treatment (76%) and patients' hesitancy to change (57 %) were the factors for not prescribing faster aspart. The factors in favor of using faster aspart for physicians were dosing flexibility at-meal (66%) and post-meal (71%), improved postprandial glycemic levels (66%), and faster onset (61%). More than 50% of the physicians were assured of reaching HbA1c target levels with faster aspart.

Limitations: Recall bias could have affected the findings as the survey was based on personal experiences.

COMMENT

What was Known Prior to this Study?

The pharmacological profile of faster aspart has been shown to be different to insulin aspart, in that onset of action occurred earlier, early glucose-lowering effect was 74% greater, and offset of glucose-lowering effect occurred earlier versus insulin aspart. The clinical impact of faster aspart was evaluated in the onset clinical program in people with type 1 diabetes mellitus (T1DM) and type 2 diabetes mellitus (T2DM), where it showed promising results in terms of hemoglobin A1c (HbA1c) reduction and control of postprandial glucose (PPG) excursions, without an increased risk of overall hypoglycemia compared with insulin aspart.[73]

What this Study Adds?

This survey helped in understanding the characteristics of patients who were initiated on faster aspart and the experiences, perceptions, and behaviors of physicians who have used faster aspart for the treatment of T1DM and T2DM. This real-world data on prescribers' clinical experiences with faster aspart adds to, and complements, the current body of evidence for its use in the management of diabetes.

Major Strengths of the Study

Real-world studies are useful because they enable assessment of a wider, more representative, disease population in terms of age, comorbidities, treatment adherence, and other important factors. This study included broad range of physicians [general practitioners (GPs) and specialists] from the United Kingdom, Denmark, Switzerland, Finland, and Canada who were treating people with diabetes.

Limitations of the Study

The findings of this survey are based heavily on physicians' experiences, and could therefore be subject to recall bias.

Implications of the Findings for the Clinicians

The main prescription drivers for faster aspart were faster onset of action, improved PPG control, and dosing flexibility. These attributes of faster aspart are likely to improve glycemic management around meals. With adequate support and monitoring, the results of this study support switching of patients from a variety of other mealtime insulins to faster aspart.

Knowledge Gaps Identified and Scope for Future Research

A similar study with a larger sample size including both, patient and physicians' perception, along with a cost-effectiveness analysis regarding the use of faster aspart should be conducted in India.

---

16. A Randomized Trial Evaluating the Efficacy and Safety of Fast-acting Insulin Aspart Compared with Insulin Aspart, Both in Combination with Insulin Degludec with or without Metformin, in Adults with Type 2 Diabetes (Onset 9)

Ref: Lane WS, Favaro E, Rathor N, Jang HC, Kjærsgaard MIS, Oviedo A, et al. A Randomized Trial Evaluating the Efficacy and Safety of Fast-Acting Insulin Aspart Compared With Insulin Aspart, Both in Combination With Insulin Degludec With or Without Metformin, in Adults With Type 2 Diabetes (ONSET 9). Diabetes Care. 2020;43(8):1710-6.

ABSTRACT

Objective: To assess the effectiveness and safety profile of fast-acting insulin aspart (faster aspart) and insulin aspart (IAsp), administered along with insulin degludec regardless of cotreatment with metformin, in type 2 diabetes mellitus (T2DM).[74]

Research design and methods: A multicenter, double-blind, treat-to-target trial was conducted wherein 546 and 545 participants were randomly administered faster aspart and IAsp, respectively. For efficacy evaluation, all the relevant available information were assessed, irrespective of discontinuation or use of additional drugs.

Results: Change in hemoglobin A1c (HbA1c) values from baseline after 16 weeks was taken as primary endpoint. Faster aspart was found noninferior compared to IAsp with estimated treatment difference (ETD) of 20.04% [(95% CI 20.11, 0.03); 20.39 mmol/mol (21.15; 0.37); $p < 0.001$]. However, it was superior to IAsp for change in 1-hour postprandial glucose (PPG) from baseline [ETD 20.40 mmol/L (20.66; 20.14); 27.23 mg/dL (211.92; 22.55); $p = 50.001$ for superiority], and self-measured 1-hour PPG increment for the mean over all meals [ETD 20.25 mmol/L (20.42; 20.09); 24.58 mg/dL (27.59; 21.57); $p = 0.003$]. Furthermore, incidence of treatment-emergent severe or blood glucose (BG)-confirmed hypoglycemia was lower for faster aspart compared to IAsp [estimated treatment ratio 0.81 (95% CI 0.68, 0.97)].

Conclusion: The faster aspart along with insulin degludec was effective in providing better glycemic control, superior PPG control, and was associated with a lower rate of severe or BG-confirmed hypoglycemia.

COMMENT

What was Known Prior to this Study?

Rapid acting insulin analogs (RAIAs) aim to mimic the physiological action of endogenous insulin secreted in response to meals to reduce postprandial glucose (PPG) excursions. However, current RAIAs have a delayed onset and a longer duration of action compared with endogenous insulin in individuals without diabetes and there is an unmet need for mealtime insulins that more closely mimic physiological prandial insulin secretion.

What this Study Adds?

In combination with insulin degludec, faster aspart provided effective overall glycemic control, superior PPG control, and a lower rate of severe or blood glucose (BG)-confirmed hypoglycemia versus insulin aspart (IAsp) in adults with type 2 diabetes mellitus (T2DM), not optimally controlled with a basal-bolus regimen.

Major Strengths of the Study

The strengths of the study include the positive efficacy and safety findings in a difficult-to-treat population of people with a mean diabetes duration of >19 years, along with a relatively high trial completion rate (>95%). The study also employed a double-blind design and used a meal test, which, although not fully representative of a real-life setting, standardized macronutrient composition between participants, to measure PPG control at baseline and 16 weeks.

Limitations of the Study

A limitation of the trial was the need for participants to perform frequent capillary BG monitoring for dose titration, which, in the real-world setting, many patients may be unwilling to do.

Implications of the Findings for the Clinicians

Targeting PPG excursions is important for achieving overall glycemic control and reducing the risk of the macrovascular and microvascular complications of diabetes. Compared with IAsp, faster aspart has been shown to improve 1-hour PPG control in bolus-naïve patients treated with basal insulin and oral antidiabetic drug (OADs).

Knowledge Gaps Identified and Scope for Future Research

These patients were selected for inclusion in a randomized trial setting and may therefore not be representative of a real-world patient cohort. Real-world studies along with randomized control trial (RCT) data will provide robust evidence.

17. Oral Semaglutide versus Empagliflozin in Patients with Type 2 Diabetes Uncontrolled on Metformin: The PIONEER 2 Trial

Ref: Rodbard HW, Rosenstock J, Canani LH, Deerochanawong C, Gumprecht J, Lindberg SØ, et al. Oral Semaglutide Versus Empagliflozin in Patients With Type 2 Diabetes Uncontrolled on Metformin: The PIONEER 2 Trial. Diabetes Care. 2019;42(12):2272-81.

ABSTRACT

Objective: To assess the efficacy and safety of oral semaglutide, a glucagon-like peptide-1 (GLP-1) analog and empagliflozin, a sodium-glucose cotransporter-2 inhibitor in type 2 diabetes mellitus (T2DM) where metformin fails to achieve the adequate glycemic levels.

Research design and methods: A 52-week trial was conducted wherein subjects with T2DM were randomly administered oral semaglutide 14 mg ($n = 412$) or empagliflozin 25 mg ($n = 410$) once daily. Change in hemoglobin A1c (HbA1c) levels from baseline was taken as the primary endpoint, while change in body weight was confirmatory secondary endpoint. Queries related to efficacy of the drugs—treatment policy (irrespective of drug discontinuation or escape medication) and trial product (on trial product without rescue medication) was discussed.

Results: HbA1c reduction was more in semaglutide compared to empagliflozin group at week 26 {treatment policy −1.3% vs. −0.9% [−14 vs. −9 mmol/mol], estimated treatment difference [ETD] −0.4% [95% CI −0.6, −0.3] [−5 mmol/mol (−6, −3)]; $p < 0.0001$}. With respect to weight loss, oral semaglutide fared better at week 52 (trial product 24.7 vs. 23.8 kg; $p = 0.0114$), compared to empagliflozin. Incidence of adverse events, specifically gastrointestinal, was more in semaglutide group.

Conclusion: Decrease in HbA1c was more in oral semaglutide group compared to empagliflozin group at week 26 in type 2 diabetic patients who were on metformin but had inadequate glycemic levels. However, no such pattern was seen with body weight reduction. At week 52, body weight along with HbA1c, showed significant decrease in oral semaglutide group. Moreover, oral semaglutide had good tolerability like other GLP-1 receptor agonists.

COMMENT

Critical Appraisal

What was Known Prior to this Study?

In the management of type 2 diabetes mellitus (T2DM), glucagon-like peptide-1 (GLP-1) receptor agonists (RAs) are considered to be an effective option as compared to other antidiabetic medications due to their superior glycemic control, low risk of hypoglycemia, weight benefits, and cardiovascular risk reduction. Despite their multiple benefits, the utilization of these drugs is low and a major factor for this underutilization is the injectable formulation. An oral GLP-1RA may lead to initiation of GLP-1RAs earlier in the continuum of diabetes and improve acceptance and adherence for many patients, overcoming the therapeutic inertia.

Semaglutide is a human GLP-1 analog, recommended in a few countries, except India for once-weekly injection. It is associated with a good hemoglobin A1c (HbA1c) reduction, weight loss, and fewer cardiovascular events in T2DM. Oral semaglutide, an oral formulation, is coformulated with the absorption enhancer sodium N-[8-(2-hydroxybenzoyl)amino] caprylate (SNAC), which facilitates semaglutide absorption across the gastric mucosa. It has demonstrated a significant reduction in HbA1c and body weight compared to placebo in patients with T2DM uncontrolled with diet and exercise or oral antidiabetic medication, including in patients with moderate renal impairment.

What this Study Adds?

This study compares oral semaglutide with empagliflozin which is a widely used oral. Sodium-glucose cotransporter-2 (SGLT-2) inhibitor, shown to improve glycemic control, body weight, and associated with a reduced risk of cardiovascular in patients at high cardiovascular risk. This is the first head to head study with direct comparison of oral semaglutide with empagliflozin, in T2DM uncontrolled with metformin monotherapy.[75]

Major Strengths of the Study

This study showed a superior HbA1c reduction with significantly higher proportion of patients reaching the HbA1c target of <7%. The trial product estimand of change in body weight also showed a significantly greater reduction with oral semaglutide.

Additionally, the C-reactive protein, which was also monitored showed a significantly lower values in oral semaglutide arm as compared to empagliflozin.

These being the major findings from the study, the major strengths include the incorporation of both treatment policy estimand and trial product estimand, making the results more robust and easier to interpret, giving the clinician a choice to look at both estimand outcomes.

Limitations of the Study

With a robust trial design, involving 822 randomized patients, into oral semaglutide and empagliflozin arm, the limitation of this study would be the open-label design.

Implications of the Findings for the Clinicians

This study helps the practicing physicians in India, with their choice of newer oral antidiabetic medication in T2DM patients who are uncontrolled on metformin. Oral semaglutide molecule which is the only oral formulation of GLP-1RA, will open new arenas of bringing GLP-1RA therapies early in the management of diabetes, breaking the barrier of injectable therapies.

Knowledge Gaps Identified and Scope for Future Research

We see that the current study shows a higher number of diabetic retinopathy related effects with oral semaglutide as compared to empagliflozin, although the frequency was low in both the groups and none required treatment discontinuation. The possible effects of subcutaneous semaglutide on diabetic retinopathy are being investigated in the ongoing FOCUS trial. A similar study involving oral semaglutide may be needed to have a more clear perspective, in terms of oral semaglutide and diabetic retinopathy.

18. Efficacy, Safety, and Tolerability of Oral Semaglutide versus Placebo Added to Insulin with or without Metformin in Patients with Type 2 Diabetes: The PIONEER 8 Trial

Ref: Zinman B, Aroda VR, Buse JB, Cariou B, Harris SB, Hoff ST, et al. Efficacy, safety, and tolerability of oral semaglutide versus placebo added to insulin with or without metformin in patients with type 2 diabetes: The PIONEER 8 trial. Diabetes Care. 2019;42(12):2262-71.

ABSTRACT

Objective: To determine the efficacy, safety, and tolerability of oral semaglutide in type 2 diabetic patients who are on insulin with or without metformin.

Research design and methods: Type 2 diabetic patients who are on insulin with or without metformin but have inadequately controlled glycemic levels were randomly divided into four groups that received oral semaglutide at doses of 3 mg (N5184), 7 mg (N5182), or 14 mg (N5181) or to placebo (N5184) in double-blind trial. Change in hemoglobin A1c (HbA1c) level from baseline to week 26 was taken as primary endpoint, while change in body weight from baseline to week 26. Two estimands were treatment policy (impact irrespective of trial product discontinuation or escape medication) and trial product (impact on assumption that trial product was continued without escape medication).

Results: Decrease in HbA1c and body weight was more in oral semaglutide groups at week 26. Estimated treatment difference for HbA1c was –0.5% (95% CI –0.7, –0.3), –0.9% (–1.1, –0.7), and –1.2% (–1.4, –1.0) for 3 mg, 7 mg, and 14 mg, respectively; $p < 0.001$; and for body weight was 20.9 kg (95% CI –1.8, –0.0), –2.0 kg (–3.0, –1.0), and –3.3 kg (–4.2, –2.3); $p = 0.0392$ for 3 mg, $p \leq 0.0001$ for 7 mg and 14 mg, respectively (treatment policy estimand). Nausea was the most frequently occurring adverse effect with oral semaglutide (11.4–23.2% of patients vs. 7.1% with placebo).

Conclusion: Hemoglobin A1c and body weight reduction was more with oral semaglutide compared to placebo as an add-on to insulin with or without metformin in subjects with type 2 diabetes mellitus (T2DM) having uncontrolled glycemic levels.[76] The safety profile was similar to other drugs of its group.

COMMENT

Critical Appraisal

What was Known Prior to this Study?

Glucagon-like peptide-1 (GLP-1) analogs are a class of drugs with unique properties such as superior glycemic control and low risk of hypoglycemia attributed to their glucose-dependent actions. With the paradigm changing results from the LEADER trial, these drugs have also earned their spot in international cardiology guidelines for the management of type 2 diabetes mellitus (T2DM) patients with concomitant cardiovascular (CV) disorders, especially atherosclerotic disease.

Insulin therapies have been gold standards when it comes to management of T2DM, who have failed on multiple oral antidiabetic drug (OADs). With best in class glycemic control, insulin therapies still had a few major disadvantages which was risk of hypoglycemia and weight gain. In such patients, using GLP-1 receptor agonists (GLP-1RA) as an add-on therapy may prove to be beneficial due to their low risk of hypoglycemia and lowering the body weight. Insulin requirement may also come down with this combination therapy.

What this Study Adds?

The PIONEER 8 phase 3 clinical trial looks at the oral semaglutide as an add-on therapy to insulin (basal, basal-bolus, or premixed) with or without metformin in patients with uncontrolled T2DM. It gives us a closer look at the outcomes such as efficacy, safety, and tolerability of oral semaglutide when added to insulin therapies.

Major Strengths of the Study

The strength of this trial would be a robust design and use of appropriate statistical tests and representing the results in terms of both treatment policy and trial product estimand.

When we look at the consecutive insulin dosing stages, capped at baseline values and adjusted moving forward, it has given us practical results of effects of oral semaglutide, similar to what can be observed in clinical practice. With a good number of randomized participants, 731 from across the world, and a long duration of the study of 52 weeks, the results obtained will be more robust, reflecting its usefulness in clinical practice. With no increase in the risk of hypoglycemia, oral semaglutide improved the glycemic control and reduced body weight at 26 weeks, with a significant difference maintained at 52 weeks.

Limitations of the Study

Oral semaglutide has been added to a diverse variety of insulins, be it basal, bolus, or premix insulins in different regimens. This may make it difficult for us to look at the effect and interactions of oral semaglutide with individual types of insulin and different regimens. Additionally, adding an active comparator instead of a placebo would have given us insights at the results of oral semaglutide in comparison with commonly used OADs.

Implications of the Findings for the Clinicians

This study would help the practicing physicians to look at the effects of oral semaglutide as an add-on therapy to insulin and incorporate the same into their clinical practice. Furthermore, clinical guidelines may also reposition the GLP-1RAs higher mitigating a few disadvantages seen with insulins.

Knowledge Gaps Identified and Scope for Future Research

A closer look at the combination therapy of oral semaglutide with individual insulins may give us an overview of what can be good insulin to be combined with oral semaglutide molecule.

19. Effectiveness and Safety of Insulin Glargine 300 U/mL in Insulin-naïve Patients with Type 2 Diabetes after Failure of Oral Therapy in a Real-world Setting

Ref: Pfohl M, Jornayvaz FR, Fritsche A, Pscherer S, Anderten H, Pegelow K, et al. Effectiveness and safety of insulin glargine 300 U/mL in insulin-naïve patients with type 2 diabetes after failure of oral therapy in a real-world setting. Diabetes Obes Metab. 2020;22(5):759-66.

ABSTRACT

Objective: To assess the effectiveness and safety of starting insulin glargine as add on therapy, in insulin naïve type 2 diabetic patients who have inadequately controlled glycemic levels with oral antidiabetic therapy.

Methods: We conducted a multicenter, prospective, observational study on adult type 2 diabetic patients who were never treated with insulin and are only on oral antidiabetic drugs (OADs). Their hemoglobin A1c (HbA1c) ranged from 7.5% to 10%. These patients were administered insulin glargine 300 U/mL (Gla-300). The rate of achieving the predefined target of HbA1c levels was the primary endpoint of the study.

Results: Of 721 patients whose complete treatment course could be determined, 49.9% achieved their HbA1c target after 12 months of starting Gla-300, the mean duration of achieving being 341 days. There was 81% probability for these patients to stay at that level after 6 months. The mean (± SD) decrease in HbA1c and fasting plasma glucose levels was −1.22% (±1.05%) to 7.28% (± 0.92%) and −51.5 (± 48.63) mg/dL to 132.9 (± 33.0) mg/dL, respectively. Not only the incidence of hypoglycemia stayed low after 1 year of Gla-300 treatment, no episode of severe hypoglycemia was noted at night during sleep. Body weight remains unaffected.

Conclusion: Glargine-300 can be added to the oral regimen to achieve the target level of HbA1c as observed in around 50% of such patients after a year of treatment, without any increased risk of weight gain or severe episodes of hypoglycemia.

COMMENT

What was Known Prior to this Study?
There exists several randomized controlled trials (RCTs) and retrospective real-world evidences (RWEs) demonstrating efficacy and safety of glargine 300 U/mL (Gla-300).

What this Study Adds?
Beneficial effects of Gla-300 found in RCTs translate into conditions of routine clinical practice.

Major Strengths of the Study
Prospective real-world study with clinical outcomes using Gla-300.

Limitations of the Study
Noninterventional design and absence of comparator arm.

Implications for Clinicians
Gla-300 is a second-generation basal insulin that can be initiated in insulin naïve oral antidiabetic drugs (OADs) uncontrolled adult type 2 diabetes mellitus (T2DM) for good glycemic control with minimal safety concerns.[77-84]

Knowledge Gaps and Future Research
Real-world evidences in countries outside Europe and United States demonstrating effectiveness and safety of second-generation basal insulin.[85]

20. An Assessment of Physician Reasons for Prescribing Insulin Lispro 200 units/mL in Germany

Ref: Chen J, Perez-Nieves M, Piras De Oliveira C, Spaepen E, Osumili B, Poon JL, et al. An assessment of physician reasons for prescribing Insulin Lispro 200 units/mL in Germany. Postgrad Med. 2020;132(8):727-36.

ABSTRACT

Objective: To assess physicians' ground for preferring insulin Lispro 200 units/mL (IL200) and their experience of using it.

Methods: A set of 28 questions were prepared for the physicians and were rated on a scale of 0 ("not at all important"/"strongly disagree") to 4 ("absolutely important"/"strongly agree").

The questions were based on physicians' profile, justifications for prescribing IL200 and patients characteristics.

Results: Mean (SD) experience of physicians in treating diabetes was 18.1 (7.0) years, who gave consultation to around 226.8 patients. IL200 was prescribed to 56.1% of them as mealtime insulin (MTI). About, were overweight/obese, and those who received >20 units/day of MTI constituted 80.0% of IL200 patients who were type 2 diabetic patients and either obese or overweight. The choice of insulin prescribed was governed by clinical and behavioral factors. Clinical factors included patient's insulin dose, pattern of self-measured glucose levels, hemoglobin A1c (HbA1c) levels while adherence, knowledge about clinical features of hypoglycemia, patients' willingness for lifestyle modifications, and nonpreference to injections, were major behavioral factors.

Conclusion: A physician's decision to prescribe IL200 is influenced by various clinical and nonclinical factors and is patient centric.

COMMENT

What was Known Prior to this Study

Humalog® 200 units/mL KwikPen™ is commercial name of concentrated insulin Lispro 200 units/mL (IL200). It is administered prandially in type 1 and type 2 diabetic patients due to its short acting action. IL200 is expected to have similar clinical efficacy and safety profile to IL100 units/mL as both are bioequivalent. Although, the shape and size of pens of IL200 and the Humalog 100 units/mL are similar but IL200 delivers the same dose of insulin in half of the volume as compared to the Humalog as it contains twice as many units of insulin per unit volume. No dose calculations or adjustments are required by the patient experience of dialing a dose when moving from 100 units/mL insulin pen to IL200 as it has been designed to be dosed in 1 unit increments. Additionally, a significant lower glide force and glide force variability is exhibited by the IL200 pen as compared to the 100 units/mL insulin pen leading to less efforts of the patients in self-injecting with smoother insulin delivery with a positive impact on the ease of administration. A simulated injection (noninjecting) study also support this among caregivers and diabetic patients indicating the IL200 pen to be a preferred option over the 100 U/mL insulin pen.

What this Study Adds?

Valuable practice information was provided by the surveyed experienced clinicians in prescribing IL200 in Germany which was helpful to understand the current clinical decision-making. IL200 was prescribed mostly in the obese and overweight type 2 diabetic patients although one-fifth of the patients had type 1 diabetes mellitus (T1DM). The main challenge was the significant injection burden among IL200 candidates. IL200 was considered to be a relevant treatment option by the physicians surveyed in view of known treatment attributes of IL200, i.e., reduced injection volume with injection burden, fewer split doses, and requirement of fewer pens. A patient centered perspective was followed by the physicians through the alignment of medical decisions of IL200 prescriptions with patient's medical needs and nonclinical preferences. The advantages of IL200 also helped physicians to encourage and counsel patients to improve adherence to the insulin therapy. The total daily insulin dose, pattern of self-measured glucose levels, and hemoglobin A1c (HbA1c) level were the most frequently selected clinical considerations for prescribing IL200 in this survey. Furthermore, from the physicians who were surveyed in this study, the key patient behavioral aspects to prescribe IL200 were identified to be adherence, knowledge about hypoglycemia, motivation to improve lifestyle, desire to reduce insulin injection volume, and emotional struggle to keep HbA1c under control.

Major Strengths of the Study

The physicians' perception regarding IL200 and the reasons for its prescription among diabetic patients were reported in the study.

Limitations of the Study

The present was the first study to survey the physicians regarding prescription practices of IL200 and focusing to understand their experience and opinion in Germany. This study may not be completely generalizable due to its descriptive nature. Additionally, generalizability of the results may also be impacted by the often seen the low response rate (4.5%) in this type of research. The various reasons for physicians' low response are variable and may be time constraints, perceived value of the research/confidentiality issues and design of the survey. Although, the response rate was low initially, but the higher results were yielded from the screening of willing physicians (38.6% screened-in). All the included physicians completed the survey. The study included the physicians from the specialities which involved seeing the diabetic patients regularly and having experience of concentrated insulin prescription. The physicians also considered the unique characteristics of the German health system possibly affecting certain factors, especially nonclinical factors while prescribing IL200. The study questionnaire did not explore the certain factors evaluated by physicians in depth to make the survey feasible. For example, the specific comorbidities considered important by the physicians for IL200 introduction were not explored in the questionnaire. All the relevant factors may not be covered in the survey questionnaire developed for this study. Although additional free text comments collected from the surveyed physicians addressed this limitation to some degree. However, no additional meaningful factor was noted to be worthy beyond the factors evaluated in this survey. Participation of few endocrinologists constraining the ability of the study to explore the prescribing differences by physician specialty was another limitation of the study. Another future study may be to explore differences in the treatment pattern between type 1 and type 2 diabetic patients on IL200.

Implications of the Findings for the Clinicians

The present study demonstrated the physicians' consideration of IL200 to be a promising treatment option decreasing the injection burden for patients on mealtime insulin (MTI). A patient's centered perspective was adopted by physicians by aligning decisions of IL200 prescription with each patient's medical needs and nonclinical preferences aiming to counsel and encourage the diabetic patients to adhere with the treatment with IL200s advantageous attributes.

Knowledge Gaps Identified and Scope for Future Research

Similar study in an Indian setting and identifying the reasons behind the preference of Humalog 200 in Indian Patients would be an ideal approach in the coming days.

21. Cardiovascular and Kidney Outcomes of Linagliptin Treatment in Older People with Type 2 Diabetes and Established Cardiovascular Disease and/or Kidney Disease: A Prespecified Subgroup Analysis of the Randomized, Placebo-controlled CARMELINA® Trial

Ref: Cooper ME, Rosenstock J, Kadowaki T, Seino Y, Wanner C, Schnaidt S, et al. Cardiovascular and kidney outcomes of linagliptin treatment in older people with type 2 diabetes and established cardiovascular disease and/or kidney disease: A prespecified subgroup analysis of the randomized, placebo-controlled CARMELINA® trial. Diabetes Obes Metab. 2020;22(7):1062-73.

ABSTRACT

Aim: To analyze the effectiveness and safety profile of linagliptin, a dipeptidyl peptidase-4 inhibitor, in older individuals with type 2 diabetes mellitus (T2DM) who participated in CARMELINA® (Cardiovascular and Renal Microvascular Outcome Study with Linagliptin)[86] trial with high risk of renal and cardiovascular diseases (CVD).

Materials and methods: Adults (>18 years) with T2DM and with known history of CVD having urinary albumin-to-creatinine ratio (UACR) >30 mg/g, and/or renal disease were randomly administered linagliptin or placebo. The occurrence of death due to CVD, and nonfatal myocardial infarction or nonfatal stroke, 3-point major adverse CV events (3P-MACE), was taken as the primary endpoint. Evaluation of primary and the other outcomes was done across the two groups.

Results: The hazard ratio (HR) for 3P-MACE with linagliptin versus placebo was 1.02 [95% confidence interval (CI) 0.89, 1.17]. There was no increased risk of unfavorable renal outcomes or hospitalization for heart failure, associated with linagliptin across age groups. Though the adverse events, including hypoglycemia, increased with age but were similar with linagliptin and placebo despite glycated hemoglobin (HbA1c) reduction with linagliptin.

Conclusion: Use of linagliptin was not associated with increased risk of adverse outcome related to cardiovascular or renal diseases, compared to placebo.

COMMENT

What was Known Prior to this study?

- Linagliptin has demonstrated conclusive evidence of cardiovascular and renal safety, across a broad spectrum of patients with type 2 diabetes mellitus (T2DM).[86,87]
- An analysis in 2013 found that only 0.6% of interventional trials in diabetes had specifically targeted patients >65 years, while 31% had actively excluded them. Furthermore, most trials had excluded individuals >75 years.[88]
- There is limited evidence on cardiorenal safety in elderly patients, especially aged ≥75 years, across most Cardiovascular Outcome Trial (CVOTs).

What this Study[89] Adds?

In CARMELINA, patient's ≥65 years old (n = 4011; 57.4% of total study population) were evaluated in a prespecified subgroup analysis.[89] The findings were consistent with overall study, as follows:

- Linagliptin demonstrated cardiovascular [including heart failure (HF)] safety, as well as renal safety
- Linagliptin improved hemoglobin A1c (HbA1c) significantly (0.46% vs. placebo at 12 weeks), without any increase in risk of hypoglycemia
- Linagliptin demonstrated an overall safety profile (including risk of hypoglycemia), comparable to placebo

Major Strengths of the Study

- More than half of the patients (≈57%) in the study were ≥65 years old.
- Including T2DM patients with ≥75 years old (17.4%), even with ≥80 years old (around 6%)
- Around 10% of patients included in the study were Asians.
- Unlike other CVOTs, hard renal outcomes were analyzed in a prespecified manner
- Albuminuria benefits were consistent among older patients and interestingly, risk reduction was more pronounced with the advanced age group in the study.

Limitations of the Study

- Being an event driven trial with only 2.2 years median follow-up duration, linagliptin could not show statistical superiority for hard renal outcomes.
- Relatively lesser Asian patients and lesser geography covered (could have been much more relevant if more Asian patients included particularly from India)

Implications of the Findings for Clinicians

- In older patients even with established atherosclerotic cardiovascular disease (ASCVD) or chronic kidney disease (CKD) or high/very high risk, clinicians may consider using linagliptin safely.
- Frequent hypoglycemia is a major concern in older patients and linagliptin did not increase the risk of hypoglycemia.

Knowledge Gaps and Future Area of Research

- With the available armamentarium of antidiabetic medications with promising newer classes of drugs, the life expectancy of T2DM patients are on the rise.
- Hence, studies focusing on safe use of various classes of antidiabetic medications in older patients may become feasible in future.
- As of now, one such study has provided us a reassurance regarding linagliptin's safety in older patients.

22. Linagliptin and Cardiorenal Outcomes in Asians with Type 2 Diabetes Mellitus and Established Cardiovascular and/or Kidney Disease: Subgroup Analysis of the Randomized CARMELINA® Trial

Ref: Inagaki N, Yang W, Watada H, Ji L, Schnaidt S, Pfarr E, et al. Linagliptin and cardiorenal outcomes in Asians with type 2 diabetes mellitus and established cardiovascular and/or kidney disease: subgroup analysis of the randomized CARMELINA® trial. Diabetol Int. 2019;11(2):129-41.

ABSTRACT

Objective: To determine the effects of linagliptin on cardiovascular and renal outcomes in Asians having type 2 diabetes mellitus (T2DM) and history of cardiovascular disease (CVD) with albuminuria and/or renal disease.

Methods: Asian subjects with T2DM having HbA1c values 6.5–10.0% and known CVD with urinary albumin-to-creatinine ratio (UACR) >30 mg/g, and/or coexisting renal disease, were included in the study. Renal disease was defined by estimated glomerular filtration rate (eGFR) of 15 <45 mL/min/1.73 m^2 or ≥45–75 mL/min/1.73 m^2 along with UACR >200 mg/g. These subjects were randomly divided into two groups, one received linagliptin, and the other received placebo. The first event of death due to cardiovascular cause, myocardial infarction and stroke, which are not fatal [3-point major adverse CV events (MACE)], were taken as primary endpoints, death from renal failure, progression to end-stage kidney disease, or ≥40% eGFR decrease.

Results: The incidence of 3-point MACE occurred in 10.7% and 11.7% of linagliptin and placebo subjects, respectively during the follow-up period [hazard ratio (HR) 0.90; 95% confidence interval (CI) 0.55–1.48]. We observed similar rates for secondary endpoints. Risk of hospitalization for HR decreased but insignificantly, in linagliptin group (HR 0.47; 95% CI 0.24–0.95).

Conclusion: Linagliptin did not show any significant increase in adverse cardiorenal outcomes in Asian subjects with T2DM and known CVD with albuminuria and/or renal disease.

COMMENT

What was Known Prior to the Trial?

- Diabetes has been associated with higher rates of hospitalization for heart failure (hHF) and all-cause death in Asian patients.[90]
- South-Asians have an increased risk end-stage diabetic nephropathy.[90]
- Asians have higher plasma dipeptidyl peptidase-4 (DPP-4) levels, hence DPP-4 inhibitors can help.[91]
- Saxagliptin showed an increase in hHF in SAVOR TIMI 53 (Saxagliptin Assessment of Vascular Outcomes Recorded in Patients with Diabetes Mellitus-Thrombolysis in Myocardial Infarction 53).[92]
- Linagliptin had a lower risk of hHF compared to glimepiride in a real-world evidence from South Korea.[93]

Present Study-linagliptin in Asian Subgroup[5]

This analysis involved evaluation of outcomes in Asian patients from CARMELINA (Cardiovascular and Renal Microvascular Outcome Study with Linagliptin) study, including sites from Japan, China, South Korea, Taiwan, and Malaysia.[94]

- The study enrolled patients with high cardiovascular (CV) and renal risk at baseline.
- Linagliptin demonstrated no increase in the risk of CV, heart failure (HF) or renal events as compared to placebo.
- With linagliptin, less patients initiated or required an increased insulin dose.
- Similar incidence of adverse events (AEs) was found with linagliptin or placebo.
- The outcome was consistent with overall study results.

Major Strength of the Study

- This study provides evidence on cardiorenal safety profile of linagliptin in Asian patients.
- The patients enrolled in the study, had high risk for CV and renal events, including heart failure events, at baseline.

Major Limitations of the Study

- The overall trial was not statistically designed, to detect differences in treatment effects in the subgroups.
- The CARMELINA study did not include participants from India.

Implications of the Findings for the Clinicians

- Heart failure is a safety aspect.
- This analysis provides further conviction for safe clinical use of linagliptin, in patients with type 2 diabetes mellitus (T2DM) from Asian ethnicity, who may have increased CV or renal risk.

Knowledge Gaps Identified and Scope for Future Research

- Study focussing ethnic groups are limited.
- Subgroup analysis have certain limitations too, hence the findings should not be over-interpreted.
- Large scale, long-term investigations in Asians would be much more insightful.

23. Efficacy and Safety of Remogliflozin Etabonate, a New Sodium-glucose Cotransporter-2 Inhibitor, in Patients with Type 2 Diabetes Mellitus: A 24-Week, Randomized, Double-blind, Active-controlled Trial

Ref: Dharmalingam M, Aravind SR, Thacker H, Paramesh S, Mohan B, Chawla M, et al. Efficacy and Safety of Remogliflozin Etabonate, a New Sodium Glucose Co-Transporter-2 Inhibitor, in Patients with Type 2 Diabetes Mellitus: A 24-Week, Randomized, Double-Blind, Active-Controlled Trial. Drugs. 2020;80(6):587-600.

ABSTRACT

Objective: To determine the safety and efficacy of a novel elective sodium-glucose cotransporter-2 inhibitor, remogliflozin etabonate (RE), by comparing it with dapagliflozin in type 2 diabetic patients in whom monotherapy with metformin could not achieve the target hemoglobin A1c (HbA1c) level.

Methods: A multicenter, phase III study conducted over 24 weeks included subjects of age group 18–65 years who had uncontrolled type 2 diabetes mellitus (T2DM) in spite of being treated with metformin ≥1,500 mg/day. It was a randomized, double-blind, double-dummy, active-controlled, three-arm study where subjects with HbA1c 7–10% were screened and categorized into three groups. The subjects in the groups received either 100 mg twice daily (BID) (group 1) or 250 mg BID (group 2) of RE or dapagliflozin 10 mg once daily (QD) in the morning and placebo QD in the evening (group 3). Follow-up at weeks 1 and 4 and then at 4-week intervals till week 24, was done. The mean change in HbA1c from baseline was the primary endpoint. The secondary endpoints included change in fasting plasma glucose (FPG), postprandial plasma glucose (PPG), body weight, blood pressure, and fasting lipids. Assessment of treatment emergent adverse events (TEAEs), safety laboratory values, electrocardiogram, and vital signs was also done.

Results: Difference in mean HbA1c ± standard error (SE) from baseline to week 24 was −0.72 ± 0.09, −0.77 ± 0.09, and −0.58 ± 0.12% in groups 1, 2, and 3, respectively. The difference in change in secondary endpoints, FPG, PPG and body weight across the groups. The overall incidence of TEAEs, which were mostly mild to moderate, was 32.6%, 34.4%, and 29.5%, in the groups, respectively.

Conclusion: Our results showed that RE 100 mg and 250 mg is noninferior to dapagliflozin in terms of efficacy and is also well tolerated.

COMMENT

What was Known Prior to this Study?

Two phase II dose ranging studies had been conducted with remogliflozin etabonate (RE) in multinational trials. The dosing regimens of once and twice daily (BID) administration in drug naïve type 2 diabetes mellitus (T2DM) patients was compared against placebo as well as pioglitazone. These studies showed the BID regimen to be more effective which could be attributed to pharmacokinetic profile of RE. Among the doses tested, the dose of 100 mg BID and 250 mg BID showed clinically significant and most consistent effects on the glycemic as nonglycemic parameters with no additional risk identified, thereby providing with most suitable risk benefit ratio.

What this Study Adds?

This study is the first report of efficacy and safety of RE in a representative sample of an Indian T2DM population. The study demonstrated the RE to be efficacious and safe therapeutic agent for management of T2DM among Indian T2DM patients. It also established RE to be comparable to already approved agent (dapagliflozin) in same class of drug.

Major Strengths of the Study

This study is first of the report globally that compares two sodium-glucose cotransporter-2 (SGLT-2) inhibitors in head to head comparison in single clinical trial. This study included only Indian T2DM patients in both the treatment arms as compared to pivotal studies of other SGLT-2 inhibitors which largely included Caucasian population. Hence, the results of this study can be better extrapolated to Indian population than studies of other SGLT-2 inhibitors due to phenotypic variations in disease progression and drug response on background of genetic, racial, and ethic differences between Indians and Caucasians.

Limitations of the Study

The study suffered limitation of higher withdrawals than expected of approximately 28% of the subjects that were not included in the primary polydipsia (PP) analysis. The most common reason was consent withdrawal that can be attributed to need of administration of six tablets daily (including placebo) to maintain blinding. A post hoc power estimation has not been performed due to its limited utility. However, mean difference in hemoglobin A1c (HbA1c) change from baseline of −0.14% in favor of RE, and upper level of confidence interval (CI) of the mean difference extended up to 0.10% (far from the noninferiority margin of 0.35, $p < 0.001$) demonstrated results to be definitive rather than borderline.

Implications of the Findings for the Clinicians

Remogliflozin etabonate was demonstrates to be well-tolerated and effective, noninferior to dapagliflozin in efficacy when tested in exclusively Indian population. Hence, clinicians would be provided with additional therapeutic agent in SGLT-2 inhibitors class of drugs during management of their T2DM patients.

Knowledge Gaps Identified and Scope for Future Research

Remogliflozin etabonate was shown to have comparable efficacy to dapagliflozin during 24 weeks duration of study. The long-term efficacy and durability of glycemic response with RE (>24 weeks) and efficacy assessment on varied clinical scenarios of background or concomitant therapy would help assess the response in these scenarios. Additionally there is scope for future research to assess effect of RE on cardiovascular (CV) and renal outcomes among Indian T2DM patients. The real-world evidence/surveillance would help assess the effectiveness and safety in settings of clinical practice.

24. An Open-label, Single-period, Two-stage, Single Oral Dose Pharmacokinetic Study of Remogliflozin Etabonate Tablet 100 and 250 mg in Healthy Asian Indian Male Subjects Under Fasting and Fed Conditions

Ref: Joshi S, Gudi G, Menon VCA, Tandon M, Joshi V, Suryawanshi S, et al. An Open-Label, Single-Period, Two-Stage, Single Oral Dose Pharmacokinetic Study of Remogliflozin Etabonate Tablet 100 and 250 mg in Healthy Asian Indian Male Subjects Under Fasting and Fed Conditions. Clin Pharmacokinet. 2020;59(3):349-57.

ABSTRACT

Aim: To investigate the pharmacokinetic (PK) properties and safety profile of remogliflozin etabonate (RE), a renal sodium-glucose cotransporter-2 (SGLT-2) administered to healthy male subjects under fasting and fed conditions at doses 100 mg and 250 mg.

Methods: An open-label, two-stage study was conducted on 65 healthy Indian males, where a validated liquid chromatography-tandem mass spectrometry (LC-MS/MS) technique was used to determine the concentrations of remogliflozin, remogliflozin etabonate-its prodrug, and the metabolite GSK279782 in plasma. Safety assessment was done by monitoring of unfavorable events. Descriptive statistics were determined for all parameters.

Results: Remogliflozin etabonate is rapidly converted to the active moiety, remogliflozin, which is then further metabolized to GSK279782, as observed in plasma concentration profiles. At the 100 mg and 250 mg dose of RE, fed/fasted ratio for geometric mean maximum concentration (C_{max}) ranged from 0.77 to 1.44, and from 0.80 to 1.12, respectively. The fed/fasted ratio for plasma concentration-time curve (AUC) was 1.22 and 1.35 at 100 mg and 250 mg, respectively. There was a dose-proportional increase in the C_{max} and AUC_{last} for the three analytes in both states. The terminal half-life for remogliflozin ranged from 1.53 to 2.07 hour. The terminal half-lives of the three analytes were comparable irrespective of dose levels or dietary conditions.

Conclusion: Remogliflozin etabonate had favorable PKs with no relevant meal effects on at 100 mg or 250 mg dose. It also has good tolerability and safety profile.

COMMENT

What was Known Prior to this Study?

The phase I pharmacokinetic (PK) study of remogliflozin etabonate (RE) using various doses, formulations, and dosing regimens were conducted prior in Caucasian population. The PKs of RE was well-characterized in the Caucasian population on basis of these phase I clinical studies. The PK of RE was not independently tested in Indian patients.

What this Study Adds?

This study is the first report of PKs of RE in Indian healthy volunteers which helped to not only characterize the PK in Indian population but assess adequate plasma exposure of RE and its metabolites in Indian subjects that is required for drug effect. This study also demonstrated no impact of food on the drug absorption of RE as well as linearity of plasma exposure of active drug and its metabolites with increase in dose.

Major Strengths of the Study

This study characterized the PK of RE in Indian population using validated liquid chromatography-tandem mass spectrometry (LC-MS/MS) method. The study was adequately designed to assess two dose levels of RE as well as the effect of food on PK/plasma exposure at both the dose levels.

Limitations of the Study

The study had no limitation in terms of study design and study conduct. However, the terminal rate constant (λz) could not be estimated based on obtained concentration data and hence, the plasma concentration-time curve (AUC) and other elimination phase dependent parameters could not be calculated for some subjects. The known but lower exposure metabolites were not considered for assessment in this study due to lack of clinical significance as per previous PK studies on RE.

Implications of the Findings for the Clinicians

This study demonstrates adequate plasma exposure of RE in Indian subjects and linear proportional increase in the plasma concentration suggestive nonsaturation PKs over the dosing range. The presence of food having no clinically relevant effect on drug concentration achieved in plasma provides with ease of administration of drug without relation of meals.

Knowledge Gaps Identified and Scope for Future Research

The PK of RE has been demonstrated basis identified analytes. However, the metabolic profile of other known or unknown drug metabolites in Indian population can be tested. Likewise, the pharmacodynamics assessment of RE in Indian population and comparison to Caucasian population to demonstrated any variation in drug response on background of genetic and ethnic differences provides potential scope for future research.

25. Efficacy of Empagliflozin on Heart Failure and Renal Outcomes in Patients with Atrial Fibrillation: Data from the EMPA-REG OUTCOME Trial

Ref: Böhm M, Slawik J, Brueckmann M, Mattheus M, George JT, Ofstad AP, et al. Efficacy of empagliflozin on heart failure and renal outcomes in patients with atrial fibrillation: Data from the EMPA-REG OUTCOME trial. Eur J Heart Fail. 2020;22(1):126-35.

ABSTRACT

Aim: To determine the effect of empagliflozin, a sodium-glucose cotransporter-2 (SGLT-2) inhibitor on cardiovascular (CV) and renal outcomes in type 2 diabetic subjects with atrial fibrillation (AF).

Methods and results: Analyses from EMPA-REG OUTCOME (Empagliflozin Cardiovascular Outcome Event Trial in Type 2 diabetes Mellitus Patients-Removing Excess Glucose) trial were conducted on subjects with or without AF at baseline. There was reduced incidence of CV death and hospitalization due to heart failure (HF) in empagliflozin group compared to placebo in subjects with AF [hazard ratio (HR) 0.58; 95% confidence interval (CI) 0.36–0.92] as well as without AF (HR 0.67; 95% CI 0.55–0.82; *p* value for interaction = 0.56). Further, there were larger absolute treatment effects of empagliflozin. However, introduction of new loop diuretics led to higher rates of ensuing events but the rates were lower in empagliflozin group.

Conclusion: In type 2 diabetic patients with known CV disease, unfavorable outcomes of HF were seen more in those with AF at baseline than those without AF. Empagliflozin led to decreased incidence of HF-related and renal events, in presence or absence of AF. Also, subjects with AF had higher absolute number of prevented events.

COMMENT

What was Known Prior to this Study?

Presence of atrial fibrillation (AF) is associated with poor cardiovascular (CV) and mortality outcomes, and may stimulate cardiac remodeling.[95-97] Sodium-glucose cotransporter-2 (SGLT-2) inhibitors have been hypothesized to reduce central sympathetic afferent tone.[98] In EMPA-REG OUTCOME (Empagliflozin Cardiovascular Outcome Event Trial in Type 2 Diabetes Mellitus Patients-Removing Excess Glucose) study, empagliflozin had demonstrated reduction in risk of sudden cardiac death.[99]

What this Study Adds?

This was a post-hoc analysis from EMPA-REG OUTCOME study. This analysis explored whether the effects of empagliflozin versus placebo, in patients with AF. In addition to that, this analysis also looks at the effect of empagliflozin on early signs of heart failure (HF) like first new-onset edema, or need for first initiation of loop diuretics.

In the EMPA-REG OUTCOME trial, at baseline 389 patients had history of AF. The event rates were considerably higher in patients with AF compared to participants without AF. Empagliflozin has shown consistent reduction in the CV death, hospitalization for heart failure (hHF), a composite of CV death and hHF, all-cause mortality, and new or worsening nephropathy outcomes, in patients with or without AF.

The incidence of extended HF outcomes (new initiation of loop diuretics, new-onset edema, and the composite of new initiation of loop diuretics or new edema) increased the frequency of subsequent outcomes like CV death, hHF and all-cause mortality. The incident rate for these outcomes was less in patients on empagliflozin. Empagliflozin consistently reduced the incidence of new initiation of loop diuretics, new-onset edema and a composite of new initiation of loop diuretic and new-onset edema, in participants with or without AF.

Major Strengths of the Study

- Proves the consistency of evidence with empagliflozin on mortality and major cardiorenal outcomes, in patients with type 2 diabetes mellitus (T2DM) and atherosclerotic cardiovascular disease (CVD), with AF.
- The extended HF outcomes, new initiation of loop diuretics, new edema and the composite of new initiation of loop diuretics or new edema are captured in this analysis providing more insight into the effects of these outcomes on CV events.

Limitations of the Study

- Hypothesis generating post-hoc analysis
- Less number of patients with AF in the analysis
- Since, it is a post-hoc analysis, data on ejection fraction, atrial size or strain, characterization of diastolic function, duration or burden of AF and antiarrhythmic therapies, is not available.

Implications of the Findings for the Clinicians

This analysis adds that the consistency of benefits of empagliflozin even in patients with greater risk such as the presence of AF. As AF is one of the most common rhythm disturbances in patients with T2DM mellitus and HF, seen by clinicians in their practice, this analysis boosts the confidence of physicians in the use of empagliflozin in wider group of patients. Patients with T2DM and AF will benefit from the use of empagliflozin.

Knowledge Gaps Identified and Scope for Future Research

Effects of empagliflozin and other SGLT-2 inhibitors, on risk of new-onset AF, can be analyzed in further studies. The mechanisms supporting such possible effect, and their implications on associated diseases like nocturnal hypertension, reverse cardiac remodeling, etc., may be more robustly evaluated.

26. Effect of Empagliflozin on Left Ventricular Mass in Patients with Type 2 Diabetes Mellitus and Coronary Artery Disease: The EMPA-HEART CardioLink-6 Randomized Clinical Trial

Ref: Verma S, Mazer CD, Yan AT, Mason T, Garg V, Teoh H, et al. Effect of Empagliflozin on Left Ventricular Mass in Patients With Type 2 Diabetes Mellitus and Coronary Artery Disease: The EMPA-HEART CardioLink-6 Randomized Clinical Trial. Circulation. 2019;140(21):1693-702.

ABSTRACT

Aim: To determine the effect of empagliflozin, a sodium-glucose cotransporter-2 (SGLT-2) inhibitor on left ventricular (LV) mass in type 2 diabetics patients with known coronary artery disease (CAD).

Methods: A total of 97 subjects of age group 40–80 years and hemoglobin A1c (HbA1c) levels 6.5–10.0%, with known CAD and estimated glomerular filtration rate (eGFR) ≥ 60 mL/min/1.73 m², were included in the study. The subjects were randomly allocated two groups of which, one received 10 mg empagliflozin, and the other placebo for 6 months. Change in LV mass-indexed (LVMi) to body surface area (BSA) at the end of 6 months from baseline was calculated using magnetic resonance imaging, and was the primary outcome. LV end-diastolic and -systolic volumes indexed to BSA (LVEDVi and LVESVi), left ventricular ejection fraction (LVEF), 24-hour ambulatory blood pressure, hematocrit values, and N-terminal pro B-type natriuretic peptide (NT-proBNP) were also observed after 6 months.

Results: Mean reduction in LVMi was 2.6 g/m² and 0.01 g/m² for empagliflozin and placebo groups, respectively (adjusted difference −3.35 g/m², 95% CI −5.9 to −0.81 g/m², $p = 0.01$). 24 hour-ambulatory systolic (adjusted difference −6.8 mm Hg, 95% CI, −11.2 to −2.3 mm Hg, $p = 0.003$) and diastolic blood pressure (adjusted difference −3.2 mm Hg, 95% CI −5.8 to −0.6 mm Hg, $p = 0.02$), along with elevation of hematocrit was observed ($p = 0.0003$).

Conclusion: Use of empagliflozin in type 2 diabetic patients with CAD was associated with significant LVMi regression at the end of 6 months. This can partly explain the favorable cardiovascular outcomes noted in EMPA-REG OUTCOME (Empagliflozin Cardiovascular Outcome Event Trial in Type 2 Diabetes Mellitus Patients-Removing Excess Glucose) trial.

COMMENT

What was Known Prior to this Study?

In patients with type 2 diabetes mellitus (T2DM) and cardiovascular disease (CVD), the use of empagliflozin had demonstrated significant and meaningful risk-reduction for major adverse cardiovascular events, and mortality [EMPA-REG OUTCOME (Empagliflozin Cardiovascular Outcome Event Trial in Type 2 Diabetes Mellitus Patients-Removing Excess Glucose) study].[100]

However, there was limited evidence to suggest a possible improvement in cardiac structure, with the use of empagliflozin in such patients.

What this Study Adds?

- This was a double-blind, randomized, placebo-controlled trial, involving patients with T2DM and coronary artery disease (CAD), with relatively normal left ventricular mass index (LVMi). Majority of patients did not have heart failure (HF) or left-ventricular dysfunction.
- Empagliflozin use demonstrated significant reduction in LVMi (adjusted difference of −3.35 g/m² vs. placebo, $p < 0.05$), over a span of 6-month.
- This LVMi regression was demonstrated independently of reductions in 24-hour blood pressure and blood volume.

- A separately published analysis of this study also demonstrated significant reduction in myocardial extracellular volume (adjusted difference of –1.4% vs. placebo, $p < 0.05$); this is indicative of improvement in extracellular matrix remodeling, with empagliflozin.[101]
- This study also demonstrated early increase in erythropoietin production, stimulation of erythropoiesis, and increase in circulating vascular progenitor as well as anti-inflammatory cells with M2 macrophage polarization, in empagliflozin group ($p < 0.05$ vs. placebo).[102,103]
- These effects suggest possible reverse cardiac remodeling with empagliflozin, in patients with T2DM and CAD, largely without HF or left ventricular (LV) dysfunction.

Major Strengths of the Study

- A robust, experimental study-design, with conclusive demonstration of empagliflozin-related salutary effect on cardiac structure, in patients with CAD and T2DM.
- Use of cardiac magnetic resonance, to provide reliable assessments of LV parameters.
- The study findings compliment the clinical outcomes demonstrated in the EMPA-REG OUTCOME study, in a similar group of patients.

Limitations of the Study

- The study does not represent patients with HF, LV dysfunction, or chronic kidney disease.
- Majority (>90%) of study participants were male patients.
- About 29 patients had experienced changes in background therapy during the study; this aspect may be possibly balanced across the study groups, due to randomization.

Implications of the Findings for the Clinicians

The decrease in LVMi associated with empagliflozin, may contribute to the CV benefits observed in patients with T2DM and CAD, who are treated with sodium-glucose co-transporter-2 (SGLT-2)-inhibitors.

Presence of T2DM and structural heart disease, without symptoms, represents the Stage B of HF [ACCF-AHA (American College of Cardiology Foundation/American Heart Association) staging]. Possible risk-modification with the use of SGLT-2-inhibitor empagliflozin at this stage, may be relevant in preventing the progression of CV disease, and improving long-term clinical outcomes along the CV risk continuum.

Knowledge Gaps Identified and Scope for Future Research

- Majority of study participants did not have HF or LV dysfunction; thus, changes in LV volumes, ejection fraction, or N-terminal pro B-type natriuretic peptide (NT-proBNP) levels were not expected in this population. Studies like EMPA-TROPISM, REFORM, DAPA LVH, SUGAR DM-HF, and EMPA-VISION, are relevant in providing further insights on reverse LV remodeling with SGLT-2-inhibition, in patients with HF or LV dysfunction.
- The 6-month duration of study does not provide conclusive evidence, for long-term sustenance of salutary effect on cardiac structure. Longer duration studies may provide further insights in this regard.
- The possibility of such an effect in patients with different phenotypes of LV remodeling, like age-related or hypertension-related structural heart disease, may be worthy of further exploration.

27. Suboptimal Glycemic Control among Subjects with Diabetes Mellitus in India: A Subset Analysis of Cross-sectional Wave-7 (2016) Data from the International Diabetes Management Practices Study (IDMPS)

Ref: Ramachandran A, Jain SM, Mukherjee S, Phatak S, Pitale S, Singh SK, et al. Suboptimal glycemic control among subjects with diabetes mellitus in India: a subset analysis of cross-sectional wave-7 (2016) data from the International Diabetes Management Practices Study (IDMPS). Ther Adv Endocrinol Metab. 2020;11:2042018820937217.

ABSTRACT

Objective: To assess the practices of subjects with type 1 diabetes mellitus (T1DM) and type 2 diabetes mellitus (T2DM) responsible for suboptimal glycemic control in India.

Methods: Adult diabetic patients attending physicians during a defined 2 week period were included in this cross-sectional study which was a part of wave-7 (2016) of the International Diabetes Management Practices Study (IDMPS).

Results: Out of 539 subjects, 495 had T2DM. Among them, 303 took only with oral glucose lowering drugs (OGLDs), while 158 received both OGLD and insulin. Twenty-seven subjects were treated with only insulin. T1DM was treated with insulin and OGLD in 29.5% subjects. Only 31.8% of subjects with T1DM and 32.1% with T2DM achieved glycemic targets. In subjects with T2DM who received only insulin, hemoglobin A1c (HbA1c) < 7% was in only 50% subjects. Further, approximately 30% of subjects receiving only OGLD. The reasons behind the poor rates can be due to inexperience in self-management of insulin dose and lack of awareness about diabetes.

Conclusion: Optimum insulin dosing, and educating and creating awareness about diabetes in improving the glycemic control in Indian subjects with diabetes.

COMMENT

What was Known Prior to this Study?

Glycemic control remains inadequate in developing countries and contributes to the high diabetes-related complication rates.[104] The consequent diabetes-related mortality and morbidity can be avoided by measures like early insulinization and continued self-management education, as specified by major guidelines.[105,106] However, the distinct Indian diabetes phenotype characterized by lower body mass index (BMI), lower adiponectin concentrations, higher levels of highly sensitive C-reactive protein, significant procoagulant affinities, and a greater propensity to develop cardiovascular complications, necessitates an India-specific diabetes management guideline.[107-112] Despite the availability and widespread acceptance of the Research Society for the Study of Diabetes in India (RSSDI) 2015 guidelines, diabetes management in India has been hampered by multiple factors like socioeconomic disparity, geographical diversity, inadequate disease awareness, lack of access to glycated hemoglobin (HbA1c) testing and clinical inertia leading to delayed insulinization.[107,108,112-114]

What this Study Adds?

This study provides insights into the real-world diabetes management practices in Indian settings. This study showed that the overall rate of glycemic control [25.2% in type 2 diabetes mellitus (T2DM) and 7.3% in type 1 diabetes mellitus (T1DM)] was not in line with the observations from previous studies conducted in developing nations as well as earlier studies from India. Better glycemic control was seen with insulin use, either alone or in combination with oral glucose lowering drugs (OGLDs). Basal insulin was observed to be the most used insulin across both T1DM and T2DM. Lack of experience in self-management of insulin dosing, lack of insulin titration, and lack of diabetes education were the major reasons for suboptimal glycemic control. Cost of testing strips was one of the major factors for poor self-monitoring of blood glucose (SMBG) in about one-third of the patients.

Major Strengths of the Study

This study addresses the unmet need for the India-specific data on diabetes management practices, disease prevalence, and associated complications.

Limitations of the Study

This study had a few limitations due to its observational nature, such as bias, confounding factors, and the inability to ascertain cause-and-effect relationships between variables, lack of long-term follow-up for examining associations between other factors. Further this study did not scrutinize the factors preventing glycemic control or examine patient reported outcomes (PROs) like quality of life which have grown in significance for guiding diabetes management decisions.

Implications for Clinicians

To minimize the strain on economic resources, an improved access to cheaper glucometers and test strips, timely insulinization as well as adequate dose titration, continued diabetes management education, and patient empowerment for self-management of diabetes may help improve diabetes treatment and the outcomes in India.

Knowledge Gaps and Future Research

Subsequent studies may be designed to discern the cause-effect relations of the variables like diabetes education status, self-management practices, etc., affecting glycemic control in the patients. Further, longitudinal studies may be developed to understand the long-term impact of these variables pertaining to the diabetes management practices on the glycemic control. Newer therapeutic endpoints like PROs need to be evaluated for their association with glycemic control and the impact of the identified variables on these PROs.

---

28. A Practitioner's Toolkit for Insulin Motivation in Adults with Type 1 and Type 2 Diabetes Mellitus: Evidence-based Recommendations from an International Expert Panel

Ref: Kalra S, Bajaj S, Sharma SK, Priya G, Baruah MP, Sanyal D, et al. A Practitioner's Toolkit for Insulin Motivation in Adults with Type 1 and Type 2 Diabetes Mellitus: Evidence-Based Recommendations from an International Expert Panel. Diabetes Ther. 2020;11(3):585-606.

ABSTRACT

An international expert panel consisting of endocrinologists from all over the world met to discuss the issue of insulin distress, which is a hindrance in using insulin for the management of diabetes mellitus. Insulin distress is a psychological reaction of a patient when advised to use insulin as a part of diabetes management. Insulin motivation is an essential step to accomplish the target of maintaining adequate glycemic control in such population that includes dealing with factors related to patient, physician, and drug. Building up of efficient communication between diabetic patients and their physicians is of utmost importance so that the patients are comfortable with insulin use. The expert panel after reviewing existing evidences and extensive discussions recommended various strategies in the form of toolkits for insulin motivation. To eliminate insulin distress, behavioral changes should be brought in the patients so that the compliance to treatment is increased and proper diabetic care can be provided.

COMMENT

What was Known Prior to this Expert Opinion?

Insulin distress indicates patient's emotional response when insulin is advised. Its major characteristics are severe apprehension, discomfort, dejection, or denial due to a perceived inability to adjust with the demands of insulin therapy leading to diabetes distress.[115]

Although the high efficacy of insulin enables achievement of tight glycemic control, insulinization is often delayed in type 2 diabetic patients due to psychologic insulin resistance (PIR) at the levels of physician as well as patient. As a result of association of several myths with insulin therapy, the essential decision to initiate insulin as well as path of treatment often presents as psychologic barriers, leading to resistance to treatment.[116]

Almost 25% of type 2 diabetic patients hesitate to start insulin and consider it the "last-resort" option.[117] The prevalence of refusal and rejection to insulin is between 20% and 40% among insulin naïve type 2 diabetic patients. Even, adherence to insulin therapy is suboptimal among one-third of the existing insulin using patients with type 2 diabetes mellitus (T2DM).[118] As timely insulin initiation reduces the risk of micro- and macrovascular complications, it is essential to identify its barriers.[119]

Insulin distress has become a major concern in diabetic patients as it acts as a hindrance to effective management. Various advances in treatment in the form of modern analog insulin, more discrete delivery systems for insulin and digital technology have been introduced to reduce insulin distress and improve treatment outcomes.[120]

Problem areas in the diabetes (PAID) scale and diabetes distress scale (DDS) are the common tools to evaluate diabetes distress. DDS is a 17-item scale, measuring treatment regimen distress, interpersonal distress, physician distress, and emotional burden.[121,122] PAID is a self-administered 20-item scale that measures emotional distress, such as depressed mood, guilt, anger, worry, and fear, in individuals with diabetes.[123,124]

What this Expert Opinion Adds?

This initiative by a panel of endocrinologists through an international meeting provided insights for minimizing PIR among diabetic patients, identifying the factors associated with PIR and utilizing intervention strategies to address these factors to aid in timely initiation of insulin therapy at the appropriate time. The panel has developed a tool kit to aid a practitioner in implementing insulin motivation strategies at different stages of insulin therapy. Bringing in positive behavioral change by motivating the patient to improve treatment adherence helps overcome insulin distress and achieve treatment goals. Recommendations have been laid down to apply the biopsychosocial model of health rather than a purely glucocentric or biomedical approach, to initiate sequential motivational conversation and counseling and using easy-to-understand analogies to help diabetic patients overcome insulin distress.

The recommendation emphasizes on positive behavioral changes in the patients, conducting motivational interviews (MI) being empathetic and supportive and using separate toolkits at different stages—at diagnosis, pre-initiation, initiation, titration, and intensification—to achieve *"euthymia"* (positive mental health, psychologic well-being, and eustress). The panel has also suggested ways of improving insulin acceptance, compliance, and adherence by switching to pens from vials/syringes, preferring simple, single-prick only basal insulin and using advanced technology and effective communication strategies.

Major Strengths of the Expert Opinion

This recommendation addresses the unmet need of minimizing a very common roadblock in managing diabetes in the form of insulin distress. The study provides systematic, innovative, patient-centric recommendations, and toolkits to counter the hesitation of patients toward insulin and improve acceptance and adherence to insulin therapy.

Limitations of the Expert Opinion

The major limitation is applicability of the recommendations and toolkits in real world and need for individualization *as one size does not fit all*. The entire procedure recommended can be complex, time consuming, and would require intense coordination among clinician, health educators, and patients as well as it would need greater level of motivation on the part of both clinician and patient. Successful application of the toolkits will also depend on the level of awareness, literacy, and will-power of the patients. The recommendations were laid down through consensus by the expert panel and the results and usefulness of applying those in real world is still unknown.

Implications for Clinicians

These recommendations and toolkits will improve acceptance of insulin by patients, help the clinician in timely initiation, titration, and intensification of insulin therapy and in choosing appropriate regimen for individualized patients so that compliance and adherence to the therapy improves which in turn would help in achieving better glycemic control and minimizing risk of complications. Also, the intense empathetic conversations on insulin and motivational interviewing will help in developing stronger emotional bond and mutual trust between the clinician and patient.

Knowledge Gaps and Future Research

Subsequent studies may be designed to apply the toolkits and the entire recommended procedure in patients in the form of randomized controlled trials as well as real-world studies to confirm the utility of the recommendations in clinical practice.

29. Impact of Baseline Characteristics and Beta-cell Function on the Efficacy and Safety of Subcutaneous Once-weekly Semaglutide: A Patient-level, Pooled Analysis of the SUSTAIN 1-5 Trials

Ref: Aroda VR, Capehorn MS, Chaykin L, Frias JP, Lausvig NL, Macura S, et al. Impact of baseline characteristics and beta-cell function on the efficacy and safety of subcutaneous once-weekly semaglutide: A patient-level, pooled analysis of the SUSTAIN 1-5 trials. Diabetes Obes Metab. 2020;22(3):303-14.

ABSTRACT

Aim: To assess the impact of patient characteristics at baseline and beta cell function on the efficacy and safety of semaglutide in type 2 diabetic patients.

Materials and methods: A pooled analysis of SUSTAIN 1–5 (phase 3a) trials which were randomized, controlled trials was conducted. The change in hemoglobin A1c (HbA1c) from baseline and body weight (BW) were the endpoints. A composite endpoint was taken as HbA1c < 7.0% (53 mmol/mol), without weight gain or severe/blood glucose-confirmed symptomatic hypoglycemia at week 30 with semaglutide (0.5/1.0 mg). Patients were divided into subgroups on the basis of baseline HbA1c level, background medications, duration of disease, and function of beta cell of pancreas. Baseline HbA1c was subgroup as ≤7.5%, >7.5–8.0%, >8.0–8.5%, >8.5–9.0% and >9.0%.

Results: Mean reductions in HbA1c and BW were more in semaglutide 1.0 mg compared to 0.5 mg across defined subgroups. Reduction in HbA1c in its subgroups was −0.9%, −1.2%, −1.5%, −1.7%, and −2.3% (effect of subgroup within treatment: $p = 0.247$) and −1.1%, −1.4%, −1.9%, −2.1%, and −2.7% ($p = 0.045$) for semaglutide 0.5 mg and 1.0 mg, respectively. The corresponding BW reductions was −4.4, −3.9, −3.9, −3.3, and −2.9 kg ($p = 0.004$), and −6.4, −5.9, −5.2, −4.5, and −4.8 kg ($p < 0.001$), respectively.

Conclusion: Semaglutide was effective across wide range of patients with varying characteristics.

COMMENT

What was Known Prior to this Study?

The efficacy and safety of semaglutide, a subcutaneous (SC), once-weekly (OW) glucagon-like peptide-1 (GLP-1) analogue for type 2 diabetes mellitus (T2DM) treatment has been reported by the global phase 3a and 3b Semaglutide Unabated Sustainability in Treatment of Type 2 Diabetes (SUSTAIN) clinical trial development program. It has shown higher reductions in hemoglobin A1c (HbA1c) and body weight (BW) as compared to placebo and other active comparators. The full spectrum of diabetes care with treatment-naïve subjects on the oral antidiabetic drugs (OADs) and on insulin background has been represented by the SUSTAIN 1–5 trials ($n = 3,918$) with differences in baseline characteristics.

What this Study Adds?

The efficacy and safety of GLP-1 receptor agonists (GLP-1RA) therapy may be impacted by certain clinical indicators of disease status in heterogeneous populations of T2DM adults including glycemic control (HbA1c), duration of diabetes, background antidiabetic medications, and pancreatic beta-cell function. The impact of these clinical indicators on the efficacy and safety of semaglutide SC. OW was assessed in T2DM patients with inadequately controlled diabetes by post-hoc exploratory analyses of data from the SUSTAIN trials. The consistent efficacious effect of treatment with semaglutide SC. OW was shown across subgroups by disease severity and progression in subjects with uncontrolled T2DM in the study with clinically important reduction in HbA1c and BW. Semaglutide was reported to be well-tolerated and a low risk of hypoglycemia was seen.

Major Strengths of the Study

The large number of subjects with a range of treatments, i.e., from drug naïve to insulin therapy with different baseline characteristics were taken for analysis (SUSTAIN 1–5 phase 3a trials) from across the continuum of T2DM care.

Limitations of the Study

- The analysis was carried out without including comparator data due to nature of pooled semaglutide data.
- The comparison was done across post hoc-defined subgroups which was not a randomized comparison.
- The confounding effects from underlying differences including additive effects of different background therapies were present.
- No adjustments were made in the analysis for potential confounders, e.g., differences in baseline characteristics across homeostatic model assessment-β (HOMA-B) tertiles requiring the data to be interpreted cautiously although HOMA-B analyses

can be considered suitable for use in the presence of insulinotropic compounds.
- Trial inclusion/exclusion criteria may result in some selection bias.

Implications of the Findings for the Clinicians

The efficacy and safety profile of semaglutide remains same and is not affected by patient characteristics, disease severity and further support patient-centered decision-making in the treatment of T2DM.

Knowledge Gaps Identified and Scope for Future Research

Studies in subpopulations with similar parameters as primary endpoints to reach conclusive evidences.

30. Efficacy and Safety of Once-weekly Semaglutide versus Daily Canagliflozin as Add-on to Metformin in Patients with Type 2 Diabetes (SUSTAIN 8): A Double-blind, Phase 3b, Randomized Controlled Trial

Ref: Lingvay I, Catarig AM, Frias JP, Kumar H, Lausvig NL, le Roux CW, et al. Efficacy and safety of once-weekly semaglutide versus daily canagliflozin as add-on to metformin in patients with type 2 diabetes (SUSTAIN 8): A double-blind, phase 3b, randomised controlled trial. Lancet Diabetes Endocrinol. 2019;7(11):834-44.

ABSTRACT

Aim: To determine and compare the efficacy and safety of semaglutide, a glucagon-like peptide-1 (GLP-1) receptor agonist at a weekly dose and daily canagliflozin, a sodium-glucose cotransporter-2 (SGLT-2) inhibitor in type 2 diabetic patients, who are already on metformin.

Methods: A double-blind, parallel-group, phase 3b, randomized controlled trial was conducted on adult subjects with type 2 diabetes mellitus (T2DM), uncontrolled on metformin. Randomization of the subjects was done using interactive web response system, and the two groups formed were given semaglutide 1.0 mg by subcutaneous route once in a week, or canagliflozin 300 mg, orally once in a day. At week 52, change in HbA1c from baseline was the primary endpoint, while change in body weight from baseline, was the confirmatory secondary endpoint.

Findings: A greater reduction in HbA1c from baseline and body weight, was observed in subjects who received semaglutide than those who received canagliflozin [HbA1c estimated treatment difference (ETD) −0.49% points, 95% CI −0.65 to −0.33; −5.34 mmol/mol, 95% CI −7.10 to −3.57; $p < 0.0001$; and body weight ETD −1.06 kg, 95% CI −1.76 to −0.36; $p = 0.0029$]. Nausea was the most commonly observed adverse events with semaglutide seen in 47% subjects; whereas among infections and infestations, urinary tract infections were most frequently observed and observed mostly with canagliflozin. Due to occurrence of adverse effects, treatment was discontinued 10% of the subjects who were treated with canagliflozin. There was report of one fatal adverse effect in the semaglutide group which was unlikely to be due to the drug.

Interpretation: Semaglutide (1.0 mg) given by subcutaneous route once in a week was found to be better in reducing HbA1c and body weight in type 2 diabetic patients as an add on to metformin, compared to oral canagliflozin given daily.

COMMENT

What was Known Prior to this Study?

The SUSTAIN (Semaglutide Unabated Sustainability in Treatment of Type 2 Diabetes) clinical trial program has demonstrated the efficacy of semaglutide, a glucagon-like peptide-1 (GLP-1) receptor agonist (GLP-1RA) across the continuum of diabetes care. Similarly, another once-daily oral sodium-glucose co-transporter-2 (SGLT-2) inhibitor, canagliflozin has also been reported to have glycemic control and weight loss efficacy as compared to placebo and active comparators. Cardiovascular benefits have been reported to be provided by both semaglutide and canagliflozin in high risk type 2 diabetic patients.

What this Study Adds?

The comparative data on the efficacy of GLP-1 RAs versus SGLT-2 inhibitors is not sufficient but both the groups are being used as second-line agents. In this regard, SUSTAIN 8 study was carried out to compare the efficacy of semaglutide 1.0 mg with canagliflozin 300 mg in reducing hemoglobin A1c (HbA1c) and body weight in type 2 uncontrolled diabetic patients. The higher efficacy of once-weekly semaglutide 1.0 mg was demonstrated by SUSTAIN 8 in reducing HbA1c and body weight than daily canagliflozin 300 mg on a background of metformin treatment. Both the drug regimen were well tolerated and with low rates of hypoglycemia.

Major Strengths of the Study

- Substantial size
- Global population
- Double-blind nature
- Relatively long treatment period
- Being a relevant head-to-head comparison with a well-established glucose-lowering medication

Limitations of the Study

- Although not specific to this study, results from strictly implemented randomized controlled trials (RCTs) may not be reflective of outcomes in heterogenous patient population in regular clinical practice.
- Long-term effects, i.e., persistence and potential complications and comorbidities could not be assessed in this study requiring longer studies to explore them.
- The double-blind, double-dummy trial design meant that patients receiving oral canagliflozin also received a weekly injection of semaglutide-mimicking placebo. While this minimized study bias, it also limited the true effect of each treatment on patient-reported outcomes, particularly diabetes treatment satisfaction questionnaire (DTSQ) (which assesses treatment satisfaction, flexibility, and convenience), because of receipt of an injection in both treatment groups.

Implications of the Findings for the Clinicians

The evidence from the SUSTAIN clinical trial program of semaglutide of being effective glucose-lowering medication with additional benefits of weight loss and cardiovascular-protective effects are supported be the results of the present study. The results may be useful in guiding to make decisions to intensify the treatment after metformin therapy in this group of patients.

Knowledge Gaps Identified and Scope for Future Research

- Real-world evidence and pragmatic clinical trials which compare GLP-1RAs versus SGLT-2 inhibitors
- A combination of these two classes of drugs compared to each separately and with placebo in a multi-arm parallel group clinical trials.
- A similar study design can be implemented to evaluate cardiovascular safety in real world too.

REFERENCES (Drugs and Therapeutics)

1. McMurray JJV, Solomon SD, Inzucchi SE, Køber L, Kosiborod MN, Martinez FA, et al; Dapagliflozin in patients with heart failure and reduced ejection fraction. N Engl J Med. 2019;381(21):1995-2008.
2. Petrie MC, Verma S, Docherty KF, Inzucchi SE, Anand I, Belohlávek J, et al. Effect of Dapagliflozin on Worsening Heart Failure and Cardiovascular Death in Patients With Heart Failure With and Without Diabetes. JAMA. 2020;323(14):1353-1368.
3. Neal B, Arnott C. A novel cardioprotective therapy that also improves glycemia. JAMA. 2020;323(14):1349-50.
4. Consoli A, Formoso G, Baldassarre MPA, Febo F. A comparative safety review between GLP-1 receptor agonists and SGLT2 inhibitors for diabetes treatment. Expert Opin Drug Saf. 2018;17(3):293-302.
5. Fulcher G, Matthews DR, Perkovic V, de Zeeuw D, Mahaffey KW, Mathieu C, et al. Efficacy and safety of canagliflozin when used in conjunction with incretin-mimetic therapy in patients with type 2 diabetes. Diabetes Obes Metab. 2016;18(1):82-91.
6. Frias JP, Guja C, Hardy E, Ahmed A, Dong F, Öhman P, et al. Exenatide once weekly plus dapagliflozin once daily versus exenatide or dapagliflozin alone in patients with type 2 diabetes inadequately controlled with metformin monotherapy (DURATION-8): A 28 week, multicentre, double-blind, phase 3, randomised controlled trial. Lancet Diabetes Endocrinol. 2016;4(12):1004-16.
7. Ludvik B, Frias JP, Tinahones FJ, Wainstein J, Jiang H, Robertson KE, et al. Dulaglutide as add-on therapy to SGLT2 inhibitors in patients with inadequately controlled type 2 diabetes (AWARD-10): A 24-week, randomised, double-blind, placebo-controlled trial. Lancet Diabetes Endocrinol. 2018;6(5):370-81.
8. Patoulias D, Stavropoulos K, Imprialos K, Katsimardou A, Kalogirou MS, Koutsampasopoulos K, et al. Glycemic efficacy and safety of glucagon-like peptide-1 receptor agonist on top of sodium-glucose co-transporter-2 inhibitor treatment compared to sodium-glucose co-transporter-2 inhibitor alone: A systematic review and meta-analysis of randomized controlled trials. Diabetes Res Clin Pract. 2019;158:107927.
9. Zinman B, Bhosekar V, Busch R, Holst I, Ludvik B, Thielke D, et al. Semaglutide once weekly as add-on to SGLT-2 inhibitor therapy in type 2 diabetes (SUSTAIN 9): A randomised, placebo-controlled trial. Lancet Diabetes Endocrinol. 2019;7(5):356-67.
10. Mantsiou C, Karagiannis T, Kakotrichi P, Malandris K, Avgerinos I, Liakos A, et al. Glucagon-like peptide-1 receptor agonists and sodium-glucose co-transporter-2 inhibitors as combination therapy for type 2 diabetes: A systematic review and meta-analysis. Diabetes Obes Metab. 2020;22(10):1857-68.
11. American Diabetes Association. Classification and diagnosis of diabetes: Standards of Medical Care in Diabetes-2020. Diabetes Care. 2020;43(Suppl 1):S14-S31.
12. Rosenstock J, Bajaj HS, Janež A, Silver R, Begtrup K, Hansen MV, et al. Once-weekly insulin for type 2 diabetes without previous insulin treatment. N Engl J Med. 2020;383(22):2107-16.
13. Gottlieb PA, Michels AW. Advances in Diabetes Treatment-Once-Weekly Insulin. N Engl J Med. 2020;383(22):2171-2.
14. Gilon P. The Role of α-Cells in Islet Function and Glucose Homeostasis in Health and Type 2 Diabetes. J Mol Biol. 2020;432(5):1367-94.
15. Gilon P, Cheng-Xue R, Lai BK, Chae HY, Gomez-Ruiz A. Physiological and pathophysiological control of glucagon secretion by pancreatic α-cells, In: Islets of Langerhans. Springer. Dordrecht, Heidelberg, New York, London. 2015:175-245.
16. Christensen M, Bagger JI, Vilsbøll T, Knop FK. The alpha-cell as target for type 2 diabetes therapy. Rev Diabet Stud. 2011;8(3):369-81.
17. Okamoto H, Cavino K, Na E, Krumm E, Kim SY, Cheng X, et al. Glucagon receptor inhibition normalizes blood glucose in severe insulin-resistant mice. Proc Natl Acad Sci U S A. 2017;114(10):2753-8.
18. Okamoto H, Kim J, Aglione J, Lee J, Cavino K, Na E, et al. Glucagon Receptor Blockade With a Human Antibody Normalizes Blood Glucose in Diabetic Mice and Monkeys. Endocrinology. 2015;156(8):2781-94.
19. Kazda CM, Ding Y, Kelly RP, Garhyan P, Shi C, Lim CN, et al. Evaluation of efficacy and safety of the glucagon receptor antagonist LY2409021 in patients with type 2 diabetes: 12- and 24-week phase 2 studies. Diabetes Care. 2016;39:1241-9.
20. Kazierad DJ, Bergman A, Tan B, Erion DM, Somayaji V, Lee DS, et al. Effects of multiple ascending doses of the glucagon receptor antagonist PF-06291874 in patients with type 2 diabetes mellitus. Diabetes Obes Metab. 2016;18(8):795-802.
21. Lefebvre PJ, Paquot N, Scheen AJ. Inhibiting or antagonizing glucagon: Making progress in diabetes care. Diabetes Obes Metab. 2015;17(8):720-5.
22. Vajda EG, Potter SC, Fujitaki JM, Reddy RK, Van Poelje PD, Lee YH, et al. LGD-6972, a potent, orally-bioavailable, small molecule glucagon receptor antagonist for the treatment of type 2 diabetes (Abstract). Diabetes. 2012;61(Suppl 1):A252.
23. Vajda EG, Logan D, Lasseter K, Armas D, Plotkin DJ, Pipkin JD, et al. Pharmacokinetics and pharmacodynamics of single and multiple doses of the glucagon receptor antagonist LGD-6972 in healthy subjects and subjects with type 2 diabetes mellitus. Diabetes Obes Metab. 2017;19(1):24-32.
24. Pettus JH, D'Alessio D, Frias JP, Vajda EG, Pipkin JD, Rosenstock J, et al. Efficacy and Safety of the Glucagon Receptor Antagonist RVT-1502 in Type 2 Diabetes Uncontrolled on Metformin Monotherapy: A 12-Week Dose-Ranging Study. Diabetes Care. 2020;43(1):161-8.

25. Kazierad DJ, Chidsey K, Somayaji VR, Bergman AJ, Calle RA. Efficacy and safety of the glucagon receptor antagonist PF-06291874: A 12-week, randomized, dose-response study in patients with type 2 diabetes mellitus on background metformin therapy. Diabetes Obes Metab. 2018;20(11):2608-16.
26. Jun LS, Millican RL, Hawkins ED, Konkol DL, Showalter AD, Christe ME, et al. Absence of glucagon and insulin action reveals a role for the GLP-1 receptor in endogenous glucose production. Diabetes. 2015;64(3):819-27.
27. Sivitz WI, Phillips LS, Wexler DJ, Fortmann SP, Camp AW, Tiktin M, et al. Optimization of Metformin in the GRADE Cohort: Effect on Glycemia and Body Weight. Diabetes Care. 2020;43(5):940-7.
28. McGovern A, Tippu Z, Hinton W, Munro N, Whyte M, de Lusignan S. Comparison of medication adherence and persistence in type 2 diabetes: a systematic review and meta-analysis. Diabetes Obes Metab. 2018;20(4):1040-43.
29. Schauer PR, Bhatt DL, Kirwan JP, Wolski K, Aminian A, Brethauer SA, et al. Bariatric surgery versus intensive medical therapy for diabetes-5-year outcomes. N Engl J Med. 2017;376(7):641-51.
30. Falken Y, Hellström PM, Holst JJ, Näslund E. Changes in glucose homeostasis after Roux-en-Y gastric bypass surgery for obesity at day three, two months, and one year after surgery: Role of gut peptides. J Clin Endocrinol Metab. 2011;96(7):2227-35.
31. Wewer Albrechtsen NJ, Hornburg D, Albrechtsen R, Svendsen B, Toräng S, Jepsen SL, et al. Oxyntomodulin Identified as a Marker of Type 2 Diabetes and Gastric Bypass Surgery by Mass-spectrometry Based Profiling of Human Plasma. EBioMedicine. 2016;7:112-20.
32. Dar MS, Chapman WH 3rd, Pender JR, Drake AJ 3rd, O'Brien K, Tanenberg RJ, et al. GLP-1 response to a mixed meal: What happens 10 years after Roux-en-Y gastric bypass (RYGB)? Obes Surg. 2012;22(7):1077-83.
33. Tan T, Behary P, Tharakan G, Minnion J, Al-Najim W, Albrechtsen NJW, et al. The Effect of a Subcutaneous Infusion of GLP-1, OXM, and PYY on Energy Intake and Expenditure in Obese Volunteers. J Clin Endocrinol Metab. 2017;102(7):2364-72.
34. Behary P, Tharakan G, Alexiadou K, Johnson N, Wewer Albrechtsen NJ, Kenkre J, et al. Combined GLP-1, Oxyntomodulin, and Peptide YY Improves Body Weight and Glycemia in Obesity and Prediabetes/Type 2 Diabetes: A Randomized, Single-Blinded, Placebo-Controlled Study. Diabetes Care. 2019;42(8):1446-53.
35. Alexiadou K, Tan TMM. Gastrointestinal Peptides as Therapeutic Targets to Mitigate Obesity and Metabolic Syndrome. Curr Diab Rep. 2020;20(7):26.
36. Afrezza. MannKind Corporation, Danbury, CT. [online] Available from https://www.accessdata.fda.gov/drugsatfda_docs/label/2018/022472s018lbl.pdf [Last accessed March, 2021].
37. FIASP. [online] Available from https://www.novo-pi.com/fiasp.pdf [Last accessed March, 2021].
38. Bode BW, McGill JB, Lorber DL, Gross JL, Chang PC, Bregman DB, et al. Inhaled Technosphere Insulin compared with injected pranidal insulin in type 1 diabetes: A randomized 24-week trial. Diabetes Care. 2015;38(12):2266-73.
39. International Hypoglycaemia Study Group. Glucose concentrations of less than 3.0 mmol/L (54 mg/dL) should be reported in clinical trials: A joint position statement of the American Diabetes Association and the European Association for the Study of Diabetes. Diabetes Care. 2017;40(1):155-7.
40. Seaquist ER, Blonde L, McGill JB, Heller SR, Kendall DM, Bumpass JB, et al. Hypoglycaemia is reduced with use of inhaled Technosphere® Insulin relative to insulin aspart in type 1 diabetes mellitus. Diabet Med. 2020;37(5):752-9.
41. Elraiyah T, Tsapas A, Prutsky G, Domecq JP, Hasan R, Firwana B, et al. A systematic review and meta-analysis of adjunctive therapies in diabetic foot ulcers. J Vasc Surg. 2016;63(2 Suppl):46S-58S.e1-2.
42. Kranke P, Bennett MH, Martyn-St James M, Schnabel A, Debus SE, Weibel S. Hyperbaric oxygen therapy for chronic wounds. Cochrane Database Syst Rev. 2015:2015(6):CD004123.
43. Zhao D, Luo S, Xu W, Hu J, Lin S, Wang N. Efficacy and Safety of Hyperbaric Oxygen Therapy Used in Patients With Diabetic Foot: A Meta-analysis of Randomized Clinical Trials. Clin Ther. 2017;39(10):2088-94.
44. Santema KTB, Stoekenbroek RM, Koelemay MJW, Reekers JA, van Dortmont LMC, Oomen A, et al. Hyperbaric oxygen therapy in the treatment of ischemic lower extremity ulcers in patients with diabetes: Results of the DAMO2CLES multicenter randomized clinical trial. Diabetes Care. 2018;41(1):112-9.
45. Golledge J, Singh TP. Systematic review and meta-analysis of clinical trials examining the effect of hyperbaric oxygen therapy in people with diabetes-related lower limb ulcers. Diabet Med. 2019;36(7):813-26.
46. Duzgun AP, Satir HZ, Ozozan O, Saylam B, Kulah B, Coskun F. Effect of hyperbaric oxygen therapy on healing of diabetic foot ulcers. J Foot Ankle Surg. 2008;47(6):515-9.
47. Zweck E, Roden M. GLP-1 receptor agonists and cardiovascular disease: drug-specific or class effects? Lancet Diabetes Endocrinol. 2019;7(2):89-90.
48. Cooke CE, Lee HY, Tong YP, Haines ST. Persistence with injectable antidiabetic agents in members with type 2 diabetes in a commercial managed care organization. Curr Med Res Opin. 2010;26(1):231-8.
49. Husain M, Birkenfeld AL, Donsmark M, Dungan K, Eliaschewitz FG, Franco DR, et al. Oral Semaglutide and Cardiovascular Outcomes in Patients with Type 2 Diabetes. N Engl J Med. 2019;381(9):841-51.
50. Marso SP, Bain SC, Consoli A, et al. Semaglutide and cardiovascular outcomes in patients with type 2 diabetes. N Engl J Med. 2016;375(19):1834-44.
51. Cosentino F, Grant PJ, Aboyans V, Bailey CJ, Ceriello A, Delgado V, et al. 2019 ESC Guidelines on diabetes, pre-diabetes, and cardiovascular diseases developed in collaboration with the EASD. Eur Heart J. 2020;41(2):255-323.

52. Crusell MKW, Hansen TH, Nielsen T, Allin KH, Rühlemann MC, Damm P, et al. Gestational diabetes is associated with change in the gut microbiota composition in third trimester of pregnancy and postpartum. Microbiome. 2018;6(1):89.
53. Luoto R, Laitinen K, Nermes M, Isolauri E. Impact of maternal probiotic-supplemented dietary counselling on pregnancy outcome and prenatal and postnatal growth: A double-blind, placebo-controlled study. Br J Nutr. 2010;103(12):1792-9.
54. Wickens KL, Barthow CA, Murphy R, et al. Early pregnancy probiotic supplementation with Lactobacillus rhamnosus HN001 may reduce the prevalence of gestational diabetes mellitus: A randomized controlled trial. Br J Nutr. 2017;117(6):804-13.
55. Lindsay KL, Kennelly M, Culliton M, Smith T, Maguire OC, Shanahan F, et al. Probiotics in obese pregnancy do not reduce maternal fasting glucose: A double-blind, placebo-controlled, randomized trial (Probiotics in Pregnancy Study). Am J Clin Nutr. 2014;99(6):1432-9.
56. Dallanora S, Medeiros de Souza Y, Deon RG et al. Do probiotics effectively ameliorate glycemic control during gestational diabetes? A systematic review. Arch Gynecol Obstet. 2018;298(3):477-85.
57. Pan J, Pan Q, Chen Y, Zhang H, Zheng X. Efficacy of probiotic supplement for gestational diabetes mellitus: a systematic review and meta-analysis. J Matern Fetal Neonatal Med. 2019;32(2):317-23.
58. Taylor BL, Woodfall GE, Sheedy KE, O'Riley ML, Rainbow KA, Bramwell EL, et al. Effect of Probiotics on Metabolic Outcomes in Pregnant Women with Gestational Diabetes: A Systematic Review and Meta-Analysis of Randomized Controlled Trials. Nutrients. 2017;9(5):461.
59. Masulli M, Vitacolonna E, Fraticelli F, Della Pepa G, Mannucci E, Monami M. Effects of probiotic supplementation during pregnancy on metabolic outcomes: A systematic review and meta-analysis of randomized controlled trials. Diabetes Res Clin Pract. 2020;162:108111.
60. McMurray JJV, Solomon SD, Inzucchi SE, Køber L, Kosiborod MN, Martinez FA, et al. Dapagliflozin in Patients with Heart Failure and Reduced Ejection Fraction. N Engl J Med. 2019;381(21):1995-2008.
61. Sullivan K, Van Spall HGC. Dapagliflozin reduced worsening HF or CV death in HF with reduced ejection fraction. Ann Intern Med. 2020;172(4):JC16.
62. Neal B, Arnott C. A Novel Cardioprotective Therapy that also improves Glycemia. JAMA. 2020;323(14):1349-50.
63. Vieira JL, Mehra MR. Dapagliflozin in Patients with Heart Failure and Reduced Ejection Fraction. N Engl J Med. 2020;382(10):972-3.
64. Liu Q, Li S, Quan H, Li J. Vitamin B12 status in metformin treated patients: Systematic review. PLoS One. 2014;9(6):e100379.
65. Ahmed MA. Metformin and vitamin B12 deficiency: Where do we stand? J Pharm Pharm Sci. 2016;19(3):382-98.
66. Yang W, Cai X, Wu H, Ji L. Associations between metformin use and vitamin B12 levels, anemia, and neuropathy in patients with diabetes: A meta-analysis. J Diabetes. 2019;11(9):729-43.
67. de Groot-Kamphuis DM, van Dijk PR, Groenier KH, Houweling ST, Bilo HJ, Kleefstra N. Vitamin B12 deficiency and the lack of its consequences in type 2 diabetes patients using metformin. Neth J Med. 2013;71(7):386-90.
68. Karamanos B, Thanopoulou A, Drossinos V, Charalampidou E, Sourmeli S, Archimandritis A; et al. Study comparing the effect of pioglitazone in combination with either metformin or sulphonylureas on lipid profile and glycaemic control in patients with type 2 diabetes (ECLA). Curr Med Res Opin. 2011;27(2):303-13.
69. Reinstatler L, Qi YP, Williamson RS, Garn JV, Oakley GP Jr. Association of biochemical B12 deficiency with metformin therapy and vitamin B12 supplements: The National Health and Nutrition Examination Survey, 1999-2006. Diabetes Care. 2012;35(2):327-33.
70. Adetunji OR, Mani H, Morgan C, Gill GV. Metformin and anaemia: myth or reality? Practical Diabetes Int. 2009;26(7):265-6.
71. Heller S, Lingvay I, Marso SP, Philis Tsimikas A, Pieber TR, Poulter NR, et al. Risk of severe hypoglycaemia and its impact in type 2 diabetes in DEVOTE. Diabetes, Obesity and Metabolism. 2020;22(12):2241-7.
72. de Valk HW, Feher M, Hansen TK, Jendle J, Koefoed MM, Rizi EP, et al. Switching to Degludec is Associated with Reduced Hypoglycaemia, Irrespective of Definition Used or Patient Characteristics: Secondary Analysis of the ReFLeCT Prospective, Observational Study. Diabetes Ther. 2020;11(9):2159-67.
73. Baru A, Amir S, Ekelund M, Montagnoli R, Da Rocha Fernandes JD. A survey of physician experience and treatment satisfaction using fast-acting insulin aspart in people with type 1 or type 2 diabetes. Postgrad Med. 2020;132(4):320-7.
74. Lane WS, Favaro E, Rathor N, Jang HC, Kjærsgaard MIS, Oviedo A, et al. A Randomized Trial Evaluating the Efficacy and Safety of Fast-Acting Insulin Aspart Compared With Insulin Aspart, Both in Combination With Insulin Degludec With or Without Metformin, in Adults With Type 2 Diabetes (Onset 9). Diabetes Care. 2020;43(8):1710-6.
75. Rodbard HW, Rosenstock J, Canani LH, Deerochanawong C, Gumprecht J, Lindberg SO, et al. Oral Semaglutide Versus Empagliflozin in Patients With Type 2 Diabetes Uncontrolled on Metformin: The PIONEER 2 Trial. Diabetes Care. 2019;42(12):2272-81.
76. Zinman B, Aroda VR, Buse JB, Cariou B, Harris SB, Hoff ST, et al. Efficacy, Safety, and Tolerability of Oral Semaglutide Versus Placebo Added to Insulin With or Without Metformin in Patients With Type 2 Diabetes: The PIONEER 8 Trial. Diabetes Care 2019;42(12):2262-71.
77. Davies MJ, D'Alessio DA, Fradkin J, Kernan WN, Mathieu C, Mingrone G, et al. Management of hyperglycaemia in type 2 diabetes, 2018. A consensus report by the American Diabetes Association (ADA) and the European Association for the study of Diabetes (EASD). Diabetologia. 2018;61(12):2461-98.
78. Sutton G, Minguet J, Ferrero C, Bramlage P. U300, a novel long-acting insulin formulation. Expert Opin Biol Ther. 2014;14(12):1849-60.

79. Bolli GB, Riddle MC, Bergenstal RM, Ziemen M, Sestakauskas K, Goyeau H, et al. New insulin glargine 300 U/mL compared with glargine 100 U/mL in insulin-naïve people with type 2 diabetes on oral glucose-lowering drugs: A randomized controlled trial (EDITION 3). Diabetes Obes Metab. 2015;17(4):386-94.
80. Rosenstock J, Cheng A, Ritzel R, Bosnyak Z, Devisme C, Cali AMG, et al. More similarities than differences testing insulin glargine 300 units/mL versus insulin degludec 100 units/mL in insulin-naive type 2 diabetes: The randomized head-to-head BRIGHT trial. Diabetes Care. 2018;41(10):2147-54.
81. Sullivan SD, Nicholls CJ, Gupta RA, Menon AA, Wu J, Westerbacka J, et al. Comparable glycaemic control and hypoglycaemia in adults with type 2 diabetes after initiating insulin glargine 300 units/mL or insulin degludec: The DELIVER Naïve D real-world study. Diabetes Obes Metab. 2019;21(9):2123-32.
82. Bailey TS, Zhou FL, Gupta RA, Preblick R, Gupta VE, Berhanu P, et al. Glycaemic goal attainment and hypoglycaemia outcomes in type 2 diabetes patients initiating insulin glargine 300 units/mL or 100 units/mL: Real-world results from the DELIVER Naïve cohort study. Diabetes Obes Metab. 2019;21(7):1596-1605.
83. Howe CJ, Cole SR, Lau B, Napravnik S, Eron JJ Jr. Selection bias due to loss to follow up in cohort studies. Epidemiology. 2016;27(1):91-7.
84. Home PD, Dain MP, Freemantle N, Kawamori R, Pfohl M, Brette S, et al. Four-year evolution of insulin regimens, glycaemic control, hypoglycaemia and body weight after starting insulin therapy in type 2 diabetes across three continents. Diab Res Clin Pract. 2015;108(2):350-9.
85. Chiesa M, Hobbs S. Making sense of social research: How useful is the Hawthorne Effect? Eur J Soc Psychol. 2008;38(1):67-74.
86. Rosenstock J, Perkovic V, Johansen OE, Cooper ME, Kahn SE, Marx N, et al. Effect of Linagliptin vs Placebo on Major Cardiovascular Events in Adults With Type 2 Diabetes and High Cardiovascular and Renal Risk: The CARMELINA Randomized Clinical Trial. JAMA. 2019;321(1):69-79.
87. Rosenstock J, Kahn SE, Johansen OE, Zinman B, Espeland MA, Woerle HJ, et al. Effect of Linagliptin vs Glimepiride on Major Adverse Cardiovascular Outcomes in Patients with Type 2 Diabetes: The CAROLINA Randomized Clinical Trial. JAMA. 2019; 322(12):1155-66.
88. Lakey WC, Barnard K, Batch BC, Chiswell K, Tasneem A, Green JB. Are current clinical trials in diabetes addressing important issues in diabetes care? Diabetologia. 2013;56(6):1226-35.
89. Cooper, ME, Rosenstock, J, Kadowaki, T, Seino Y, Wanner C, Schnaidt S, et al. Cardiovascular and kidney outcomes of linagliptin treatment in older people with type 2 diabetes and established cardiovascular disease and/or kidney disease: A prespecified subgroup analysis of the randomized, placebo-controlled CARMELINA® trial. Diabetes Obes Metab. 2020;22(7):1062-73.
90. Chawla R, Jaggi S. Implications of CVD-REAL 2 study for Indian diabetic population. J Diabetology. 2019;10:57-61.
91. Singh AK. Incretin response in Asian type 2 diabetes: Are Indians different? Indian J Endocrinology Metabolism. 2015;19(1):30-8.
92. Scirica BM, Bhatt DL, Braunwald E, Steg PG, Davidson J, Hirshberg B, et al. Saxagliptin and Cardiovascular Outcomes in Patients with Type 2 Diabetes Mellitus. N Engl J Med. 2013;369(14):1317-26.
93. Kim YG, Yoon D, Park S, Han SJ, Kim DJ, Lee KW, et al. Dipeptidyl Peptidase-4 Inhibitors and Risk of Heart Failure in Patients with Type 2 Diabetes Mellitus: A Population-Based Cohort Study. Circ Heart Fail. 2017;10(9):e003957.
94. Inagaki N, Yang W, Watada H, Ji L, Schnaidt S, Pfarr E, et al. Linagliptin and cardiorenal outcomes in Asians with type 2 diabetes mellitus and established cardiovascular and/or kidney disease: Subgroup analysis of the randomized CARMELINA® trial. Diabetol Int. 2019;11(2):129-41.
95. Lubitz SA, Benjamin EJ, Ellinor PT. Atrial fibrillation in congestive heart failure. Heart Fail Clin. 2010;6(2):187-200.
96. Anter E, Jessup M, Callans DJ. Atrial Fibrillation and Heart Failure: treatment considerations for a dual epidemic. Circulation. 2009;119(18):2516-25.
97. Slawik J, Adrian L, Hohl M, Lothschütz S, Laufs U, Böhm M. Irregular pacing of ventricular cardiomyocytes induces pro-fibrotic signalling involving paracrine effects of transforming growth factor beta and connective tissue growth factor. Eur J Heart Fail. 2019;21(4):482-91.
98. Verma S. Are the Cardiorenal Benefits of SGLT2 Inhibitors Due to Inhibition of the Sympathetic Nervous System? JACC Basic Transl Sci. 2020;5(2):180-2.
99. Zinman B, Wanner C, Lachin JM, Fitchett D, Bluhmki E, Hantel S, et al. Empagliflozin, cardiovascular outcomes, and mortality in type 2 diabetes. N Engl J Med. 2015;373(22):2117-28.
100. Verma S, Mazer CD, Yan AT, Mason T, Garg V, Teoh H, et al. Effect of Empagliflozin on Left Ventricular Mass in Patients With Type 2 Diabetes Mellitus and Coronary Artery Disease: The EMPA-HEART CardioLink-6 Randomized Clinical Trial. Circulation. 2019;140(21):1693-702.
101. Mason T, Verma S, Yan AT, Chowdhury B, Zuo F, Thorpe KE, et al. The Effect of Empagliflozin on Myocardial Extracellular Matrix Expansion in Patients With Type 2 Diabetes and Coronary Artery Disease. Circulation. 2019;140(Suppl 1): A13456.
102. Mazer CD, Hare GMT, Connelly PW, Gilbert RE, Shehata N, Quan A, et al. Effect of Empagliflozin on Erythropoietin Levels, Iron Stores, and Red Blood Cell Morphology in Patients With Type 2 Diabetes Mellitus and Coronary Artery Disease. Circulation. 2020;141(8):704-7.
103. ESC Congress 2019 together with World Congress of Cardiology (ESC-WCC 2019-World Heart Federation). France, 2019.
104. Aschner P, Gagliardino JJ, Ilkova H, et al. Persistent poor glycaemic control in individuals with type 2 diabetes in developing countries: 12 years of real-world evidence of the International Diabetes Management Practices Study (IDMPS). Diabetologia. 2020;63(4):711-21.

105. Roy MP. Diabetes and health awareness in India. J Family Community Med. 2018;25(1):52.
106. Unnikrishnan IR, Anjana R and Mohan V. Importance of controlling diabetes early-the concept of metabolic memory, legacy effect, and the case for early insulinisation. J Assoc Physicians India. 2011;59(Suppl 8–12).
107. Bajaj S. RSSDI clinical practice recommendations for the management of type 2 diabetes mellitus 2017. Int J Diabetes Dev Ctries. 2018;38(Suppl 1):1-115.
108. Kaveeshwar SA and Cornwall J. The current state of diabetes mellitus in India. Australas Med J. 2014;7(1):45-8.
109. Anjana RM, Deepa M, Pradeepa R, Mahanta J, Narain K, Das HK, et al. Prevalence of diabetes and prediabetes in 15 states of India: Results from the ICMR-INDIAB population-based cross-sectional study. Lancet Diabetes Endocrinol. 2017;5(8):585-96.
110. Rajadhyaksha V. Managing diabetes patients in India: Is the future more bitter or less sweet? Perspect Clin Res. 2018;9(1):1-3
111. Inzucchi SE, Bergenstal RM, Buse JB, Diamant M, Ferrannini E, Nauck M, et al. Management of hyperglycemia in type 2 diabetes, 2015: A patient-centered approach. Update to a position statement of the American Diabetes Association and the European Association for the Study of Diabetes. Diabetes Care. 2015; 38(8): 140-149.
112. Lim LL, Tan AT, Moses K, Rajadhyaksha V, Chan SP. Place of sodium-glucose cotransporter-2 inhibitors in East Asian subjects with type 2 diabetes mellitus: Insights into the management of Asian phenotype. J Diabetes Complications. 2017;31(2): 494-503.
113. Ma RCW, Chan JCN. Type 2 diabetes in East Asians: similarities and differences with populations in Europe and the United States. Ann N Y Acad Sci. 2013;1281(1):64-91.
114. Joshi SR. Diabetes care in India. Ann Glob Health. 2015; 81(6): 830-8.
115. Kalra S, Balhara YPS. Insulin distress. US Endocrinol. 2018;14(1):27-9.
116. Home P, Riddle M, Cefalu WT, Bailey CJ, Bretzel RG, Del Prato S, et al. Insulin therapy in people with type 2 diabetes: Opportunities and challenges? Diabetes Care. 2014;37(6):1499-508.
117. Bai X, Liu Z, Li Z, Yan D. The association between insulin therapy and depression in patients with type 2 diabetes mellitus: A meta-analysis. BMJ Open. 2018;8(11):e020062.
118. Luk A. Psychological insulin resistance: Scope of the problem. Hong Kong Med J. 2016;22(4):304-5.
119. Russell-Jones D, Pouwer F, Khunti K. Identification of barriers to insulin therapy and approaches to overcoming them. Diabetes Obes Metab. 2018;20(3):488-96.
120. Sorli C, Heile MK. Identifying and meeting the challenges of insulin therapy in type 2 diabetes. J Multidiscip Healthc. 2014;7:267-82.
121. Polonsky WH, Fisher L, Guzman S, Villa-Caballero L, Edelman SV. Psychological insulin resistance in patients with type 2 diabetes: the scope of the problem. Diabetes Care. 2005;28(10):2543-5.
122. Behavioral Diabetes Institute (BDI). Tools to face the psychological demands of diabetes. [online] Available from https://behavioraldiabetes.org/scales-and-measures/#1448435050704-6e22e4b0-81ec [Last accessed March, 2021].
123. Venkataraman K, Tan LS, Bautista DC, Griva K, Zuniga YL, Amir M, et al. Psychometric properties of the problem areas in diabetes (PAID) instrument in Singapore. PLoS One. 2015;10(9):e0136759.
124. Welch GW, Jacobson AM, Polonsky WH. The problem areas in diabetes scale. An evaluation of its clinical utility. Diabetes Care. 1997;20(5):760-6.

Section 8: Newer Technologies and Future Directions

Partha P Chakraborty, Sanjay Reddy, Jothydev Kesavade, Sanjay Agarwal

1. Effects of Continuous Glucose Monitoring on Metrics of Glycemic Control in Diabetes: A Systematic Review with Meta-analysis of Randomized Controlled Trials

Ref: Maiorino MI, Signoriello S, Maio A, Chiodini P, Bellastella G, Scappaticcio L, et al. Effects of Continuous Glucose Monitoring on Metrics of Glycemic Control in Diabetes: A Systematic Review With Meta-analysis of Randomized Controlled Trials. Diabetes Care. 2020;43:1146-56.

ABSTRACT

Background: Continuous glucose monitoring (CGM) offers important information to help in achieving glycemic targets in patients with diabetes.

Purpose: Authors carried out a meta-analysis of randomized controlled trials (RCTs) comparing CGM with usual care for glycemic control parameters in both type 1 diabetes mellitus (T1DM) and type 2 diabetes mellitus (T2DM).

Data sources: Various electronic databases were searched for articles published from inception until 30 June, 2019.

Study selection: Authors selected RCTs that evaluated both changes in glycated hemoglobin (HbA1c) and time in range (TIR), in conjunction with time below range (TBR), time above range (TAR), and glucose variability expressed as coefficient of variation (CV).

Data extraction: Two investigators extracted data from each trial.

Data synthesis: All results were examined by a random effects model to estimate the weighted mean difference (WMD) with the 95% confidence interval (CI). Authors included 15 RCTs with duration of 12–36 weeks and involving 2,461 patients. Considering overall data, compared with the usual care (overall data), CGM was associated with modest decrease in HbA1c (WMD −0.17%, 95% CI −0.29 to −0.06, I^2 = 96.2%), increase in TIR (WMD 70.74 min, 95% CI 46.73–94.76, I^2 = 66.3%), and lesser TAR, TBR, and CV, with heterogeneity between studies. A significant and robust increase in TIR was found independently of diabetes type, method of insulin delivery, and reason for CGM use. In preplanned subgroup analyses, real-time CGM resulted in a greater improvement in mean HbA1c (WMD −0.23%, 95% CI −0.36 to −0.10, $p < 0.001$), TIR (WMD 83.49 min, 95% CI 52.68–114.30, $p < 0.001$), and TAR. On the other hand, both intermittent-scanned continuous glucose monitoring and sensor-augmented pump were associated with a higher decline in TBR.

Conclusion: In both T1DM and T2DM, CGM improves glycemic control by improving TIR and reducing TBR, TAR, and glucose variability.

COMMENT

What was Known Prior to this Study?

Glycated hemoglobin (HbA1c), though has long been used as a predictor of diabetes-related complications, does not provide information about glycemic variability (GV) and episodes of acute hyperglycemia or hypoglycemia. In patients with significant endogenous insulin deficiency, diabetes control is often brittle, and such patients are best evaluated by a combination of self-monitoring of blood glucose (SMBG) or continuous glucose monitoring (CGM) and HbA1c. Use of CGM is associated with a reduction in HbA1c of ≈ 0.2–0.3%, with less hypoglycemia compared with usual care. Time in range (TIR) (70–180 mg/dL), time above range (TAR) (>180 mg/dL) and time below range (TBR) (<70 mg/dL) are useful metrics of glucose patterns, and TIR correlates with the risk of diabetes complications. For adults with T1DM and T2DM, the CGM-based target for TIR is >70% (>16 h 48 min), TAR is <25% (<6 h), and TBR is <4% (<58 min). Each 5% increase in TIR is clinically beneficial. The target for %CV is ≤36%. None of the earlier meta-analyses evaluated the efficacy of CGM on TIR, TBR, TAR, and CV.

What this Study Adds?

Use of CGM led to a modest reduction in HbA1c (0.17%) in this study, which was significant in patients with T1DM, but not in T2DM. TIR increased significantly (≈71 min; 5%) along with reduction in TBR (27 min; 1.9%), TAR (≈30 min for glucose value 180–250 mg/dL and ≈28 min for glucose value >250 mg/dL), and %CV (≈3%) with CGM use. Moreover, increase in TIR was evident across prespecified subgroup analysis, including type of diabetes, background therapy, CGM modality [real-time CGM (rtCGM) or intermittently-scanned glucose monitoring (iCGM) or sensor-augmented pump (SAP)], and reason for its use, with moderate to low or null heterogeneity in most cases.

Major Strengths of the Study

Only randomized controlled trials (RCTs), where CGM was used for >50% of the total follow-up time, were included in this meta-analysis. Extension studies from previous trials, observational studies or publications without original data or with incomplete data were not considered. In addition, studies using retrospective CGM without real-time reading of glucose values, and trials where the insulin regimen differed between intervention and control groups were also excluded. Both children and adults including pregnant patients with T1DM or T2DM, treated with intensive insulin regimen, were evaluated. Different modes of CGM (rtCGM, iCGM, or SAP) were compared with the standard care (usually SBGM). The strengths of this analysis are the comprehensive systematic literature search, the inclusion of studies with different technical and clinical factors, the use of valuable emerging metrics of glycemic control as primary or secondary outcomes, and the conduction of preplanned subgroup analyses.

Limitations of the Study

Heterogeneity was high for most of the study outcomes; all studies were sponsored by industry, had short duration, and used an open-label design. Participants were not blinded to the intervention; hence, performance biases are high for all studies. Adequate assessment of detection bias was limited due to insufficient information relative to the blinding of outcome assessors or data analysts to the data assessment.

Implications of the Findings for the Clinicians

This systematic review and meta-analysis showed that use of CGM improves the TIR and reduces the time spent in hypoglycemia or hyperglycemia, in patients with both T1DM and T2DM having modestly elevated HbA1c. All patients treated with either multiple subcutaneous insulin injection or continuous subcutaneous insulin infusion should be advised to use CGM, if possible, irrespective of their prevailing HbA1c.

Knowledge Gaps Identified and Scope for Future Research

Further studies with longer follow-up are needed to assess the effectiveness of CGM systems in the long-term, and its relationship with diabetes-related complications. Effectiveness of CGM in patients on oral agents should also be looked for.

2. Clinical Targets for Continuous Glucose Monitoring Data Interpretation: Recommendations from the International Consensus on Time in Range

Ref: Battelino T, Danne T, Bergenstal RM, Amiel SA, Beck R, Biester T, et al. Clinical Targets for Continuous Glucose Monitoring Data Interpretation: Recommendations From the International Consensus on Time in Range. Diabetes Care. 2019;42:1593-603.

ABSTRACT

The continuous glucose monitoring (CGM) has been made feasible due to technological improvements in sensor accuracy, greater convenience and ease of use. But, its use in routine clinical practices is relatively low due to the lack of clear and defined glycemic targets. Three peer-reviewed articles have provided summary of recommendations for use of key CGM metrics, but diabetes professional organizations are yet to adopt it and develop guidance for the practical application of these metrics in clinical practice. In February, 2019, an international panel of physicians, researchers, and individuals with diabetes who are expert in CGM technologies convened by Advanced Technologies and Treatments for Diabetes (ATTD) Congress addressed this issue. Here, we summarize the consensus recommendations of ATTD for utilization and reporting of various aspects of CGM data.

COMMENT

What was Known Prior to this Study?

Continuous glucose monitoring (CGM) is increasingly being used in patients with type 1 diabetes mellitus (T1DM) over the past few years. However, successful utilization of CGM data in routine clinical practice remains relatively low. This is attributed to the lack of clear and agreed-upon glycemic metrics obtained from CGM data between different consensus statements. An analysis of the 7-point self-monitored blood glucose (SMBG) data from the Diabetes Control and Complications Trial (DCCT) showed that diabetes complications (progression of diabetic retinopathy and development of microalbuminuria) correlate with time in target range (70–180 mg/day). Correlation between time in range (TIR) and diabetic retinopathy has also been observed in type 2 diabetes mellitus (T2DM). The core metrics (14 in number) for assessing CGM data were defined in 2017.

What this Study Adds?

Ten metrics that may be most useful in clinical practice have been standardized. More than 70% of data from the most recent 14 days are to be interpreted retrospectively. This is obtained from use of ambulatory glucose profile (AGP) for CGM report. Targets have been set for most adults with T1DM and T2DM, elderly people/high-risk people with T1DM and T2DM, and pregnant women with pregestational T1DM and T2DM and with gestational diabetes mellitus (GDM) (**Table 1**).

A correlation between TIR and glycated hemoglobin (HbA1c) has also been proposed. TIR of 70% and 50% corresponds with an HbA1c of 6.7–7% and 7.9–8.3%, respectively. An increase in TIR of 10% (2.4 h/day) leads to a decrease in HbA1c of approximately 0.5–0.8%.

Limitations of the Study

Targets in pregnant women with pregestational T1DM are based on limited evidence

TABLE 1: CGM-based targets in different populations with diabetes.

Glucose value	Time spent			
	T1DM* and T2DM	Elderly patients/high-risk patients with T1DM or T2DM	Pregnant patient with T1DM	Pregnant patient with T2DM or GDM
>250 mg/dL	<5% (<1 h 12 min)	<10% (<2 h 24 min)		
>180 mg/dL	<25% (<6 h)	<50%		
>140 mg/dL			<25% (<6 h)	<5%
70–180 mg/dL	>70% (>16 h 48 min)	>50% (>12 h)		
63–140 mg/dL			>70% (>16 h 48 min)	>95%
<70 mg/dL	<4% (<1 h)	<1% (<15 min)		
<63 mg/dL			<4% (<1 h)	<4%
<54 mg/dL	<1% (<15 min)		<1% (<15 min)	<1%

*TIR target is ≈60% in patients younger than 25 years of age and HbA1c goal of 7.5%.
>250 mg/dL: Level 2 hyperglycemia
181–250 mg/dL: Level 1 hyperglycemia
54–69 mg/dL: Level 1 hypoglycemia
<54 mg/dL: Level 2 hypoglycemia

(CGM: continuous glucose monitoring; GDM: gestational diabetes mellitus; HbA1c: glycated hemoglobin; T1DM: type 1 diabetes mellitus)

obtained from a Swedish trial and the Continuous Glucose Monitoring in Women With Type 1 Diabetes in Pregnancy Trial (CONCEPTT). Data is very sparse for pregnant women with pregestational T2DM and GDM.

Implications of the Findings for the Clinicians

Increasing TIR is as important as reduction in HbA1c. The hazard rates for progression of retinopathy and development of microalbuminuria are increased by 64% and 40%, respectively for each 10% reduction in TIR. Using CGM-based metrics is more useful to motivate people with diabetes. The goals are specific, defines exactly what is to be achieved, and can be measured by patients, themselves. High-risk patients can also be provided with small targets (i.e., 5% increase in TIR), which need to be achieved in short term. In addition, women contemplating pregnancy and pregnant women, know the targets, that to be reached as soon as possible.

3. Diabetes Digital App Technology: Benefits, Challenges, and Recommendations. A Consensus Report by the European Association for the Study of Diabetes (EASD) and the American Diabetes Association (ADA) Diabetes Technology Working Group

Ref: Fleming GA, Petrie JR, Bergenstal RM, Holl RW, Peters AL, Heinemann L. Diabetes digital app technology: benefits, challenges, and recommendations. A consensus report by the European Association for the Study of Diabetes (EASD) and the American Diabetes Association (ADA) Diabetes Technology Working Group. Diabetologia. 2020;63:229-41.

ABSTRACT

With the help of rapid developing digital health technology, people with diabetes find it easy to manage their diabetes. Numerous digital and health applications ("apps") available on smartphones and other wireless devices provide glucose-monitoring data, and are useful for those who need to adopt either lifestyle interventions or medication adjustments in response to that data. However, these apps have not been reviewed and monitored for patient safety and clinical validity as per the regulations and guidelines. The available evidence on the safety and effectiveness of mobile health apps, remains limited. A joint review was conducted by the European Association for the Study of Diabetes (EASD) and the American Diabetes Association (ADA) for assessment of practices of regulatory authorities and organizations in relation to these diabetes apps, where it was discovered that these apps were highly unregulated. International organizations, including the International Medical Device Regulators Forum and the World Health Organization, have been working toward classifying different types of digital health technology and integrating digital health technology into the field of medical devices. Here, we focus on several issues that the diabetes community, including regulatory authorities, policy makers, professional organizations, researchers, people with diabetes, and healthcare professionals (HCPs), need to address to ensure that diabetes health technology can meet its full potential in terms of safety and efficacy.

COMMENT

What was Known Prior to this Study?

The last three decades have witnessed a revolution in digital and wireless technology. People, all over the world, are using endless numbers of apps, including different health-related apps. Among almost half a million health-related apps available for wireless devices (usually smartphones), apps designed to help manage diabetes are among those most commonly available. The use is more frequent in people with or at risk for diabetes, and these apps, perhaps need to be incorporated as a component of comprehensive diabetes care. However, not every app is useful or good. There are very few data on long-term benefits, and even high-quality short- term data are limited.

What this Study Adds?

This consensus statement has provided a list of recommendations for the regulatory agencies, manufacturing companies, international and national professional societies, international and national research funding bodies, researchers/academics, healthcare professionals (HCPs), and consumers of digital health apps (people with diabetes, family members, and caregivers). It includes systematic and structured guidelines for digital health app development and assessment, improved consistency and accessibility of safety reports and app documentation, greater investment in gathering of clinical data to provide evidence on digital health interventions, increased accessibility for all consumer populations to use diabetes mobile apps confidentially and securely, increased communication and cooperation across stakeholder groups.

Knowledge Gaps Identified and Scope for Future Research

A realistic assessment of all the diabetes-related apps needs to be done to know what is safe and truly beneficial for people with diabetes. The different regulatory agencies and manufacturing companies should start working collaboratively with health professionals, researchers, and people with diabetes to create an environment in which diabetes can be managed safely and effectively, bringing benefits to all stakeholders and the entire diabetes community.

4. Systematic Review of Randomized Controlled Trials Evaluating Glycemic Efficacy and Patient Satisfaction of Intermittent-scanned Continuous Glucose Monitoring in Patients with Diabetes

Ref: Cowart K, Updike W, Bullers K. Systematic Review of Randomized Controlled Trials Evaluating Glycemic Efficacy and Patient Satisfaction of Intermittent-Scanned Continuous Glucose Monitoring in Patients with Diabetes. Diabetes Technol Ther. 2020;22:337-45.

ABSTRACT

Introduction: For self-management of diabetes, the intermittent-scanned continuous glucose monitoring (isCGM) helps in greater personalization. This systematic review included studies conducted among patients who had type 1 diabetes mellitus (T1DM) and type 2 diabetes mellitus (T2DM) with the aim of providing an updated analysis of the efficacy as well as patient satisfaction of isCGM.

Methods: This systematic review included research library search in PubMed, EMBASE, and Cochrane Library; keywords and subject headings were used for identifying studies that evaluated efficacy as well as applications of isCGMs among patients who had T1DM and T2DM.

Results: This systematic review included a total of nine randomized controlled trials (RCTs) including patients who had T1DM and T2DM and used isCGM. On the basis of existing RCT evidence that evaluated isCGM among patients who had diabetes, this was found that isCGM may result in a small reduction in glycated hemoglobin (HbA1c) levels in particular subgroups of patients who had uncontrolled T2DM (i.e., patients ≤65 years receiving multiple insulin injections daily). In patients who had uncontrolled T1DM and receiving insulin, isCGM is beneficial in combination with structured diabetes education programs. There is mixed evidence in relation to the effect on improvement in time in glycemic variability (GV), glycemic range, and hypoglycemia. In comparison with usual care, the isCGM showed more patient satisfaction and less diabetes distress.

Conclusion: The isCGM may be beneficial in improving HbA1c among particular subgroups of patients. Presently, extra advantages with isCGM on time regarding hypoglycemia, GV, and glycemic range are still not clear. Further clinical trials should be conducted for evaluating the role of isCGM among patients who have uncontrolled T2DM and receiving insulin as well as oral antidiabetic drugs.

COMMENT

What was Known Prior to this Study?

Frequent daily use of self-monitoring of blood glucose (SMBG) is associated with improved glycemic control in patients on intensive insulin therapy. However, repeated SMBG is painful, inconvenient and difficult to adhere with in the long run. Continuous glucose monitoring (CGM) is an effective alternative to SMBG and provides additional information like time in range (TIR), time above range (TAR), and time below range (TBR). Two types of CGM devices are currently available: (1) real-time CGM (rtCGM) and (2) intermittent-scanned CGM (isCGM). Unlike rtCGM, isCGM devices do not have alarm features to adjust insulin infusion immediately, and to obtain information "intermittently". All the studies, performed so far on CGM included patients on either rtCGM or isCGM. There is paucity of studies evaluating effects of isCGM solely in patients with diabetes. Existing evidences suggest nonsignificant reduction in glycated hemoglobin (HbA1c) at 6 months among patients with insulin-treated type 2 diabetes mellitus (T2DM) (REPLACE trial) or type 1 diabetes mellitus (T1DM) (IMPACT trial) with isCGM compared to SMBG.

What this Study Adds?

The effects of isCGM on HbA1c, glycemic variability (GV), TIR, and TBR are variable. Positive outcomes regarding hypoglycemia with use of isCGM have been seen in two randomized controlled trials (RCTs) (IMPACT, REPLACE), and not in others. Structured diabetes education program related to isCGM failed to decrease hypoglycemia in adolescents and adults with uncontrolled T1DM and T2DM in the FLASH study. Similarly, significant increase in TIR along with reduction in GV was seen in the IMPACT trial that included patients with well-controlled T1DM and excluded those with hypoglycemia unawareness. Additionally, when a structured diabetes education program was provided with isCGM use (FLASH trial), TIR improved as compared with usual medical care. However, there was no change in TIR with isCGM used in other RCTs. isCGM use is consistently associated with significant reduction in HbA1c in patients with T2DM, who are <65 years of age and are being treated with multiple daily insulin injections (MDIs) for uncontrolled diabetes. Patients with uncontrolled T1DM using insulin may also benefit from isCGM, when combined with a structured diabetes education program.

Major Strengths of the Study

A key strength to this systematic review is that multiple databases were searched to identify studies relevant to the research question. Additionally, validated search filters to identify RCTs were applied to Embase and PubMed. It also sought to answer a focused research question on isCGM, since many previous systematic reviews and meta-analyses have combined isCGM and rtCGM data. Furthermore, at the study level, it utilized the Cochrane risk of bias assessment to evaluate the RCTs.

Limitations of the Study

Limitations to the available RCTs were inconsistent inclusion criteria (i.e., age, diabetes type, and medication use) and use of different diabetes technologies and comparators. Some RCTs had an active comparator (i.e., rtCGM and others used SMBG). Additionally, many studies were small and had low generalizability. Furthermore, the long-term impact of isCGM on glycemic efficacy is unknown, since most currently published RCTs were short in duration.

Implications of the Findings for the Clinicians

In comparison to SMBG, isCGM is associated with significant reduction in HbA1c in a selected group of patients. isCGM device does not have an alarm feature as compared with rtCGM devices, and should better be avoided in patients with hypoglycemic unawareness.

Knowledge Gaps Identified and Scope for Future Research

Continuous glucose monitoring (CGM) is not well studied in those with 65 years of age or older, during pregnancy, or in patients with gestational diabetes. Additionally, few RCTs have included children or adolescents and report mixed findings on outcomes with isCGM use. At this time, RCT evidence is also lacking in patients with T2DM treated with oral antidiabetic agents and high-risk patients with diabetes—particularly those prone to hypoglycemia and with an HbA1c ≥ 9%. This is an important high-risk population for intervention, warranting further clinical trial investigation. As such, isCGM should be studied for a longer duration in those with T1DM and T2DM to better understand the long-term impact on glycemic measures.

5. Serum Tenascin-C is Independently Associated with Increased Major Adverse Cardiovascular Events and Death in Individuals with Type 2 Diabetes: A French Prospective Cohort

Ref: Gellen B, Thorin-Trescases N, Thorin E, Gand E, Sosner P, Brishoual S, et al. Serum tenascin-C is independently associated with increased major adverse cardiovascular events and death in individuals with type 2 diabetes: a French prospective cohort. Diabetologia. 2020;63:915-23.

ABSTRACT

Aim: To establish an association between serum tenascin-C (TN-C) levels and risk of major adverse cardiovascular events (MACE) and death in people with type 2 diabetes mellitus (T2DM).

Methods: Type 2 diabetic subjects from the SURDIAGENE cohort [SUivi Rénal, DIAbète de type 2 et GENEtique] were included in this prospective study. The primary endpoint was all-cause death and MACE [cardiovascular (CV) death, nonfatal myocardial infarction, or stroke] was the secondary endpoint. The incremental predictive value of TN-C was assessed using proportional hazard model and relative integrated discrimination improvement (rIDI).

Results: A total of 1,321 individuals with a mean age of 64 ± 11 years were observed for a median of 89 months. Death occurred in 442 individuals and an increased risk of death [hazard ratio (HR) per 1 standard deviation (SD): 1.27 (95% CI 1.17, 1.38); $p < 0.0001$] was found to be associated with serum TN-C concentrations. About 497 had MACE during follow-up. MACE occurred in 497 individuals during follow-up which was again associated with serum TN-C concentrations [HR per 1 SD: 1.23 (95% CI 1.13, 1.34); $p < 0.0001$]. There was a modest and significant improvement in prediction of the risk of all-cause death (rIDI: 8.2%; $p = 0.0006$) and MACE (rIDI: 6.7%; $p = 0.0014$) when serum TN-C levels were used along with traditional risk factors.

Conclusion/interpretation: An increased serum TN-C concentration is independently associated with death and MACE in individuals with T2DM. Therefore, TN-C can be treated as a prognostic biomarker for risk stratification in such patients.

COMMENT

What was Known Prior to this Study?

The major causes of morbidity and mortality in patients with type 2 diabetes mellitus (T2DM) are cardiovascular (CV) complications. T2DM is associated with chronic low-grade inflammation, and different proinflammatory markers are elevated in patients with T2DM. Tenascin-C (TN-C), a damage-associated molecular pattern (DAMP) protein, is an extracellular matrix (ECM) circulating glycoprotein that is highly expressed in inflammatory conditions and CV diseases. TN-C is associated with CV morbidity and/or death in patients with prediabetes and chronic kidney disease (CKD). A significant positive association between increased TN-C levels and severity of proliferative diabetic retinopathy has also been reported. Chronic inflammation in diabetes seems to promote ECM remodeling and to induce the expression of "diabetic-specific ECM proteins", including TN-C, which are not normally present in healthy individuals.

What this Study Adds?

Adding TN-C concentrations to the already established prognostic factors [age, sex, active smoking, statin treatment, hypertension, insulin treatment, estimated glomerular filtration rate (eGFR), and history of CV disease] in T2DM modestly, but significantly improves the accuracy of the risk modeling for all-cause death and major adverse cardiovascular events (MACE). The associations were robust, and remained unchanged for each outcome even after adjusting for body mass index (BMI), glycated hemoglobin (HbA1c), diabetes duration, low-density lipoprotein (LDL) levels, systolic blood pressure (SBP), other inflammatory markers, and the presence of diabetic retinopathy. TN-C, thus, seems to be independently associated with CV disease in patients with T2DM.

Major Strengths of this Study

The strengths of this study include prospective design, an extended follow-up period and independent adjudication for outcomes. Samples were collected and handled under standardized conditions.

Limitations of the Study

Participants from the SURDIAGENE study were recruited from a hospital-based monocentric cohort and this design may limit its application in the general population.

Implications of the Findings for the Clinicians

Tenascin-C could be a promising biomarker for risk stratification in individuals with T2DM.

Knowledge Gaps Identified and Scope for Future Research

Tenascin-C may be considered as a biomarker for risk stratification in patients with T2DM. In the recent past, a number of glucose lowering agents such as sodium-glucose cotransporter-2 (SGLT-2) inhibitors and glucagon-like peptide-1 receptor agonist (GLP-1 RA) have been associated with reduced MACE, CV death, and even all-cause death. However, the underlying mechanism(s) of these beneficial effects have not been clearly defined. Effects of these agents on circulatory TN-C may be evaluated. Studies with TN-C as a potential therapeutic target in individuals with T2DM are also warranted. Moreover, the potential role of TN-C as an etiological or predictive factor for diabetes deserves further study.

6. Diabetes Screening: Detection and Application of Saliva 1,5-Anhydroglucitol by Liquid Chromatography-mass Spectrometry

Ref: Jian C, Zhao A, Ma X, Ge K, Lu W, Zhu W, et al. Diabetes Screening: Detection and Application of Saliva 1,5-Anhydroglucitol by Liquid Chromatography-Mass Spectrometry. J Clin Endocrinol Metab. 2020;105:dgaa114.

ABSTRACT

Context: In patients with diabetes mellitus (DM), saliva detection helps in prevention of patients from suffering physical uneasiness unlike other widely used invasive methods of monitoring blood glucose. But, there is scarcity of studies related to saliva 1,5-anhydroglucitol (1,5-AG) in such patients.

Objective: The aim of this study is to assess the effectiveness of saliva 1,5-AG in screening of diabetes in a Chinese population.

Methods: This population-based cross-sectional study recruited 641 participants without a valid diabetic history from September, 2018 to June, 2019. Liquid chromatography–mass spectrometry was used for measuring salivary 1,5-AG. DM was defined according to the definition given by American Diabetes Association criteria. Receiver operating characteristic curves were used for evaluating the efficiency of saliva 1,5-AG for diabetes screening. Optimal cut-off point was evaluated as per the Youden index.

Results: Participants with DM had lower levels of saliva 1,5-AG compared to those without DM (both $p < 0.05$). There was positive correlation between saliva 1,5-AG and serum 1,5-AG and negative correlation between saliva 1,5-AG and blood glucose and glycated hemoglobin (HbA1c) (all $p < 0.05$). For diabetes screening, the optimal cut-off points of saliva 1,5-AG 0 was 0.436 µg/mL (sensitivity: 63.58%, specificity: 60.61%), and for saliva 1,5-AG 120 was 0.438 µg/mL (sensitivity: 62.25%, specificity: 60.41%). Fasting plasma glucose (FPG) in combination with fasting saliva 1,5-AG decreased the number of participants who needed an oral glucose tolerance test by 47.22% in comparison to FPG alone.

Conclusion: Combination of saliva 1,5-AG with FPG or HbA1c resulted in improvement of the efficiency of diabetes screening. In nonfasting measurements, saliva 1,5-AG is helpful, and is a noninvasive as well as convenient method for screening of diabetes.

COMMENT

What was Known Prior to this Study?

Serum 1,5-anhydroglucitol (1,5-AG) is an approved marker for evaluating short-term glycemic control (preceding 1 week) in patients with diabetes. 1,5-AG shares structural similarity with glucose except in C1 position, where a hydrogen atom replaces hydroxyl group of glucose. 1,5-AG competes with glucose in proximal renal tubules for reabsorption by sodium glucose transporters. In long-standing hyperglycemia, large amounts of glucose are continuously filtered out, which competitively inhibits the reabsorption of 1,5-AG, resulting in urinary loss of 1,5-AG. Thus, patients with diabetes have lower 1,5-AG levels. Serum 1,5-AG combined with fasting blood glucose improves the efficiency of diabetes screening and decreases the need for cumbersome oral glucose tolerance test (OGTT). 1,5-AG in serum is measured by gas/liquid chromatography–mass spectrometry or enzymatic methods. Salivary estimation of different biomarkers is increasingly being used in a variety of disorders (Cushing's syndrome, cancers, infections, and cardiovascular diseases). Salivary glucose, amylase, and protein glycosylation products have been evaluated in patients with diabetes. Salivary estimation of 1,5-AG by enzymatic methods is inappropriate due to cross-reaction of the substance with salivary galactose.

What this Study Adds?

Salivary 1,5-AG correlates well with serum 1,5-AG. This particular study is the first of its kind to propose the optimal cut-off point of saliva 1,5-AG for diabetes screening (0.44 µg/mL). A combination of salivary 1,5-AG with fasting plasma glucose (FPG) or glycated hemoglobin (HbA1c) enhances the efficiency of diabetes screening and reduces the need for OGTT.

Major Strengths of the Study

The study utilized mass spectrometry for estimating 1,5-AG, a "gold standard" method. It has eliminated the possibility of interference of galactose, fucose, xylose, mannose, and other components in saliva with 1,5-AG estimation.

Limitations of this Study

This was a single-center study and the groups were imbalanced in terms of sample size, age, and body mass index (BMI). Only adults were included. They did not use mass spectrometry and enzymatic methods to measure saliva and serum 1,5-AG levels simultaneously for all samples.

Implications of the Findings for the Clinicians

Salivary 1,5-AG is a potential noninvasive parameter for screening of diabetes and monitors glycemic control in appropriate patients. However, the test is time-consuming, costly, technically difficult (proteins are to be removed from samples before analysis), and requires well-trained operators.

Knowledge Gaps Identified and Scope for Future Research

Serum 1,5-AG concentrations are altered in patients with advanced chronic kidney disease (CKD) (stage 4 and 5), with certain dietary habits (dairy products) and in patients using sodium-glucose cotransporter-2 (SGLT-2) inhibitors. A gender and racial differences in serum 1,5-AG have also been reported. The optimal sex-specific and ethnicity-specific cut-off for diagnosis of diabetes, particularly in presence of aforementioned confounding factors needs to be validated in larger studies. Moreover, the role of salivary 1,5-AG as a screening and monitoring tool in pediatric population has to be evaluated.

7. Circulating Retinol-binding Protein 4 is Inversely Associated with Pancreatic β-cell Function Across the Spectrum of Glycemia

Ref: Huang R, Yin S, Ye Y, Chen N, Luo S, Xia M, et al. Circulating Retinol-Binding Protein 4 Is Inversely Associated With Pancreatic β-Cell Function Across the Spectrum of Glycemia. Diabetes Care. 2020;43:1258-65.

ABSTRACT

Objective: To evaluate the association of circulating retinol-binding protein 4 (RBP4) levels with β-cell function across the spectrum of glucose intolerance.

Research design and methods: A standard 2-hour oral glucose tolerance test (OGTT) with the use of traditional measures were used to screen 291 subjects aged 35–60 years with normal glucose tolerance (NGT), newly diagnosed impaired fasting glucose or impaired glucose tolerance (IFG/IGT), and type 2 diabetes mellitus (T2DM). 74 subjects were recruited for an oral minimal model test, and β-cell function was assessed with model-derived indices. Circulating RBP4 levels were measured by a commercially available enzyme-linked immunosorbent assay (ELISA) kit.

Results: In 291 subjects across the spectrum of glycemia, the Stumvoll first-phase and second-phase insulin secretion indexes showed inverse correlation between circulating RBP4 levels with β-cell function, but homeostasis model assessment of β-cell (HOMA-β), calculated from the 2-hour OGTT did not show this. Both direct measures and model-derived measures observed inverse association in subjects involved in the oral minimal model test with β-cell function.

Conclusion: The linkage between RBP4 and the pathogenesis of T2DM can be explained by the independent, inverse correlation between circulating RBP4 levels and β-cell function across the spectrum of glycemia.

COMMENT

What was Known Prior to this Study?

Retinol-binding protein 4 (RBP4), secreted from the adipocytes and hepatocytes, is significantly elevated both in preclinical models and in patients with obesity and diabetes. Gain-of-function mutations in the RBP4 promoter region and circulating RBP4 have predictive value for incident type 2 diabetes mellitus (T2DM) in high-risk populations. RBP4 level is positively correlated with insulin resistance in animal models, but not in humans. Several studies did not find any correlation between circulating RBP4 levels and insulin resistance in patients with T2DM; hence, the underlying reason(s) of this association remains unknown.

What this Study Adds?

In subjects with normal glucose tolerance (NGT), impaired fasting glucose or impaired glucose tolerance (IFG/IGT), and drug-naive, newly diagnosed T2DM, and circulating RBP4 levels are inversely associated with pancreatic β-cell function across the spectrum of glycemia. The association remained significant even after adjusting for known risk factors for diabetes such as age, sex, physical activity, and family history of T2DM.

Major Strengths of the Study

In most of the earlier studies, β-cell function was evaluated by homeostasis model assessment of β-cell (HOMA-β), mean insulin levels, or area under the curve for insulin from intravenous glucose loading tests, which is in a way nonphysiological as it bypasses the critical effect of intestine-derived incretin hormone on insulin secretion. The current study evaluated β-cell function with both 2-hour oral glucose tolerance test (OGTT)-derived indices and estimates derived from the oral minimal model test. The latter quantitatively simulates the complex process of glucose metabolism with a mathematical model and analogs β-cell responsibility. The strength of the study is the application of several methodologies to evaluate β-cell function such as Stumvoll indexes, insulinogenic index (IGI), and C-peptide index (CPI). Second, the negative association between RBP and β-cell function was confirmed in subjects with progressively increasing glycemia, from NGT to T2DM. This finding has increased the strength of the study and may provide a reasonably accurate and unbiased estimate of the relationship. In addition, the biochemical assays were performed in a central laboratory to minimize potential bias.

Limitations of the Study

The causal relationship between RBP4 and β-cell function cannot be inferred by the cross-sectional design of the study. Moreover, the relatively small sample size does not allow for generalization of the findings to other ethnicities.

Knowledge Gaps Identified and Scope for Future Research

The dynamic association between serum RBP4 and β-cell function in the course of T2DM needs to be further verified in large-scale prospective cohort studies.

8. Positioning Time in Range in Diabetes Management

Ref: Advani A. Positioning time in range in diabetes management. Diabetologia. 2020;63:242-52.

ABSTRACT

With the emergence of continuous glucose monitoring (CGM) technologies, patients with diabetes and healthcare professionals have now been introduced to a range of new indicators of glucose control. Some of these metrics such as time in range (TIR) are useful for monitoring the quality of glucose control, which routine laboratory testing fails to capture. TIR denotes the proportion of time that a person's glucose level is within a desired target range. As this can be easily understood by the patient and discussed with the healthcare provider, adoption of standardized TIR targets becomes important. Consensus recommendations have recently been introduced to facilitate this. Although, it is a nonreliable indicator of frequency or severity of hypoglycemia due to the skewed distribution of possible glucose values outside of the target range, it is expected to play a crucial role in deciding valid endpoints in clinical trials. This is due to emerging evidence of association of TIR to risk of complications at regulatory level. Here, we review the association of TIR with risk of diabetes complications and glycated hemoglobin (HbA1c). This review also discusses guidelines for deciding on "time in range" goals for individuals with diabetes compliant with this technology. For majority of diabetic population, the targets recommended are TIR >70%, a target below range (TBR) <3.9 mmol/L of <4%, and a TBR <3.0 mmol/L of <1%. Relaxations are applicable to these targets are relaxable for older or high-risk individuals and people with diabetes of <25 years of age. However, individualization of glycemic targets should always be considered.

COMMENT

What was Known Prior to this Study?

Landmark trials in diabetes mellitus have provided robust evidences suggesting that intensive glucose lowering reduces the risk of long-term diabetes complications, intensive glucose control involved frequent daily self-monitoring of blood glucose (SMBG) and regular laboratory measurement of glycated hemoglobin (HbA1c). Emerging evidence indicates that time in range (TIR) can also predict the risk of long-term diabetes complications and pregnancy outcomes, particularly in patients treated with intensive insulin regimen. It also helps to reduce the time spent in hypoglycemia. Most clinicians are unfamiliar with interpretation of continuous glucose monitoring (CGM) data to calculate TIR, positioning TIR relative to other glucose metrics and goals of TIR in a particular patient.

What this Study Adds?

This review discusses the rationale and definitions of TIR, target above range (TAR), and target below range (TBR). Consensus recommendations on TIR on different subgroups of diabetes have also been provided. A 10% change in the TIR percent (between 50% and 60%) has been found to be associated with a 0.78% change in HbA1c. This article has also briefed the evidence linking TIR to the risk of long-term diabetes complications.

Implications of the Findings for the Clinicians

Time in range is not a substitute for HbA1c value, but they complement each other. TIR detects acute fluctuations in glucose value, hence helps to reduce glycemic variability. TIR correlates better with the patient experience and patient-reported outcomes. TIR should be measured in all patients on intensive insulin regimen, patients with brittle diabetes and in situations, when HbA1c levels are discordant with mean glucose values.

Knowledge Gaps Identified and Scope for Future Research

The current recommendation is based on CGM metrics over a 14-day period; however, the optimal time period over which TIR should be determined for predicting complications risk is currently unknown. Studies are required comparing the outcomes using TIR obtained from intermittent versus CGM wear, and between different CGM systems such as real-time CGM (rtCGM) and intermittent-scanned continuous glucose monitoring (isCGM)/"flash" CGM. Furthermore, work is needed to define achievable TIR and TBR targets in patients with type 2 diabetes mellitus (T2DM), treated with oral agents and in pregnant women with pregestational T2DM or gestational diabetes.

9. Neprilysin Inhibition: A New Therapeutic Option for Type 2 Diabetes?

Ref: Esser N, Zraika S. Neprilysin inhibition: a new therapeutic option for type 2 diabetes? Diabetologia. 2019;62:1113-22.

ABSTRACT

Neprilysin, a peptidase preferentially hydrolyses oligopeptide substrates, most of which are involved in regulation of the cardiovascular, nervous, and immune systems. Its role in glucose metabolism has also been suggested by recent studies. Glycemic control and insulin sensitivity improved with a dual angiotensin receptor-neprilysin inhibitor (ARNI) in patients with type 2 diabetes mellitus (T2DM) and/or obesity. Additionally, beneficial effects on glucose homeostasis were also observed with inhibition of neprilysin, alone or in combination with renin-angiotensin system blockers, in preclinical studies. So, neprilysin inhibitors (NIs) can be suggested as a novel therapeutic drug for treating T2DM. However, their combination with angiotensin II receptor blockers (ARBs) may be needed to avoid unfavorable outcomes of neprilysin inhibition alone. Here, we review the evidence from existing studies, with a focus on mechanisms producing glycemic effects, impact of neprilysin inhibition on diabetic complications and also the unwanted effects that limit the efficacy and safety of NIs.

COMMENT

What was Known Prior to this Study?

Neprilysin, a ubiquitous peptidase, acts upon certain substrates such as glucagon-like peptide-1 (GLP-1), natriuretic peptides, and bradykinin that modulate glucose metabolism. Both circulatory and tissue neprilysin activity are higher in mice with diet-induced obesity, and its levels correlate with decreased insulin sensitivity and reduced beta cell function. There are emerging evidences on higher plasma neprilysin levels in humans with metabolic syndrome. Beneficial metabolic effects of fixed dose combinations of the angiotensin II receptor blocker (ARB) valsartan and the neprilysin inhibitor (NI) sacubitril [termed angiotensin receptor-neprilysin inhibitor (ARNI)] have been established in prospective comparison of ARNI with angiotensin-converting enzyme (ACE) inhibitor to Determine Impact on Global Mortality and Morbidity in Heart Failure (PARADIGM-HF) and two other studies, supporting the possible role of NI in prevention and treatment of type 2 diabetes mellitus (T2DM).

What this Study Adds?

This review discusses the proposed mechanisms of favorable effects of neprilysin inhibition on glucose homeostasis. NI stimulates glucose- and GLP-1-mediated insulin secretion in a GLP-1 receptor-dependent manner and improves insulin sensitivity (by increasing bradykinin). GLP-1 concentration is increased due to reduced breakdown by neprilysin, and possibly inhibition of dipeptidyl peptidase-4 (DPP-4) enzyme. Concentrations and activities of a number of gut-derived peptides, natriuretic peptides, and different hormones are also altered. This review has also discussed the evidence with neutral/adverse effects of neprilysin inhibition on glycemic status.

Implications of the Findings for the Clinicians

Neprilysin inhibitor (as ARNI) is now approved for use in patients with heart failure, a population in which approximately 35% also have T2DM. Though NI is associated with favorable glycemic effects, neprilysin inhibition alone has been shown to increase angiotensin II levels, which in turn may promote insulin resistance and β-cell dysfunction. Hence NI monotherapy may not be appropriate as an antihyperglycemic agent or may even have some undesirable effects. In addition, the effect may wane off when NI is used for prolonged periods.

Knowledge Gaps Identified and Scope for Future Research

Neprilysin also cleaves islet amyloid polypeptide (IAPP), and neprilysin inhibition increases amyloid formation and subsequent β-cell apoptosis. There is a possibility that, despite initial favorable effects, chronic use of NI in patients with T2DM may promote β-cells loss, and therefore may lead to deterioration of glycemic status over time. So long-term studies are required focusing on changes in glycemic parameters. In the PARADIGM-HF trial, ARNI use was associated with nephroprotection compared with RAS inhibition alone. Such a finding suggests possible role of neprilysin inhibition in preventing or delaying end organ damage in T2DM, and should be studied prospectively. Both NI and DPP-4 inhibitors prevent breakdown of GLP-1; hence the effect of combining both these agents on circulatory GLP-1 levels and glycemic parameters need to be studied. Moreover, the effects of combining NI with other glucose lowering agents are to be looked for.

10. Early Pregnancy Prediction of Gestational Diabetes Mellitus Risk using Prenatal Screening Biomarkers in Nulliparous Women

Ref: Snyder BM, Baer RJ, Oltman SP, Robinson JG, Breheny PJ, Saftlas AF, et al. Early pregnancy prediction of gestational diabetes mellitus risk using prenatal screening biomarkers in nulliparous women. Diabetes Res Clin Pract. 2020;163:108139.

ABSTRACT

Aims: Evaluation of biomarkers for predicting risk of development of gestational diabetes mellitus (GDM) in nulliparous women during early pregnancy.

Methods: A population-based cohort study of nulliparous women who participated in the California Prenatal Screening Program from 2009 to 2011 ($n = 105,379$) was conducted. Hospital discharge records or birth certificates were used to identify GDM cases. Maternal characteristics and prenatal screening biomarkers were used to develop and validate models. We assessed the clinical utility of the biomarkers by risk stratification and reclassification.

Results: Reduced levels of pregnancy-associated plasma protein A (PAPP-A) in first trimester and elevated levels of unconjugated estriol (uE3) and dimeric inhibin A (INH) in second trimester appeared to be associated with increased risk of GDM. The area under the receiver operating characteristic curve [area under the curve (AUC)] showed a small, but significant increase on considering PAPP-A only and PAPP-A, uE3, and INH along with maternal characteristics [maternal characteristics only: AUC 0.714 (95% CI 0.703–0.724), maternal characteristics + PAPP-A: AUC 0.718 (95% CI 0.707–0.728), maternal characteristics + PAPP-A, uE3, and INH: AUC 0.722 (0.712–0.733)].

Conclusion: Biomarkers PAPP-A, uE3, and INH are not of much utility for predicting risk of development of GDM in nulliparous women during early pregnancy. More studies are warranted to evaluate other clinical biomarkers for predicting the same.

COMMENT

What was Known Prior to this Study?

Gestational diabetes mellitus (GDM) is associated with adverse fetal and maternal outcomes, both in short term and in the long run. Maternal risk factors associated with increased risk of GDM are ethnicity, age, BMI, sedentary lifestyle, polycystic ovary syndrome, family history of type 2 diabetes mellitus (T2DM), history of GDM in prior pregnancy. In most developed countries, universal screening with oral glucose tolerance test (OGTT) is performed at 24-28 weeks of gestation to identify women with GDM. However, women at high risk of developing GDM in current pregnancy should be identified as early as possible to improve clinical outcomes by reducing maternal and fetal exposure to metabolic alterations and potential epigenetic malprogramming. Numerous biomarkers, other than glycemic parameters, such as adipokines and inflammatory mediators are altered in early pregnancy, and have been evaluated as predictors of glucose intolerance in later part of pregnancy. Abnormal levels of biomarkers, performed in first and second trimester of pregnancy, such as pregnancy-associated plasma protein A (PAPP-A), human chorionic gonadotropin (hCG), alpha-fetoprotein (AFP), unconjugated estriol (uE3), and INH, have been shown to be associated with a number of adverse obstetric outcomes in addition to predicting risks of aneuploidy and fetal structural anomalies.

What this Study Adds?

Decreased levels of first trimester PAPP-A and increased levels of second trimester uE3 and INH were significantly associated with GDM development. The addition of PAPP-A only and PAPP-A, uE3, and INH to a previously validated model including maternal demographic and clinical characteristics offered minimal but significant improvements in predictive accuracy. However, no net improvement in classification of GDM was observed, indicating that these biomarkers have limited clinical utility over GDM risk prediction based on maternal characteristics alone.

Major Strengths of this Study

This study assessed the value of combining well-known clinical risk factors with serum biomarkers in GDM risk prediction. It used both first and early second trimester prenatal screening biomarkers. The sample size was large enough to build and validate adequately powered prediction models. Utilization of a racially and ethnically diverse cohort supports the generalizability of the findings. In addition, quality control related to the measurements of biomarkers was optimal.

Limitations of the Study

The study focused on nulliparous women only, so the findings may not be generalizable to multiparous women. Because the data source was administrative and medical charts were inaccessible, inaccurate reporting of demographic and clinical variables, including GDM, is possible. The authors have also mentioned that they did not have data on exactly how or when GDM was screened and diagnosed, which may have caused some misclassification.

Knowledge Gaps Identified and Scope for Future Research

Gestational diabetes mellitus is a metabolic disease. The utility of different readily accessible nonglycemic biomarkers either alone or in combination with maternal clinical characteristics in predicting GDM risks warrants investigation in future studies. Incorporating biomarkers that precede the onset of hyperglycemia into a risk prediction model for GDM may facilitate earlier risk assessment, screening, and diagnosis, particularly in high-risk women.

11. Six-month Randomized, Multicenter Trial of Closed-loop Control in Type 1 Diabetes

Ref: Brown SA, Kovatchev BP, Raghinaru D, Lum JW, Buckingham BA, Kudva YC, et al. Six-Month Randomized, Multicenter Trial of Closed-Loop Control in Type 1 Diabetes. N Engl J Med. 2019;381:1707-17.

ABSTRACT

Introduction: In patients who have type 1 diabetes mellitus (T1DM), glycemic outcomes may be improved by closed-loop systems (CLSs) which automate insulin delivery.

Methods: This was a randomized, multicenter trial, conducted for duration of 6 months. Study population included patients with T1DM who were randomized in a 2:1 ratio either to closed-loop group (who received treatment with a CLS) or a control group [who received sensor-augmented pump (SAP)]. The primary outcome considered in the study was the percentage of time that the level of the blood glucose was within the target range of 70–180 mg/dL (3.9–10.0 mmol/L); blood glucose level was measured by continuous glucose monitoring (CGM).

Results: Total 168 patients in the age range of 14–71 years were included, who were randomized to closed-loop group ($n = 112$) or control group (n = 56). The glycated hemoglobin (HbA1c) level was in the range of 5.4–10.6%. Trial was completed by all the patients. During the 6 months, the mean (±SD) percentage of time that the glucose level within the target range increased in the closed-loop group to 71 ± 12% (from 61 ± 17% at baseline) and was not changed in the control group (at 59 ± 14%) [mean adjusted difference, 11 percentage points; 95% confidence interval (CI) 9–14; $p < 0.001$]. The results in terms of the main secondary outcomes [mean glucose level, HbA1c level, percentage of time that the glucose level was >180 mg/dL, and percentage of time that the glucose level was <70 mg/dL or <54 mg/dL (3.0 mmol/L)] all fulfilled the prespecified hierarchical criterion for significance, which favored the CLS. The mean difference (closed loop minus control) in the percentage of time that the level of blood glucose was lesser than 70 mg/dL was –0.88 percentage points (95% CI –1.19 to –0.57; $p < 0.001$). After 6 months, the mean adjusted difference in HbA1c level was –0.33 percentage points (95% CI –0.53 to –0.13; $p = 0.001$). Over 6 months, in the closed-loop group, the median percentage of time that the system was in closed-loop mode was 90%. There were no serious hypoglycemic events in the study. In the closed-loop group, there was one episode of diabetic ketoacidosis.

Conclusion: In the patients who have T1DM, as compared to those who received the sensor-augmented insulin pump, CLS use was found to be associated with a higher percentage of time spent in a target glycemic range. (Funded by the National Institute of Diabetes and Digestive and Kidney Diseases; iDCLClinicalTrials.gov number, NCT03563313)

COMMENT

What was Known Prior to this Study?

Achieving glycemic targets in type 1 diabetes mellitus (T1DM) is a challenging task, and recent advancements in the insulin delivery systems have helped a higher proportion of patients reaching the glycemic goals. The CLS (also referred to as an "artificial pancreas") with automated insulin delivery is the latest addition to the advanced technologies, used in diabetes care. CLS, which modulates basal insulin delivery, but does not administer automated boluses, is referred to as "hybrid" CLS. Studies have suggested that hybrid CLS is more effective than sensor-augmented pump (SAP) therapy (open-loop system) in patients with T1DM.

What this Study Adds?

This study reported the results of the International Diabetes Closed Loop (iDCL) trial, a randomized trial assessing the efficacy and safety of a CLS (Control-IQ, Tandem Diabetes Care) as compared with a SAP. This particular CLS uses an algorithm with a dedicated hypoglycemia safety module, automated correction boluses, and overnight intensification of basal insulin delivery designed to target near-normal glycemia consistently each morning. The time in range (TIR) was higher (≈11%; 2.6 h per day) and time spent in hypoglycemia was lower (≈13 min/day) in the CLS users during the study period (6 months). Over the course of the trial, the glycated hemoglobin (HbA1c) level improved among patients who used the CLS. However, more adverse events (ketosis) were reported in the CLS group than in the control group due to pump infusion set failure.

Major Strengths of the Study

The trial population included both insulin-pump users and injection insulin users (switched to pump therapy in the run-in phase) across a wide age range (14–71 years) and baseline range of HbA1c levels (5.4–10.6%). The end results were consistent across these and other baseline characteristics of the participants. This study had 100% patient retention and a high level of adherence to the use of the assigned devices in both treatment groups. Continuous glucose monitoring (CGM) was used by both the groups, with minimal reliance on blood glucose measurements. The trial was conducted without remote monitoring, to reflect real-world use.

Limitations of the Study

Though CLS performed better than SAP in this trial, 70% of the participants were using a CGM and 79% were using an insulin pump at the time of enrollment, percentages that are substantially higher than the reported usage in the general population of patients with T1DM. So, the findings may not be applicable to patients with T1DM in general. There were more unscheduled contacts in the CLS group, which was attributed to the use of an investigational device, and the insulin pumps used by the control group did not have a feature to suspend insulin for predicted hypoglycemia, which is now available for some pumps and has been shown to reduce the amount of CGM-measured hypoglycemia.

Implications of the Findings for the Clinicians

Closed-loop system may be offered to highly motivated patients with T1DM, who are accustomed to devices, and have an interest in and willingness to use a CLS to improve their glucose metrics.

Index

A

Addison's disease 81
Adrenalitis 75
Advanced microvascular disease, development of 27
Alpha-fetoprotein 175
Ambulatory glucose profile 162
American Diabetes Association 33, 81, 128, 164
Anemia 124
Angiotensin-converting enzyme inhibitor 173
Angiotensin-receptor-neprilysin inhibitor 173
Anti-glutamic acid decarboxylase antibody 25, 80
Antihyperglycemic medications, use of 33
Anti-islet cell antibody 80
Antiretroviral therapy 98
Anti-thyroid peroxidase 81
Arginine vasopressin secretion 10
Aspartate aminotransferase 52
Association of Maternal Lactation with Diabetes and Hypertension 15
Atherosclerosis 2, 3
Atherosclerotic cardiovascular disease 139, 145
Atrial fibrillation 144, 145
Autoantibody
  loss 18
  profile of 80
  reversion 18
Autoimmune
  diseases 22, 23
  disorders 23
  thyroid disease 80

Autonomic function, parasympathetic 64

B

Beta-cell function 151
Beta-thalassemia major 1
Blood
  glucose 131
    fasting 56, 110
    self-monitoring of 85-87, 89, 149, 162, 165, 172
  pressure 59
    systolic 22, 168
Body mass index 6, 16, 17, 23, 29, 33, 35, 36, 59, 65, 148
Bone
  formation rate 68
  histomorphometry 68, 69
  mineral density 17, 68, 71
Branched chain amino acids 4
Breastfeeding 16
Brown adipose tissue 4
Bullous pemphigoid 60, 61
  risk of 60

C

Canagliflozin 33, 153
Cardiac autonomic
  dysfunction 64
  neuropathy 64
Cardiovascular death 105
Cardiovascular disease 15, 30, 31, 33, 41, 48, 49, 65, 138, 139, 146
Cardiovascular disorders 134
Cardiovascular outcome trial 138
Carotid intima-media thickness test 53, 54

Charcot's foot 64, 65, 70
Charcot's neuroarthropathy 64, 65, 70
Closed-loop systems 176
Continuous glucose monitoring 53, 54, 84-86, 88-90, 99, 100, 114, 115, 160-163, 165, 171, 172, 176, 177
  effect of 84, 160
Continuous subcutaneous insulin infusion 89, 91
Coronary artery disease 44, 45, 146
Coronavirus 37
  disease (COVID) 2019 38
C-reactive protein 78

D

Dapagliflozin 106, 122, 142
  effect of 105
Deoxyribonucleic acid 11
Depression 66, 67
Diabetes 4, 29, 44, 56, 57
  action to control cardiovascular risk in 40, 41, 51
  advanced technologies and treatments for 85, 162
  complications 66
  control and complications trial 86, 162
  digital app technology 163
  distress scale 150
  mellitus 1, 30, 32, 37, 38, 45, 49, 54, 56, 62, 68, 111, 148, 168, 172
    gestational 95-98, 121, 162, 163, 174, 175
    prevalence of 37

Index

type 1 5, 6, 12, 13, 18, 23, 25, 27, 34, 50, 58, 75, 77, 78, 80, 82, 84, 86, 88-90, 99, 101, 116, 127, 129, 128, 136, 148, 149, 160, 162, 163, 165, 176
type 2 2, 3, 5, 6, 8, 9, 12, 13, 16, 17, 21, 25, 30, 31, 33-36, 38, 39, 42, 47-51, 54, 58, 62, 64, 68, 76, 82, 101, 102, 109, 111, 113, 114, 119, 120, 122-124, 127-132, 134, 135, 138, 139, 141, 142, 145, 146, 148-150, 152, 153, 160, 162, 165-167, 170, 172, 173, 175
screening 168
Dipeptidyl peptidase-4
 enzyme 173
 inhibitor 60, 109, 111
 protein 61
Dual-energy X-ray absorptiometry 17

E

Empagliflozin 33, 131
 effect of 146
 efficacy of 144
Enzyme-linked immunosorbent assay 14
Estimated glomerular filtration rate 19, 21, 27, 50, 82, 140, 146, 168
European Association for Study of Diabetes 163, 164
Euthymia 151
Extracellular matrix 167

F

Fatty liver disease, nonalcoholic 2, 3, 52
Foot ulcers, diabetes-associated 118
Fractional flow reserve 44

G

Genome-wide
 analysis 12
 association studies 5, 6, 9
Glomerular filtration rate 50, 77, 78

Glucagon
 like peptide 6, 12, 33, 107, 114, 115, 132, 134, 173
 receptor 111
 antagonist 111
Glucokinase 25
Glucose
 homeostasis, abnormal 1
 tolerance, normal 170, 171
Glutamic acid decarboxylase 24, 25
Glycemia 113, 114
 pancreatic beta-cell function across spectrum of 170
 reduction approaches 113
Glycemic control 56, 84, 86, 148, 160
Glycemic index 7

H

Heart failure 105, 106, 122, 139, 140, 144, 145, 146
Hemoglobin, glycated 54, 59, 84, 148, 160, 163, 172
Hepatitis
 B virus 62
 C virus 62
 chronic viral 62, 63
Hepatocyte nuclear factor 25
High-density lipoprotein cholesterol 22
Highly active antiretroviral therapy 98
Homeostasis model assessment 1, 122, 170
Human chorionic gonadotropin 175
Human leukocyte antigen 81
Hyperbaric oxygen therapy 118
Hyperglucagonemia 10
 paradoxical 11
Hyperglycemia 57, 160
Hyperinsulinemia 10
Hypoglycemia 86, 90, 116, 127, 160
 severe 126
Hypophysitis 75

I

Immune checkpoint inhibitor 75, 76
Impaired glucose tolerance 1, 170

Indian Demographic Health Survey 29
Indian diabetes risk score 42
Insulin 33
 antibody 18
 autoantibody 24, 25, 80
 resistance 1-3
 secretion 59
Insulinogenic index 171
Intermittently-scanned glucose monitoring 161
International Diabetes Management Practices Study 148
Intrauterine growth restriction 31
Islet amyloid polypeptide 174
Islet autoantibodies 18
 absence of 24
Islet cell
 antibody 18
 autoantibody 80

J

Juvenile Diabetes Research Foundation 87

K

Ketoacidosis, diabetic 77
Kidney disease 138, 139
 chronic 19, 20, 46, 47, 50, 82, 119, 139, 167, 170
 diabetic 21, 47, 50, 77, 78
 nonalbuminuric chronic 49

L

Left ventricular mass index 146
Linagliptin 138, 139
Liquid chromatography-mass spectrometry 168
Liraglutide 33
Liver
 biopsy 53
 fatty acid-binding protein 83
 iron concentration 1
 transplantation 31, 32
Low-density lipoprotein 59, 168
Lower glycemic index 7
Lower high-density lipoprotein 24

M

Madras Diabetes Research Foundation 42, 43
Magnetic resonance imaging 1
Major adverse cardiovascular events 44, 45, 51, 126, 167, 168
Major histocompatibility complex 6
Maturity onset diabetes of young 24, 25
Mealtime insulin 137
Meglitinides 33
Menarche, delayed 27
Metabolic syndrome 32
Metformin 95, 109, 124, 131, 153
    monotherapy 111
Microbiota, effect of 121
Microtubule actin cross-linking factor 1 8
Microvascular diseases 48
Mixed meal test 114, 115
Multiple daily insulin injections 166
Multiple subcutaneous injections 100
Multiple-dose injection therapy 86
Mycobacterium avium 14
Myocardial infarction 44

N

National Health and Nutrition Examination Survey 27, 33, 42, 43, 48, 49
Neonatal intensive care unit 95, 100
Nephropathy, diabetic 78
Nervous system
    parasympathetic 64, 65
    sympathetic 64, 65
Neutrophil gelatinase-associated lipocalin 83
New York Heart Association 105, 122, 123
New-onset diabetes after transplantation 32

O

Obesity 114
    prevalence of 95
Oral antidiabetic drugs 131, 134, 135, 152
Oral disease 48
Oral glucose
    lowering drugs 148, 149
    tolerance test 56, 169, 171, 175
Oral semaglutide 119, 131
Osteopenia 16
Osteoporosis 16
Oxyntomodulin 114, 115

P

Pancreatic alpha-cells 111
Pancreatic islet autoantibodies 13
Pancreatic polypeptide 56
Pancreatitis, chronic 56
Paratuberculosis 14
Peptide innovation 120
Placental growth factor 102
Plasma glucose, fasting 111, 121, 141
Postprandial plasma glucose 141
Post-transplant metabolic syndrome 31, 32
Pre-eclampsia 102
Primary polydipsia analysis 142
Psychologic insulin resistance 150

Q

Quality-adjusted life years 49
Quantitative insulin sensitivity check index 1

R

Randomized controlled trials 79, 85, 87, 88, 107, 121, 124, 131, 135, 160
Randomized double-blind placebo-controled study 70
Rapid acting insulin analogs 130

Real-time continuous glucose monitoring 86, 87, 99
Recombinant human parathyroid hormone 70
Remogliflozin etabonate 141, 142
Renal disease
    end-stage 46, 47, 50, 78, 82
    progression of 82
Renal insufficiency, chronic 50
Renin-angiotensin-aldosterone system 78
Retinol-binding protein 4 170, 171
Retinopathy 58
Revised National Tuberculosis Control Program 29
Roux-en-Y gastric bypass 115

S

Semaglutide 132, 133, 153
Sensor-augmented pump 91
Sensor-integrated pump therapy, use of 90
Serum angiogenic markers 101
Serum placental growth factor 101
Single nucleotide polymorphism 6
Sodium-glucose cotransporter-2 34, 122, 123, 132, 142, 143, 170
    inhibitor 105, 107, 141, 144-147
Steatohepatitis, nonalcoholic 52, 112
Stumvoll indexes 171
Suboptimal glycemic control 148
Sulfonylureas 33, 109

T

Technosphere insulin 116
Teriparatide 70
Thiazolidinediones 33
Thyroiditis 75
Triglycerides 22
Tuberculosis 28, 29

U

Ultrasonography 37, 63
Upper gastrointestinal
    endoscopy 63
Uric acid 78
Urinary albumin excretion 78
Urine albumin-to-creatinine
    ratio 22

V

Vascular diseases 48
Vascular endothelial growth
    factor 102
Very low-calorie diet 114, 115
Vitamin
    B12 124
        deficiency 124
    D 95, 96
        supplementation 38

W

World Health Organization 17, 36

Z

Zinc transporter 13, 24, 80

EU GSPR Authorised Reprsentative
Logos Europe, 9 rue Nicolas Poussin
1700, La Rochelle, France
Phone: +33 (0) 6 67 93 73 78
E-mail: contact@logoseurope.eu

www.ingramcontent.com/pod-product-compliance
Ingram Content Group UK Ltd.
Pitfield, Milton Keynes, MK11 3LW, UK
UKHW051848210426
5322IPUK00024B/606